Emerging Strategies in Drug Development and Clinical Care in the Era of Personalized and Precision Medicine

Emerging Strategies in Drug Development and Clinical Care in the Era of Personalized and Precision Medicine

Cristina Manuela Dragoi
Alina Crenguța Nicolae
Ion-Bogdan Dumitrescu

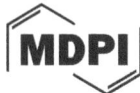

Basel • Beijing • Wuhan • Barcelona • Belgrade • Novi Sad • Cluj • Manchester

Editors

Cristina Manuela Dragoi
Department of Biochemistry
Carol Davila University of
Medicine and Pharmacy
Bucharest
Romania

Alina Crenguța Nicolae
Department of Biochemistry
Carol Davila University of
Medicine and Pharmacy
Bucharest
Romania

Ion-Bogdan Dumitrescu
Physics and Informatics
Department
Carol Davila University of
Medicine and Pharmacy
Bucharest
Romania

Editorial Office
MDPI AG
Grosspeteranlage 5
4052 Basel, Switzerland

This is a reprint of articles from the Special Issue published online in the open access journal *Pharmaceutics* (ISSN 1999-4923) (available at: www.mdpi.com/journal/pharmaceutics/special_issues/9WUD0G24J6).

For citation purposes, cite each article independently as indicated on the article page online and as indicated below:

Lastname, A.A.; Lastname, B.B. Article Title. *Journal Name* **Year**, *Volume Number*, Page Range.

ISBN 978-3-7258-2296-6 (Hbk)
ISBN 978-3-7258-2295-9 (PDF)
doi.org/10.3390/books978-3-7258-2295-9

© 2024 by the authors. Articles in this book are Open Access and distributed under the Creative Commons Attribution (CC BY) license. The book as a whole is distributed by MDPI under the terms and conditions of the Creative Commons Attribution-NonCommercial-NoDerivs (CC BY-NC-ND) license.

Contents

Preface vii

Cristina Manuela Drăgoi, Alina Crenguța Nicolae and Ion-Bogdan Dumitrescu
Emerging Strategies in Drug Development and Clinical Care in the Era of Personalized and Precision Medicine
Reprinted from: *Pharmaceutics* **2024**, *16*, 1107, doi:10.3390/pharmaceutics16081107 1

Anne Harnett, Stephen Byrne, Jennifer O'Connor, Eimear Burke, Laura South and Declan Lyons et al.
Point Prevalence Survey of Acute Hospital Patients with Difficulty Swallowing Solid Oral Dose Forms
Reprinted from: *Pharmaceutics* **2024**, *16*, 584, doi:10.3390/pharmaceutics16050584 8

Lara Marques, Bárbara Costa, Mariana Pereira, Abigail Silva, Joana Santos and Leonor Saldanha et al.
Advancing Precision Medicine: A Review of Innovative In Silico Approaches for Drug Development, Clinical Pharmacology and Personalized Healthcare
Reprinted from: *Pharmaceutics* **2024**, *16*, 332, doi:10.3390/pharmaceutics16030332 19

Sarah Dräger, Tim M. J. Ewoldt, Alan Abdulla, Wim J. R. Rietdijk, Nelianne Verkaik and Christian Ramakers et al.
Exploring the Impact of Model-Informed Precision Dosing on Procalcitonin Concentrations in Critically Ill Patients: A Secondary Analysis of the DOLPHIN Trial
Reprinted from: *Pharmaceutics* **2024**, *16*, 270, doi:10.3390/pharmaceutics16020270 58

María Del Mar Sánchez Suárez, Alicia Martín Roldán, Carolina Alarcón-Payer, Miguel Ángel Rodríguez-Gil, Jaime Eduardo Poquet-Jornet and José Manuel Puerta Puerta et al.
Treatment of Chronic Lymphocytic Leukemia in the Personalized Medicine Era
Reprinted from: *Pharmaceutics* **2023**, *16*, 55, doi:10.3390/pharmaceutics16010055 72

Young Beom Kwak, Jeong In Seo and Hye Hyun Yoo
Exploring Metabolic Pathways of Anamorelin, a Selective Agonist of the Growth Hormone Secretagogue Receptor, via Molecular Networking
Reprinted from: *Pharmaceutics* **2023**, *15*, 2700, doi:10.3390/pharmaceutics15122700 110

Hye-Young Joung, Jung-Mi Oh, Min-Suk Song, Young-Bae Kwon and Sungkun Chun
Selegiline Modulates Lipid Metabolism by Activating AMPK Pathways of Epididymal White Adipose Tissues in HFD-Fed Obese Mice
Reprinted from: *Pharmaceutics* **2023**, *15*, 2539, doi:10.3390/pharmaceutics15112539 124

Ljiljana Rakicevic
DNA and RNA Molecules as a Foundation of Therapy Strategies for Treatment of Cardiovascular Diseases
Reprinted from: *Pharmaceutics* **2023**, *15*, 2141, doi:10.3390/pharmaceutics15082141 139

Panagiotis Kanellopoulos, Berthold A. Nock, Eric P. Krenning and Theodosia Maina
Toward Stability Enhancement of NTS$_1$R-Targeted Radioligands: Structural Interventions on [^{99m}Tc]Tc-DT1
Reprinted from: *Pharmaceutics* **2023**, *15*, 2092, doi:10.3390/pharmaceutics15082092 156

Rui Silva, Helena Colom, Joana Bicker, Anabela Almeida, Ana Silva and Francisco Sales et al.
Population Pharmacokinetic Analysis of Perampanel in Portuguese Patients Diagnosed with Refractory Epilepsy
Reprinted from: *Pharmaceutics* **2023**, *15*, 1704, doi:10.3390/pharmaceutics15061704 . . . . **172**

Gemma García-Lluch, Carmen Peña-Bautista, Lucrecia Moreno Royo, Miguel Baquero, Antonio José Cañada-Martínez and Consuelo Cháfer-Pericás
Angiotensin II Receptor Blockers Reduce Tau/Aß42 Ratio: A Cerebrospinal Fluid Biomarkers' Case-Control Study
Reprinted from: *Pharmaceutics* **2023**, *15*, 924, doi:10.3390/pharmaceutics15030924 . . . . **188**

Gabriela Becker, Maria Fernanda Pessano Fialho, Indiara Brusco and Sara Marchesan Oliveira
Kinin B_1 and B_2 Receptors Contribute to Cisplatin-Induced Painful Peripheral Neuropathy in Male Mice
Reprinted from: *Pharmaceutics* **2023**, *15*, 852, doi:10.3390/pharmaceutics15030852 . . . . **204**

Mihaela Axente, Andrada Mirea, Corina Sporea, Liliana Pădure, Cristina Manuela Drăgoi and Alina Crenguța Nicolae et al.
Clinical and Electrophysiological Changes in Pediatric Spinal Muscular Atrophy after 2 Years of Nusinersen Treatment
Reprinted from: *Pharmaceutics* **2022**, *14*, 2074, doi:10.3390/pharmaceutics14102074 . . . . **225**

Jillian Marie Walker, Padraic O'Malley and Mei He
Applications of Exosomes in Diagnosing Muscle Invasive Bladder Cancer
Reprinted from: *Pharmaceutics* **2022**, *14*, 2027, doi:10.3390/pharmaceutics14102027 . . . . **234**

Preface

The advent of personalized and precision medicine has heralded a transformative era in healthcare, redefining the way we understand, diagnose, and treat diseases. *"Emerging Strategies in Drug Development and Clinical Care in the Era of Personalized and Precision Medicine"* delves into this dynamic landscape, offering a comprehensive exploration of innovative approaches that align therapeutic strategies with individual patient profiles.

This reprint brings together experienced clinicians and pioneering researchers who illuminate the complex interplay between genetics, environment, and lifestyle in shaping health outcomes. Through a series of curated chapters, we explore the cutting-edge advancements in drug development, targeted therapies, and clinical care that promise to revolutionize patient outcomes.

We hope that this reprint will serve as a useful academic resource and an inspiration for clinicians, researchers, and policymakers, fostering a deeper understanding of the potential that personalized and precision medicine holds for the future of global health.

Cristina Manuela Dragoi, Alina Crenguța Nicolae, and Ion-Bogdan Dumitrescu
Editors

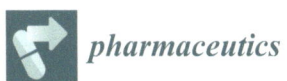

Editorial

Emerging Strategies in Drug Development and Clinical Care in the Era of Personalized and Precision Medicine

Cristina Manuela Drăgoi, Alina Crenguța Nicolae * and Ion-Bogdan Dumitrescu

Faculty of Pharmacy, "Carol Davila" University of Medicine and Pharmacy, 020956 Bucharest, Romania; cristina.dragoi@umfcd.ro (C.M.D.); ion.dumitrescu@umfcd.ro (I.-B.D.)
* Correspondence: alina.nicolae@umfcd.ro

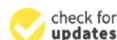

Citation: Drăgoi, C.M.; Nicolae, A.C.; Dumitrescu, I.-B. Emerging Strategies in Drug Development and Clinical Care in the Era of Personalized and Precision Medicine. *Pharmaceutics* 2024, 16, 1107. https://doi.org/10.3390/pharmaceutics16081107

Received: 5 July 2024
Accepted: 24 July 2024
Published: 22 August 2024

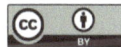

Copyright: © 2024 by the authors. Licensee MDPI, Basel, Switzerland. This article is an open access article distributed under the terms and conditions of the Creative Commons Attribution (CC BY) license (https://creativecommons.org/licenses/by/4.0/).

1. Introduction

In the ever-changing landscape of modern medicine, we face an important moment where the interplay of disease, drugs, and patients defines a new paradigm. The trajectory is shifting from conventional drug development towards personalized therapeutic strategies addressed to the unique physiology of each individual. In recent decades, remarkable efforts in preventive measures, diagnostic techniques, and treatment approaches have led to substantial enhancements in patient care. However, the achievement of personalized medicine strongly depends on a comprehensive understanding of pathogenesis, therapeutic agents, biochemical mechanisms, drug interactions, and patient-specific factors [1–3].

In this setting, the aim of this Special Issue on "Emerging strategies in drug development and clinical care in the era of personalized and precision medicine" was to assemble a compendium of the most recent pertinent research papers elucidating the current state-of-the-art knowledge and projecting future directions in drug development and clinical practice. Central to this effort was the focus on biochemical mechanisms of action, innovative drug formulations, and rigorous preclinical and clinical evaluations encompassing efficacy, pharmacokinetics, and toxicity within the framework of precision and personalized medicine.

This Special Issue addressed a significant topic by synthesizing cutting-edge research across various facets of drug development and clinical care. By consolidating insights into therapeutic strategies, drug design, and pharmacological testing, it offers a detailed pathway for crossing the bridges of medicine to the new horizons of personalized medicine. Moreover, it underscores the imperative of interdisciplinary collaboration and the integration of diverse data sources to unlock new avenues for therapeutic innovation, as in recent years, the integration of smart wearables and artificial intelligence (AI) technology into healthcare has revolutionized personalized medicine [4–6]. These advancements have the potential to enhance patient outcomes, improve disease management, and offer more tailored therapeutic interventions.

The significance of these technologies in personalized medicine and their transformative impact on the healthcare landscape comes not only from helping individuals maintain a healthier lifestyle, but also from continuously providing physiological and metabolic data essential for managing chronic diseases. They enable continuous and real-time monitoring of an individual's health status, gathering extensive data on various physiological and metabolic parameters, such as heart rate, blood pressure, glucose levels, physical activity, and sleep patterns. The integration of these data with AI algorithms allows for the development of highly personalized health interventions tailored to the specific needs of each individual [7,8].

2. A Glimpse over the Published Studies

The field of personalized and precision medicine is experiencing a profound transformation, marked by innovative approaches for drug development and clinical care. In this

Special Issue of *Pharmaceutics*, thirteen groundbreaking papers delve into diverse aspects of this evolving landscape, shedding light on novel therapeutic strategies, molecular mechanisms, and diagnostic methodologies. Through rigorous investigation and interdisciplinary collaboration, these studies contribute significantly to our understanding of personalized medicine and pave the way for future advancements in patient care.

One notable study by Dräger et al. investigates the impact of model-informed precision dosing on procalcitonin concentrations in critically ill patients. By using advanced dosing strategies, the authors demonstrate the potential to optimize antibiotic treatment and improve patient outcomes. Similarly, Kwak et al. employ molecular networking techniques to elucidate the metabolic pathways of anamorelin, offering valuable insights into the pharmacokinetics and pharmacodynamics of this growth hormone secretagogue receptor agonist.

In another study, Joung et al. approached the therapeutic potential of selegiline in modulating lipid metabolism in obese mice, highlighting the importance of targeting specific molecular pathways in the management of metabolic disorders. Furthermore, Kanellopoulos et al. propose structural interventions to enhance the stability of radioligands targeted at the neurotensin subtype 1 receptor, laying the groundwork for more effective cancer theranostics.

This Special Issue also features population pharmacokinetic analyses of perampanel in patients with refractory epilepsy by Silva et al., as well as investigations into the effects of angiotensin II receptor blockers on cerebrospinal fluid biomarkers in Alzheimer's disease by García-Lluch et al. These studies underscore the growing emphasis on individualized treatment approaches tailored to the unique characteristics of each patient.

Moreover, Becker et al. explore the role of kinin receptors in cisplatin-induced peripheral neuropathy, while Axente et al. provide insights into the clinical and electrophysiological changes in pediatric spinal muscular atrophy following nusinersen treatment. These findings contribute to a better understanding of neurological disorders and the targeted therapeutic interventions employed by clinicians.

Additionally, this Special Issue features comprehensive reviews by Marques et al., Sánchez Suárez et al., Rakicevic, and Walker et al., which offer comprehensive overviews of innovative in silico approaches for drug development, personalized treatment strategies for chronic lymphocytic leukaemia, nucleic acid-based therapies for cardiovascular diseases, and the diagnostic applications of exosomes in muscle-invasive bladder cancer, respectively.

In the last article published in this Special Issue, Anne Harnett et al. present a comprehensive study on the prevalence and management of swallowing difficulties among acute hospital inpatients. This survey reveals that a great number of patients face challenges swallowing solid oral dose forms, with significant implications for medication administration safety and efficacy. The authors emphasize the risk of inappropriate modifications, which can lead to patient harm. They advocate for a proactive approach, such as implementing screening tools, to identify patients with swallowing difficulties and ensure safer medication administration practices.

3. Novel Biomarkers in Precision Medicine

Personalized medicine represents a paradigm shift in healthcare, focusing on tailoring medical treatment to the individual characteristics of each patient. Central to this approach is the identification and application of novel biomarkers—biological molecules that serve as indicators of a biological state or condition. These biomarkers can be found in blood, tissues, or other bodily fluids, and their discovery and validation are crucial for advancing personalized medicine [9–14].

One of the key advantages of novel biomarkers in personalized medicine is their potential to enhance the specificity and sensitivity of disease diagnosis. Traditional diagnostic methods often rely on generalized criteria that may not account for individual variations in disease presentation [15–17]. Novel biomarkers enable the detection of diseases at earlier stages and with greater accuracy by reflecting the unique molecular signatures associated with different disease states. For example, the identification of specific genetic mutations, such as BRCA1 and BRCA2 in breast cancer, has revolutionized the screening and risk assessment for patients, allowing for more targeted and effective interventions [18].

Moreover, novel biomarkers play a pivotal role in the customization of therapeutic strategies. In cancer treatment, for instance, the expression levels of certain proteins or the presence of specific genetic alterations can guide the selection of targeted therapies, thereby improving treatment efficacy and minimizing adverse effects. The development of companion diagnostic tests that identify the suitability of a particular therapy for a patient based on their biomarker profile exemplifies this approach [19–21]. Personalized treatment plans based on biomarker information can lead to better outcomes, as seen with the use of HER2 inhibitors in HER2-positive breast cancer patients [22].

In addition to their diagnostic and therapeutic applications, novel biomarkers are essential for monitoring disease progression and treatment response. Biomarkers can provide real-time insights into how a disease evolves and how a patient responds to treatment, enabling dynamic adjustments to therapeutic regimens. For chronic patients with diabetes, cardiovascular, neurologic and psychiatric diseases, osteoporosis, inflammatory and autoimmune conditions, there are several biomarkers that offer valuable information on disease control and risk stratification, facilitating more proactive and individualized management strategies [14,23–30].

The future of personalized medicine hinges on the continuous discovery and validation of novel biomarkers. Advances in high-throughput technologies, such as next-generation sequencing and mass spectrometry, have accelerated the identification of potential biomarkers. Integrative approaches combining genomics, proteomics, metabolomics, and other omics data are poised to uncover a comprehensive array of biomarkers that reflect the complexity of human diseases. As our understanding of the molecular underpinnings of diseases deepens, the translation of these biomarkers into clinical practice will further refine and revolutionize personalized medicine, ultimately leading to more precise, effective, and patient-centered healthcare [2,19,31].

4. A Preview of AI-Integrated Technologies for Shaping the Future of Personalized Medicine

The nine research studies and four reviews featured in this Special Issue comprehensively outline the current practices, highlight gaps in solution-finding approaches, and present future perspectives in the field of personalized medicine. A significant advancement in this area is the integration of technology, particularly the application of artificial intelligence (AI) in patient care. Smart devices are capable of continuously collecting data on vital signs and other health metrics, providing a comprehensive and real-time overview of an individual's health status. This continuous monitoring facilitates the early detection of potential health issues, thereby enabling timely interventions and enhanced disease management [32,33].

For individuals with chronic conditions such as metabolic, cardiovascular and respiratory diseases, wearable devices offer a practical solution for ongoing health monitoring. AI algorithms play a central role by analyzing the collected data to identify trends and anomalies, allowing healthcare providers to adjust treatment plans accordingly. This data-driven approach not only improves patient outcomes but also optimizes the overall management of chronic diseases.

AI-driven analysis of data from smart devices provides personalized insights into an individual's health behaviors and their impacts. This can help people make informed decisions about their lifestyle, such as adjusting their diet, exercise routine, or medication adherence, in order to optimize their health. Another important role is in acknowledging the impact of every small intervention regarding nutrition, sleep patterns, and chronobiologic approaches intended to optimize activity versus rest outlines, on the general state of health for an individual [34–40].

By employing machine learning and predictive analytics, AI can identify patterns and predict future health risks. This proactive approach allows for the implementation of preventive measures, potentially reducing the incidence and severity of chronic diseases.

Smart devices also encourage patients to take an active role in managing their health. The feedback provided by these devices can motivate users to adhere to healthier behaviors and treatment plans, fostering a sense of empowerment and responsibility for their own well-being. The data collected by wearable devices can be integrated with electronic health records, providing healthcare professionals with a more comprehensive view of a patient's health. This holistic approach facilitates more accurate diagnoses, personalized treatment plans, and improved coordination of care.

The vast amounts of data generated by smart devices contribute to medical research by offering insights into population health trends and the effectiveness of various interventions. These data can inform the development of new treatments and healthcare policies aimed at improving public health [41].

5. Conclusions

In conclusion, the journey towards personalized and precision medicine represents a paradigm shift in healthcare, with the potential to revolutionize patient care and outcomes. This Special Issue serves as a reassurance statement, revealing the path for the future where therapeutic interventions are not only efficacious but also intricately tailored to the unique needs of each patient. As the next step forward, the integration of smart devices and AI into personalized medicine represents a significant advancement in healthcare. These technologies enable continuous health monitoring, personalized nutritional, lifestyle, chronobiological and medical interventions, and predictive analytics, which collectively enhance disease management, improve patient outcomes, and promote proactive health management.

Author Contributions: Conceptualization, C.M.D., A.C.N. and I.-B.D.; methodology, A.C.N.; software, I.-B.D.; validation, C.M.D.; formal analysis, C.M.D. and I.-B.D.; investigation, C.M.D.; resources, C.M.D. and A.C.N.; data curation, C.M.D. and A.C.N.; writing—original draft preparation, C.M.D.; writing—review and editing, C.M.D. and I.-B.D.; visualization, C.M.D.; supervision, C.M.D. and I.-B.D.; project administration, C.M.D. All authors have read and agreed to the published version of the manuscript.

Funding: This research received no external funding.

Acknowledgments: As Guest Editors of this Special Issue "Emerging Strategies in Drug Development and Clinical Care in the Era of Personalized and Precision Medicine", we would like to express our deep appreciation to all authors whose valuable work was published under this Special Issue and thus contributed to the success of the edition.

Conflicts of Interest: The authors declare no conflicts of interest.

List of Contributions:

1. Walker, J.M.; O'Malley, P.; He, M. Applications of Exosomes in Diagnosing Muscle Invasive Bladder Cancer. *Pharmaceutics* **2022**, *14*, 2027. https://doi.org/10.3390/pharmaceutics14102027.
2. Axente, M.; Mirea, A.; Sporea, C.; Pădure, L.; Drăgoi, C.M.; Nicolae, A.C.; Ion, D.A. Clinical and Electrophysiological Changes in Pediatric Spinal Muscular Atrophy after 2 Years of Nusinersen Treatment. *Pharmaceutics* **2022**, *14*, 2074. https://doi.org/10.3390/pharmaceutics14102074.
3. Becker, G.; Fialho, M.F.P.; Brusco, I.; Oliveira, S.M. Kinin B_1 and B_2 Receptors Contribute to Cisplatin-Induced Painful Peripheral Neuropathy in Male Mice. *Pharmaceutics* **2023**, *15*, 852. https://doi.org/10.3390/pharmaceutics15030852.
4. García-Lluch, G.; Peña-Bautista, C.; Royo, L.M.; Baquero, M.; Cañada-Martínez, A.J.; Cháfer-Pericás, C. Angiotensin II Receptor Blockers Reduce Tau/Aß42 Ratio: A Cerebrospinal Fluid Biomarkers' Case-Control Study. *Pharmaceutics* **2023**, *15*, 924. https://doi.org/10.3390/pharmaceutics15030924.

5. Silva, R.; Colom, H.; Bicker, J.; Almeida, A.; Silva, A.; Sales, F.; Santana, I.; Falcão, A.; Fortuna, A. Population Pharmacokinetic Analysis of Perampanel in Portuguese Patients Diagnosed with Refractory Epilepsy. *Pharmaceutics* 2023, *15*, 1704. https://doi.org/10.3390/pharmaceutics15061704.
6. Kanellopoulos, P.; Nock, B.A.; Krenning, E.P.; Maina, T. Toward Stability Enhancement of NTS$_1$R-Targeted Radioligands: Structural Interventions on [^{99m}Tc]Tc-DT1. *Pharmaceutics* 2023, *15*, 2092. https://doi.org/10.3390/pharmaceutics15082092.
7. Rakicevic, L. DNA and RNA Molecules as a Foundation of Therapy Strategies for Treatment of Cardiovascular Diseases. *Pharmaceutics* 2023, *15*, 2141. https://doi.org/10.3390/pharmaceutics15082141.
8. Joung, H.-Y.; Oh, J.-M.; Song, M.-S.; Kwon, Y.-B.; Chun, S. Selegiline Modulates Lipid Metabolism by Activating AMPK Pathways of Epididymal White Adipose Tissues in HFD-Fed Obese Mice. *Pharmaceutics* 2023, *15*, 2539. https://doi.org/10.3390/pharmaceutics15112539.
9. Kwak, Y.B.; Seo, J.I.; Yoo, H.H. Exploring Metabolic Pathways of Anamorelin, a Selective Agonist of the Growth Hormone Secretagogue Receptor, via Molecular Networking. *Pharmaceutics* 2023, *15*, 2700. https://doi.org/10.3390/pharmaceutics15122700.
10. Sánchez Suárez, M.D.M.; Martín Roldán, A.; Alarcón-Payer, C.; Rodríguez-Gil, M.Á.; Poquet-Jornet, J.E.; Puerta Puerta, J.M.; Jiménez Morales, A. Treatment of Chronic Lymphocytic Leukemia in the Personalized Medicine Era. *Pharmaceutics* 2024, *16*, 55. https://doi.org/10.3390/pharmaceutics16010055.
11. Dräger, S.; Ewoldt, T.M.J.; Abdulla, A.; Rietdijk, W.J.R.; Verkaik, N.; Ramakers, C.; de Jong, E.; Osthoff, M.; Koch, B.C.P.; Endeman, H., on behalf of the DOLPHIN Investigators. Exploring the Impact of Model-Informed Precision Dosing on Procalcitonin Concentrations in Critically Ill Patients: A Secondary Analysis of the DOLPHIN Trial. *Pharmaceutics* 2024, *16*, 270. https://doi.org/10.3390/pharmaceutics16020270.
12. Marques, L.; Costa, B.; Pereira, M.; Silva, A.; Santos, J.; Saldanha, L.; Silva, I.; Magalhães, P.; Schmidt, S.; Vale, N. Advancing Precision Medicine: A Review of Innovative In Silico Approaches for Drug Development, Clinical Pharmacology and Personalized Healthcare. *Pharmaceutics* 2024, *16*, 332. https://doi.org/10.3390/pharmaceutics16030332.
13. Harnett, A.; Byrne, S.; O'Connor, J.; Burke, E.; South, L.; Lyons, D.; Sahm, L.J. Point Prevalence Survey of Acute Hospital Patients with Difficulty Swallowing Solid Oral Dose Forms. *Pharmaceutics* 2024, *16*, 584. https://doi.org/10.3390/pharmaceutics16050584.

References

1. Marques, L.; Costa, B.; Pereira, M.; Silva, A.; Santos, J.; Saldanha, L.; Silva, I.; Magalhães, P.; Schmidt, S.; Vale, N. Advancing Precision Medicine: A Review of Innovative In Silico Approaches for Drug Development, Clinical Pharmacology and Personalized Healthcare. *Pharmaceutics* 2024, *16*, 332. [CrossRef]
2. Yamamoto, Y.; Kanayama, N.; Nakayama, Y.; Matsushima, N. Current Status, Issues and Future Prospects of Personalized Medicine for Each Disease. *J. Pers. Med.* 2022, *12*, 444. [CrossRef] [PubMed]
3. Akhoon, N. Precision Medicine: A New Paradigm in Therapeutics. *Int. J. Prev. Med.* 2021, *12*, 12. [CrossRef]
4. Gameiro, G.R.; Sinkunas, V.; Liguori, G.R.; Auler-Júnior, J.O.C. Precision Medicine: Changing the Way We Think about Healthcare. *Clinics* 2018, *73*, e723. [CrossRef] [PubMed]
5. Abdelhalim, H.; Berber, A.; Lodi, M.; Jain, R.; Nair, A.; Pappu, A.; Patel, K.; Venkat, V.; Venkatesan, C.; Wable, R.; et al. Artificial Intelligence, Healthcare, Clinical Genomics, and Pharmacogenomics Approaches in Precision Medicine. *Front. Genet.* 2022, *13*, 929736. [CrossRef] [PubMed]
6. Venne, J.; Busshoff, U.; Poschadel, S.; Menschel, R.; Evangelatos, N.; Vysyaraju, K.; Brand, A. International consortium for personalised medicine: An international survey about the future of personalised medicine. *Pers. Med.* 2020, *17*, 89–100. [CrossRef] [PubMed]
7. Steinhubl, S.R.; Muse, E.D.; Topol, E.J. The Emerging Field of Mobile Health. *Sci. Transl. Med.* 2015, *7*, 283rv3. [CrossRef]
8. Vicente, A.M.; Ballensiefen, W.; Jönsson, J.I. How personalised medicine will transform healthcare by 2030: The ICPerMed vision. *J. Transl. Med.* 2020, *18*, 180. [CrossRef]
9. Denny, J.C.; Collins, F.S. Precision Medicine in 2030—Seven Ways to Transform Healthcare. *Cell* 2021, *184*, 1415–1419. [CrossRef]
10. Baylot, V.; Le, T.K.; Taïeb, D.; Rocchi, P.; Colleaux, L. Between hope and reality: Treatment of genetic diseases through nucleic acid-based drugs. *Commun. Biol.* 2024, *7*, 489. [CrossRef]
11. Barbu, C.G.; Arsene, A.L.; Florea, S.; Albu, A.; Sirbu, A.; Martin, S.; Nicolae, A.C.; Burcea-Dragomiroiu, G.T.A.; Popa, D.E.; Velescu, B.S.; et al. Cardiovascular Risk Assessment in Osteoporotic Patients Using Osteoprotegerin as a Reliable Predictive Biochemical Marker. *Mol. Med. Rep.* 2017, *16*, 6059–6067. [CrossRef] [PubMed]

12. Kerioui, M.; Bertrand, J.; Bruno, R.; Mercier, F.; Guedj, J.; Desmée, S. Modelling the association between biomarkers and clinical outcome: An introduction to nonlinear joint models. *Br. J. Clin. Pharmacol.* **2022**, *88*, 1452–1463. [CrossRef] [PubMed]
13. Nechita, V.I.; Hajjar, N.A.; Drugan, C.; Cătană, C.S.; Moiș, E.; Nechita, M.A.; Graur, F. Chitotriosidase and Neopterin as Two Novel Potential Biomarkers for Advanced Stage and Survival Prediction in Gastric Cancer-A Pilot Study. *Diagnostics* **2023**, *13*, 1362. [CrossRef] [PubMed]
14. Rasheed, N.W.; Barbu, C.G.; Florea, S.; Branceanu, G.; Fica, S.; Mitrea, N.; Dragoi, C.M.; Nicolae, A.C.; Arsene, A.L. Biochemical Markers of Calcium and Bone Metabolism in the Monitoring of Osteoporosis Treatment. *Farmacia* **2014**, *62*, 728–736.
15. Park, S.Y.; Cho, D.-G.; Shim, B.-Y.; Cho, U. Relationship between Systemic Inflammatory Markers, GLUT1 Expression, and Maximum 18F-Fluorodeoxyglucose Uptake in Non-Small Cell Lung Carcinoma and Their Prognostic Significance. *Diagnostics* **2023**, *13*, 1013. [CrossRef]
16. Stanciu, A.E.; Zamfir-Chiru-Anton, A.; Stanciu, M.M.; Stoian, A.P.; Jinga, V.; Nitipir, C.; Bucur, A.; Pituru, T.S.; Arsene, A.L.; Dragoi, C.M.; et al. Clinical Significance of Serum Melatonin in Predicting the Severity of Oral Squamous Cell Carcinoma. *Oncol. Lett.* **2020**, *19*, 1537–1543. [CrossRef]
17. Lunke, S.; Bouffler, S.E.; Patel, C.V.; Sandaradura, S.A.; Wilson, M.; Pinner, J.; Hunter, M.F.; Barnett, C.P.; Wallis, M.; Kamien, B.; et al. Integrated multi-omics for rapid rare disease diagnosis on a national scale. *Nat. Med.* **2023**, *29*, 1681–1691. [CrossRef]
18. DeGroat, W.; Mendhe, D.; Bhusari, A.; Abdelhalim, H.; Zeeshan, S.; Ahmed, Z. IntelliGenes: A Novel Machine Learning Pipeline for Biomarker Discovery and Predictive Analysis Using Multigenomic Profiles. *Bioinformatics* **2023**, *39*, btad755. [CrossRef]
19. Laurie, S.; Piscia, D.; Matalonga, L.; Corvó, A.; Fernández-Callejo, M.; Garcia-Linares, C.; Hernandez-Ferrer, C.; Luengo, C.; Martínez, I.; Papakonstantinou, A.; et al. The RD-Connect Genome-Phenome Analysis Platform: Accelerating diagnosis, research, and gene discovery for rare diseases. *Hum. Mutat.* **2022**, *43*, 717–733. [CrossRef]
20. Niculae, D.; Dusman, R.; Leonte, R.A.; Chilug, L.E.; Dragoi, C.M.; Nicolae, A.; Serban, R.M.; Niculae, D.A.; Dumitrescu, I.B.; Draganescu, D. Biological Pathways as Substantiation of the Use of Copper Radioisotopes in Cancer Theranostics. *Front. Phys.* **2021**, *8*, 568296. [CrossRef]
21. Twilt, J.J.; van Leeuwen, K.G.; Huisman, H.J.; Fütterer, J.J.; de Rooij, M. Artificial Intelligence Based Algorithms for Prostate Cancer Classification and Detection on Magnetic Resonance Imaging: A Narrative Review. *Diagnostics* **2021**, *11*, 959. [CrossRef]
22. Stanowicka-Grada, M.; Senkus, E. Anti-HER2 Drugs for the Treatment of Advanced HER2 Positive Breast Cancer. *Curr. Treat. Options Oncol.* **2023**, *24*, 1633–1650. [CrossRef] [PubMed]
23. Chiș, I.-A.; Andrei, V.; Muntean, A.; Moldovan, M.; Mesaroș, A.; Dudescu, M.C.; Ilea, A. Salivary Biomarkers of Anti-Epileptic Drugs: A Narrative Review. *Diagnostics* **2023**, *13*, 1962. [CrossRef] [PubMed]
24. Ahmed, Z.; Zeeshan, S.; Liang, B.T. RNA-Seq Driven Expression and Enrichment Analysis to Investigate CVD Genes with Associated Phenotypes among High-Risk Heart Failure Patients. *Hum. Genom.* **2021**, *15*, 67. [CrossRef]
25. Drăgoi, C.; Nicolae, A.C.; Dumitrescu, I.-B.; Popa, D.E.; Ritivoiu, M.; Arsene, A.L. DNA targeting as a molecular mechanism underlying endogenous indoles biological effects. *Farmacia* **2019**, *67*, 367. [CrossRef]
26. Zhao, S.; Bao, Z.; Zhao, X.; Xu, M.; Li, M.D.; Yang, Z. Identification of Diagnostic Markers for Major Depressive Disorder Using Machine Learning Methods. *Front. Neurosci.* **2021**, *15*, 645998. [CrossRef] [PubMed]
27. Schaack, D.; Weigand, M.A.; Uhle, F. Comparison of Machine-Learning Methodologies for Accurate Diagnosis of Sepsis Using Microarray Gene Expression Data. *PLoS ONE* **2021**, *16*, e0251800. [CrossRef]
28. DeGroat, W.; Abdelhalim, H.; Patel, K.; Mendhe, D.; Zeeshan, S.; Ahmed, Z. Discovering Biomarkers Associated and Predicting Cardiovascular Disease with High Accuracy Using a Novel Nexus of Machine Learning Techniques for Precision Medicine. *Sci. Rep.* **2024**, *14*, 1. [CrossRef]
29. Ungurianu, A.; Zanfirescu, A.; Margina, D. Regulation of Gene Expression through Food-Curcumin as a Sirtuin Activity Modulator. *Plants* **2022**, *11*, 1741. [CrossRef]
30. Kegerreis, B.; Catalina, M.D.; Bachali, P.; Geraci, N.S.; Labonte, A.C.; Zeng, C.; Stearrett, N.; Crandall, K.A.; Lipsky, P.E.; Grammer, A.C. Machine Learning Approaches to Predict Lupus Disease Activity from Gene Expression Data. *Sci. Rep.* **2019**, *9*, 9617. [CrossRef]
31. Tang, L. Informatics for Genomics. *Nat. Methods* **2020**, *17*, 23. [CrossRef]
32. Babu, M.; Lautman, Z.; Lin, X.; Sobota, M.H.; Snyder, M.P. Wearable Devices: Implications for Precision Medicine and the Future of Health Care. *Annu. Rev. Med.* **2024**, *75*, 401–415. [CrossRef]
33. Ahmed, Z.; Mohamed, K.; Zeeshan, S.; Dong, X. Artificial Intelligence with Multi-Functional Machine Learning Platform Development for Better Healthcare and Precision Medicine. *Database* **2020**, *2020*, baaa010. [CrossRef] [PubMed]
34. Fagiani, F.; Di Marino, D.; Romagnoli, A.; Travelli, C.; Voltan, D.; Di Cesare Mannelli, L.; Racchi, M.; Govoni, S.; Lanni, C. Molecular regulations of circadian rhythm and implications for physiology and diseases. *Signal Transduct. Target. Ther.* **2022**, *7*, 41.
35. Dragoi, C.M.; Nicolae, A.C.; Ungurianu, A.; Margina, D.M.; Gradinaru, D.; Dumitrescu, I.-B. Circadian Rhythms, Chrononutrition, Physical Training, and Redox Homeostasis—Molecular Mechanisms in Human Health. *Cells* **2024**, *13*, 138. [CrossRef]
36. Esteva, A.; Robicquet, A.; Ramsundar, B.; Kuleshov, V.; DePristo, M.; Chou, K.; Dean, J. A Guide to Deep Learning in Healthcare. *Nat. Med.* **2019**, *25*, 24–29. [CrossRef] [PubMed]
37. Topol, E.J. High-Performance Medicine: The Convergence of Human and Artificial Intelligence. *Nat. Med.* **2019**, *25*, 44–56. [CrossRef] [PubMed]

38. Walker, W.H.; Walton, J.C.; DeVries, A.C.; Nelson, R.J. Circadian rhythm disruption and mental health. *Transl. Psychiatry* **2020**, *10*, 28. [CrossRef] [PubMed]
39. Dragoi, C.M.; Morosan, E.; Dumitrescu, I.B.; Nicolae, A.C.; Arsene, A.L.; Draganescu, D.; Lupuliasa, D.; Ionita, A.C.; Stoian, A.P.; Nicolae, C.; et al. Insights into chrononutrition: The innermost interplay amongst nutrition, metabolism and the circadian clock, in the context of epigenetic reprogramming. *Farmacia* **2019**, *67*, 557–571. [CrossRef]
40. Vadapalli, S.; Abdelhalim, H.; Zeeshan, S.; Ahmed, Z. Artificial Intelligence and Machine Learning Approaches Using Gene Expression and Variant Data for Personalized Medicine. *Brief. Bioinform.* **2022**, *23*, bbac191. [CrossRef]
41. Knoppers, B.M.; Thorogood, A.M. Ethics and big data in health. *Curr. Opin. Syst. Biol.* **2017**, *4*, 53–57. [CrossRef]

Disclaimer/Publisher's Note: The statements, opinions and data contained in all publications are solely those of the individual author(s) and contributor(s) and not of MDPI and/or the editor(s). MDPI and/or the editor(s) disclaim responsibility for any injury to people or property resulting from any ideas, methods, instructions or products referred to in the content.

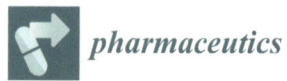 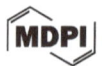

Article

Point Prevalence Survey of Acute Hospital Patients with Difficulty Swallowing Solid Oral Dose Forms

Anne Harnett [1,2,*], Stephen Byrne [2], Jennifer O'Connor [2], Eimear Burke [2], Laura South [1], Declan Lyons [1] and Laura J. Sahm [2,3,*]

1. University Hospital Limerick, Dooradoyle, V94 F858 Limerick, Ireland; laura.south@hse.ie (L.S.); declan.lyons@hse.ie (D.L.)
2. Pharmaceutical Care Research Group, School of Pharmacy, University College Cork, T12 YN60 Cork, Ireland; stephen.byrne@ucc.ie (S.B.); 119312883@umail.ucc.ie (J.O.); 119348971@umail.ucc.ie (E.B.)
3. Pharmacy Department, Mercy University Hospital, Grenville Place, T12 WE28 Cork, Ireland
* Correspondence: anne.harnett1@hse.ie (A.H.); l.sahm@ucc.ie (L.J.S.)

Abstract: The safe administration of solid oral dose forms in hospital inpatients with swallowing difficulties is challenging. The aim of this study was to establish the prevalence of difficulties in swallowing solid oral dose forms in acute hospital inpatients. A point prevalence study was completed at three time points. The following data were collected: the prevalence of swallowing difficulties, methods used to modify solid oral dose forms to facilitate administration, the appropriateness of the modification, and patient co-morbidities. The prevalence of acute hospital inpatients with swallowing difficulties was an average of 15.4% with a 95% CI [13.4, 17.6] across the three studies. On average, 9.6% of patients with swallowing difficulties had no enteral feeding tube in situ, with 6.0% of these patients receiving at least one modified medicine. The most common method of solid oral dose form modification was crushing, with an administration error rate of approximately 14.4%. The most common co-morbid condition in these patients was hypertension, with dysphagia appearing on the problem list of two (5.5%) acute hospital inpatients with swallowing difficulties. Inappropriate modifications to solid oral dose forms to facilitate administration can result in patient harm. A proactive approach, such as the use of a screening tool to identify acute hospital inpatients with swallowing difficulties, is required, to mitigate the risk of inappropriate modifications to medicines to overcome swallowing difficulties.

Keywords: solid oral dosage form (SODF); medicine administration; difficulty swallowing; dysphagia; medicine manipulation; inpatient

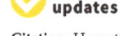

Citation: Harnett, A.; Byrne, S.; O'Connor, J.; Burke, E.; South, L.; Lyons, D.; Sahm, L.J. Point Prevalence Survey of Acute Hospital Patients with Difficulty Swallowing Solid Oral Dose Forms. *Pharmaceutics* 2024, 16, 584. https://doi.org/10.3390/pharmaceutics16050584

Academic Editors: Cristina Manuela Dragoi, Alina Crenguța Nicolae and Ion-Bogdan Dumitrescu

Received: 13 March 2024
Revised: 15 April 2024
Accepted: 19 April 2024
Published: 25 April 2024

Copyright: © 2024 by the authors. Licensee MDPI, Basel, Switzerland. This article is an open access article distributed under the terms and conditions of the Creative Commons Attribution (CC BY) license (https://creativecommons.org/licenses/by/4.0/).

1. Introduction

The oral route is the most common route for medicine administration [1]. Although solid oral dosage forms (SODFs), such as tablets and capsules, tend to be the most prevalent and preferred, modifications may be required to ease administration or to allow administration via the oral route. SODF modification can be defined as "any alteration of an oral dosage form that can be performed at the point of administration" [2]. These modifications are undertaken to allow medicine administration to patients with swallowing difficulties (SDs) regarding intact SODFs (e.g., crushing tablets or opening capsules) or to aid fractional dosing (the administration of part of an SODF to allow the administration of a lower dose, e.g., splitting tablets).

Many challenges exist around those with SDs, one of them being protecting the safety of the patient. Whilst dysphagia is a medical term used to describe dysfunction in one or more parts of the swallowing apparatus [3], patients may experience difficulty swallowing SODFs in the absence of a formal diagnosis, which may be described as pill aversion [4]. Presented with this challenge, medication modifications may be attempted, such as crushing tablets or opening capsules. This may not be appropriate legally, pharmaceutically, or therapeutically [5]. A recent review found that to optimise oral medicine modification practices, the needs of individual patients should be routinely and systematically assessed and decision-making should be supported by evidence-based recommendations with multidisciplinary input [6].

Many studies that have examined the prevalence of SDs do so in the context of specific cohorts of patients, such as community-dwelling older adults [7], cardiac surgical intensive care patients [8], those with solid cancers [9], temporomandibular joint disorders [10], and older adult inpatients [11].

Reports on the prevalence of SDs in hospital inpatients often report cohorts where the prevalence is likely to be higher, e.g., older adult care wards [11–13], and include inpatients in acute hospital settings and nursing home residents together in the study cohort [14]. A systematic search of the literature did not recover any study that reported the prevalence of swallowing difficulties in general medical and surgical acute hospital inpatients alone.

It is reported that 3% of adult inpatients in the United States of America have a diagnosis of dysphagia [15]. A formal diagnosis of dysphagia is not necessary for a patient to report difficulties in swallowing SODFs and pill aversion [4]. We consider that the true prevalence of acute hospital inpatients with difficulties in swallowing SODFs is likely to be higher than this.

The prevalence of difficulty swallowing SODFs is reported as 29.5% on older adult inpatient units in France [11]. Similarly, the prevalence of inpatients with difficulties in swallowing medicines in a care-of-the-older-adult ward or stroke unit at each of four acute hospitals in the east of England was reported as 34.2% [13]. In a systematic review, 10–34% of inpatients in hospitals, nursing homes, and long-term-stay units had difficulty swallowing SODFs [16]. The prevalence of swallowing difficulties in general medical and surgical acute hospital inpatients alone could not be established from the review of these studies.

The aim of this study was to establish the prevalence of swallowing difficulties with SODFs in hospital inpatients in an acute hospital in Ireland.

2. Materials and Methods

2.1. Study Design

This is a point prevalence survey (PPS) of swallowing difficulties in acute hospital inpatients.

2.2. Ethical Approval and Data Privacy

The study received ethical approval from the Research Ethics Committee, University Hospital Limerick in June 2022 (PPS1) and again in June 2023 (PPS2 and PPS3).

2.3. Study Setting

University Hospital Limerick is a model 4 hospital located in the Mid-West of Ireland with a catchment area of 410,000 people [17]. Model 4 refers to a hospital that admits undifferentiated acute medical and surgical patients, including tertiary referred patients, and has a category 3 intensive care unit on site and a 24 h emergency department [18].

2.4. Inclusion Criteria

Inpatients with an age greater than 18 years and hospitalised in a ward at University Hospital Limerick by 8 a.m. each day of the survey were eligible for inclusion.

2.5. Exclusion Criteria

Outpatients, cancer services patients in the inpatient or day care cancer services wards, critical care patients in the intensive care unit, high-dependency unit, or coronary care units, patients in the psychiatric unit, day patients defined as those discharged on the same day, and inpatients in the paediatric wards were all excluded. One ward with eligible patients

(29 beds) was not included in PPS1 because there was a declared outbreak of infection in the ward and access for data collection could not be justified.

2.6. Data Collection

The survey data were collected over three time periods. The first PPS was completed in September 2022 (PPS1), the second (PPS2) was completed in June 2023, and final data collection (PPS3) was completed in July 2023.

Data were collected in accordance with a modified version of the methodology established by the World Health Organisation for conducting antimicrobial point prevalence studies [19]. Patients were identified from a ward census.

For all surveys, the following data were collected:
- Total number of patients identified as eligible for inclusion from ward census;
- Total number of patients included in the survey.

2.7. Procedure

Age and sex were collected for all patients. Patients were interviewed by a research assistant to determine their swallowing status. The following question was asked: "do you have any difficulty swallowing your medicines?" Should a patient confirm that they did have a swallowing difficulty, even in the absence of a formal diagnosis, they were classified as having swallowing difficulties (SDs). In cases where patient interview was not possible, the swallowing status information was obtained from nursing staff. Swallowing status was a binary outcome (yes/no).

For any patient with a swallowing difficulty, the following data were collected: (i) the route of administration of oral medicines and (ii) description of swallowing difficulty for those patients not receiving their medication via an enteral feeding tube and those patients where patient interview was possible or, if relevant, (iii) presence and type of feeding tube. For PPS2 and PPS3, the following additional data were collected: data on their prescribed medicines and disease state(s). The method of SODF modification was obtained from the nursing staff responsible for administering the medicine.

Data were collected in hard copy for each patient and then transferred to Microsoft Excel® 2017 version 2403. All data were stored securely to ensure restricted access and full compliance with General Data Protection Regulations.

Patients with swallowing difficulties were referred to a clinical pharmacist. The pharmacist then provided input into patient care regarding alternative formulations, e.g., suspensions versus tablets.

2.8. Data Analysis

Data were analysed using Microsoft Excel® 2017, SPSS version 28 (IBM, Corp. Armonk, NY, USA) and Open Epi [20]. Median and range were reported for age, as data were not normally distributed. Association between categorical variables was assessed. A Pearson's Chi-square test was conducted to assess whether sex and swallowing difficulties were related. A Mann–Whitney U test was performed to examine whether age differed by a patient's ability to swallow their SODF medicines. p-values < 0.05 were considered to be statistically significant.

An SODF was defined as a product listed by the European Medicines Agency (EMA) as an "oral preparation—solid form" in the EMA list of pharmaceutical dosage forms, with the exception of chewable tablets, which were excluded from the definition in this study.

Each method of SODF manipulation was checked against the Summary of Product Characteristics (SmPC) to assess its appropriateness. If the method used to modify the medicine was not permitted/not described as per the SmPC, then two practice guidelines, (i) Drug administration via Enteral Feeding Tubes [21] and (ii) The NEWT Guidelines for administration of medication to patients with enteral feeding tubes or swallowing difficulties [22], were consulted. Modification practices that did not adhere to the terms of either the SmPC or practice guidelines were considered inappropriate. For these modifications, a medication administration error rate was calculated as follows: number of inappropriate modifications to SODFs/total number of instances in which SODFs were modified, similar to the error calculation method used in other studies [11,12].

If deemed appropriate, the following details were collected: (i) method of modification, (ii) vehicle used, (iii) number of instances of modification, and (iv) reasons for inappropriateness.

Disease states were classified according to the International Classification of Diseases and Related Health Problems (ICD-10) [23].

3. Results

3.1. Prevalence of Patients with Swallowing Difficulties

A total of 1120 patients, 96.9% of eligible patients, participated in the PPSs (Table 1).

Table 1. Demographics of participating inpatients.

Title of Survey	Number of Patients Eligible for Inclusion	Number of Participating Inpatients (%)	Median Age (Range) Years	Female Sex (%)
PPS1	348	328 (94.3%)	72 (18–99)	45.43%
PPS2	390	383 (98.2%)	70 (18–99)	45.43%
PPS3	418	409 (97.8%)	71 (18–99)	49.14%
Total	1156	1120 (96.9%)	71 (18–99)	

Of those with swallowing difficulties (n = 172) the median age (years), age range (years), and percentage female were as follows: PPS1 (74, 24–95, 37.8%), PPS 2 (77, 21–93, 49.3%), PPS3 (73, 21–93, 55.2%). The relationship between sex and swallowing difficulties was not significant χ^2 ([1], N = [1120]) = [1.56], p = [0.211]. However, a Mann–Whitney U test revealed a statistically significant difference in the age of those with swallowing difficulties (median age 74 with 95% confidence interval CI [73, 77], n = 172) and those without swallowing difficulties (median age 70 with a 95% CI [69, 72], n = 948), U = 69,571, z = -3.064, p = 0.002, r = -0.09, although the effect size is small as per the Cohen (1988) criteria [24].

The prevalence of swallowing difficulties in eligible acute hospital inpatients was 13.7% with a 95% CI [10.4, 17.9], 18.0% with a 95% CI [14.5, 22.2], and 14.2% with a 95% CI [11.1, 17.9], in PPS1, PPS2, and PPS3, respectively, with an average prevalence of 15.4% with a 95% CI [13.4, 17.6], (Table 2). On average, 5.8% of patients with swallowing difficulties had an enteral feeding tube in situ (Table 2).

Table 2. The prevalence of adult acute hospital inpatients with swallowing difficulties.

Title of Survey	Number PSDs (%)	Number PSDs and No EFT (%)	Number PSDs and EFT (%)	Type EFT
PPS1	45/328 (13.7%)	21/328 (6.4%)	24/328 (7.3%)	8 G, 16 NG
PPS2	69/383 (18%)	50/383 (13.0%)	19/383 (5.0%)	3 G, 16 NG
PPS3	58/409 (14.2%)	36/409 (8.8%)	22/409 (5.4%)	10 G, 12 NG
Total	172/1120 (15.4%)	107/1120 (9.6%)	65/1120 (5.8%)	21 G, 44 NG

PSDs: patients with swallowing difficulties, EFT: enteral feeding tube, G: gastrostomy tube, NG: nasogastric tube.

The majority of patients with swallowing difficulties and an enteral feeding tube received their medicines via the tube: PPS1 22/24 (92%), PPS2 17/19 (89.5%), and PPS3 18/22 (82%). Among the patients with a swallowing difficulty and an enteral feeding tube who did not receive their SODFs via the enteral feeding tube (n = 6), three patients swallowed their medicines without modification and three had their medicines crushed and administered in yoghurt. The remaining two patients were not prescribed SODFs and swallowed oral liquid medicines.

The prevalence of patients with swallowing difficulties and an enteral feeding tube requiring modification of their SODFs is recorded in Table 3, with an average prevalence of 5.3%. A patient with a swallowing difficulty and a gastrostomy tube was more likely to have medicines administered via the tube than if the patient had a nasogastric tube (Table 3).

Table 3. Prevalence of SODF modification in patients with a swallowing difficulty and enteral feeding tube.

Title of Survey	PSDs and EFT/Total Number PSDs	PSDs and EFT						Prevalence of PSDs and EFT Requiring Modification of SODF
		All SODF Modified		Some SODF Modified		No SODF Modified		
		Gast	NG	Gast	NG	Gast	NG	
PPS1	24/46 (52%)	8/8 (100%)	14/16 (87.5%)	0/8 (0%)	0/16 (0%)	0/8 (0%)	2 [a]/16 (12.5%)	22/328 (6.7%)
PPS2	19/69 (27.5%)	3/3 (100%)	15/16 (93.8%)	0/3 (0%)	0/16 (0%)	0/3 (0%)	1 [b]/16 (6.25%)	18/383 (4.7%)
PPS3	22/58 (38%)	9/10 (90%)	10/12 (83%)	0/10 (0%)	1 [c]/12 (8.3%)	1 [b]/10 (8.3%)	1 [b]/12 (8.3%)	20/409 (4.9%)
								60/1120 (5.3%)

[a] No SODF prescribed, liquid medicines taken orally. [b] SODF taken orally. [c] Some SODF crushed and taken orally in yogurt, other SODF crushed and administered via the EFT, SODF: solid oral dose form, PSDs: patients with swallowing difficulties, EFT: enteral feeding tube, Gast: gastrostomy tube, NG: nasogastric tube.

The prevalence of patients with swallowing difficulties and no enteral feeding tube requiring modification of their SODF is recorded in Table 4, with an average prevalence of 6.0%. Regarding patients with swallowing difficulties without an enteral feeding tube, PPS2 and PPS3 show that approximately half of these patients have no modification to their SODF, with 46% and 47.2%, respectively, while in PPS1, all patients with a swallowing difficulty and no enteral feeding tube required some medicines to be altered as a result. PPS2 and PPS3 record that approximately one third of patients with swallowing difficulties and no enteral feeding tube (30% and 30.6%, respectively) require all SODF to be modified, with PPS1 increasing that number to three quarters (77%). In all three PPSs, approximately one fifth of patients with swallowing difficulties and no enteral feeding tube required the modification of some, but not all, of their SODF.

Table 4. Prevalence of SODF modifications in patients with swallowing difficulties and no enteral feeding tube.

Title of Survey	PSDs No EFT	PSDs and No EFT			Prevalence of PSDs and No EFT Requiring Modification of SODF
		All SODF Modified	Some SODF Modified	No SODF Modified	
PPS1	21/46 (47.8%)	17/21 (77.3%)	4/21 (18.2%)	0/21 (0%)	21/328 (6.4%)
PPS2	50/69 (72.5%)	15/50 (30.0%)	12/50 (24.0%)	23/50 (46.0%)	27/383 (7.0%)
PPS3	36/58 (62.1%)	11/36 (30.6%)	8/36 (22.2%)	17/36 (47.2%)	19/409 (4.6%)
Average	107/1120 (9.6%)				67/1120 (6.0%)

SODF: solid oral dose form, PSDs: patients with swallowing difficulties, EFT: enteral feeding tube.

3.2. Description of Swallowing Difficulties

Patients were asked to describe their swallowing difficulties if they were not receiving their medicines via an enteral feeding tube and if a patient interview was possible. The majority of patients did not know their medications by name and could not name SODF(s) that they found difficult to swallow. Many gave a vague description like "the large white ones" or "the stomach tablets", with patients describing the difficulty using tablet sizes and textures rather than the name of the medication (Table 5). Fifty-eight patients provided a description of their swallowing difficulty (PPS1 (n = 5), PPS2 (n = 30), PPS3 (n = 23)). The most common description provided by patients was of difficulty in swallowing "large tablets", with approximately one third of patients with swallowing difficulties describing difficulty with swallowing all SODFs.

Table 5. Patient descriptions of difficulties in swallowing SODFs.

PSD Description of Size or Texture of SODF Contributing to the Swallowing Difficulty (n = 58)	PSDs Having Their Medicines Modified (n = 25)	PSDs Not Having Their Medicines Modified (n = 33)	Total Number of PSDs (Percent)
Capsules	1	1	2 (3.4)
Large tablet(s)/SODF(s)	12	19	31 (53.4)
All SODFs	10	7	17 (29.3)
Small tablet(s)/SODF(s)	1	3	4 (6.9)
"Chalky" SODFs	1	1	2 (3.4)
Not described	0	2	2 (3.4)
Total	25	33	58

SODF: solid oral dose form, PSDs: patients with swallowing difficulties.

3.3. Methods of Solid Oral Dose Form Modification

The most common method used to modify SODFs prior to administration to patients with swallowing difficulties, with or without an enteral feeding tube (Table 6), was crushing.

Table 6. Methods of SODF modification in PSDs with no EFT.

Method of Modification of SODF	Number of PSDs with No EFT Receiving Modifications to Some or All of Their SODF		
	PPS 1 n = 21 (%)	PPS 2 n = 27 (%)	PPS 3 n = 19 (%)
Crushed	18 (81.8%)	19 (70.3%)	12 (63%)
Capsule opened/pierced	0	1 (3.7%)	0
Split	2 (9%)	5 (18.5%)	5 (26%)
Chewed or halved	0	1 (3.7%)	0
Soaked in yoghurt	1 (4.5%)	1 (3.7%)	2 (10.5%)

SODF: solid oral dose form, PSDs: patients with swallowing difficulties, EFT: enteral feeding tube.

The most common vehicle used to administer modified SODFs to patients with swallowing difficulties and no enteral feeding tube in all three studies was yoghurt, while water was the most common vehicle to administer modified medicines to patients with swallowing difficulties and an enteral feeding tube.

3.4. Appropriateness of Solid Oral Dose Form Modification

The appropriateness of each SODF modification was then established for those patients with swallowing difficulties who had given consent.

In PPS2, twenty-two patients with swallowing difficulties were included, equating to 337 prescriptions (average: 15.3 per patient, range: 8–28). Nine patients received at least one modified SODF.

There were 187 different medications prescribed in PPS2, and 15.5% (n = 29) of these were modified prior to administration. As a medication may be administered more than once daily, we calculated this to be equivalent to 43 instances of medicine modification.

For these 43 instances, 74.4% were not in compliance with the SmPC and 14% were not in compliance with best-practice standards. This gave a medication administration error rate of 14%.

In PPS3, fourteen patients with swallowing difficulties were included, equating to 237 prescriptions (average: 16.9 per patient, range: 15–21). Four patients received at least one modified SODF.

There were 128 different medications prescribed in PPS3, and 15.6% (n = 20) of these were modified prior to administration. As a medication may be administered more than once daily, we calculated this to be equivalent to 27 instances of medication modification.

For these 27 instances, 77.8% were not in compliance with the SmPC and 14.8% were not in compliance with best-practice standards. This gave a medication administration error rate of 14.8%.

Errors included the crushing of enteric coated preparations, increasing the risk of reduced efficacy or increased side effects, such as with aspirin and omeprazole, destruction of the sustained-release formulation, such as with ranolazine, and a modification that was not recommended due to occupational exposure risk, such as with dutasteride. With 40% of the errors, an alternative, more appropriate pharmaceutical formulation was available. In the remaining cases, an alternative therapeutic option could have been considered.

3.5. Diseases and Related Health Problems of Patients with Swallowing Difficulties

In 36 patients with swallowing difficulties, there were a total of 151 conditions diagnosed. Hypertension was the most diagnosed condition (n = 17). Two patients had dysphagia listed in their diagnosed health conditions.

4. Discussion

These point prevalence surveys established the prevalence of swallowing difficulties in adults with an age greater than 18 years admitted as acute inpatients to general medical and surgical wards in an acute hospital. Across the three surveys, the prevalence of swallowing difficulties among adult hospital inpatients was 15.4% or approximately one in every seven inpatients. Excluding inpatients with an enteral feeding tube in situ, the prevalence of swallowing difficulties was 9.6% or approximately 1 patient in every 10.

A one-day prospective observational study of inpatients (n = 526) with swallowing difficulties in 17 geriatric units (acute geriatric care, rehabilitation unit, long-term care) of the three Paris-Sud teaching hospitals reported an overall prevalence of 29.5%, with a prevalence of 12.2% in the acute care unit [11]. The prevalence in the acute care unit was similar to the prevalence in acute inpatients in this study, with the overall prevalence being much higher than this study when the other settings are included. This is to be expected, as geriatric inpatients in a long-term care or rehabilitation setting are more likely to have a swallowing difficulty [25]. Patients were identified as having a swallowing difficulty through observation by the researchers, which differs from the method used here. It is not clear from the study whether patients with enteral feeding tubes were included, making it difficult to directly compare these populations.

A two-day prospective, observational study of inpatients with an age greater than 65 years (n = 719), in 23 geriatric units in Rouen University Hospital Centre (acute geriatric medicine, post-acute rehabilitation, nursing homes, long-term care units) reported a prevalence of 18.8%, excluding patients with enteral feeding tubes [12]. Our study found a much lower prevalence of swallowing difficulties in hospital inpatients without an enteral feeding tube (9.6%) than this. However, the populations differ in that only those greater than 65 years were included, and some patients were in long-term care, where it would be expected that a higher prevalence of swallowing difficulties would be found [26]. Furthermore, it is unclear from the study how patients with swallowing difficulties were identified for inclusion.

An undisguised direct observational study of inpatients (n = 625) in a care-of-the-older-adult ward or stroke unit at each of four acute hospitals in the east of England over a 4-month period reported a prevalence of 34.2% including those with an enteral feeding tube or 26.2% excluding enteral feeding tube patients [13]. Patients were identified as having a swallowing difficulty if (i) there was advice on fluid, food, or medicine consistency available or (ii) there was an enteral feeding tube in situ, (iii) the nurse considered that the patient had a swallowing difficulty, or (iv) the patient chewed SODFs. The prevalence was much higher than that identified in our study because patients in older adult care wards and stroke wards are more likely to have swallowing difficulties [26], so the two cohorts are not directly comparable.

A comparison of prevalence with other studies is not straightforward because of differences in the populations selected for inclusion, the methods used to identify eligible patients, and whether or not patients with enteral feeding tubes, which can be used for medicine administration, were included in the swallowing-difficulty cohort. An interesting finding in this study is that just over half of the patients with a swallowing difficulty and no enteral feeding tube had their SODF modified by a nurse prior to administration. However, when a patient is discharged home, a nurse is unlikely to be involved in the administration process and the patient may find it difficult to swallow the medicine without modification. Several authors report that patients are at risk of not taking medications that are difficult to swallow [27–29]. Hence, patients with swallowing difficulties are potentially at risk of intentional non-adherence when discharged from the acute hospital setting [4]. Additionally, only two of the thirty-six patients with swallowing difficulties had dysphagia recorded in their disease states, potentially making it challenging for health care professionals to be aware of these difficulties. This finding supports the proactive use of a screening tool such as Swallowing Difficulties with Medication Intake and Coping Strategies (SWAMECO) [30]. The SWAMECO questionnaire can be used to identify patients with difficulty swallowing SODFs. Whilst it was originally developed for patients with systemic sclerosis, it was subsequently validated in community-dwelling adult patients [31]. The current version of SWAMECO (version 5) contains 18 questions, 11 of which can be answered with "Yes" or "No". It includes questions such as "Does your doctor know about your swallowing difficulties when taking medicines?" (question 4) and "Which strategies do you use to make it easier to swallow medicine(s)?" (question 9). This questionnaire can be completed by the patient in approximately five minutes.

In keeping with other studies, the most common method of SODF modification was crushing [11–13,32–35]. Other, less common, methods have also been previously reported, such as capsule opening [35], tablet splitting [13,34,35], and mixing the SODF with food following crushing or opening [36]. This study also found that soaking of the SODF in yoghurt prior to administration, to soften it, was used as a method of administration. Yoghurt was the most popular food stuff used to administer modified SODFs. The use of yoghurt as a vehicle has also been previously reported [11,26,28]. The appropriateness of yoghurt as a vehicle has not been studied, as far as the authors are aware. Over half of the patients with swallowing difficulties reported that their difficulty occurred with large tablets, although the term "large tablet" is not defined and, as the patients could not identify their medicines by name, it is not possible to establish whether all patients with difficulties with large tablets were referring to similar-sized tablets. Size, shape, colour, surface characteristics, taste, and mouthfeel are reported to influence the ease with which an SODF can be swallowed [27,28,37]. In this study, size was the primary descriptor used to report swallowing difficulties with SODFs. The modification of SODFs prior to administration can lead to medication administration errors [13,32]. This study found an error rate of approximately 14.4%. Other studies report error rates from 3.1% [38] to 48.2% [11]; however, direct comparison of medication administration error rates in patients with swallowing difficulties with other studies is difficult due to variation in the cohort included in terms of age, setting, and the presence of an enteral feeding tube. Direct comparison is also complicated by variation in the method used to calculate the error rate, the description of a medication administration error, and the calculation of a medication administration error rate for the entire patient cohort in the study and not just patients with swallowing difficulties [12,32,39]. A prospective observational study of inpatients in three nursing homes in the Netherlands found a medication administration error rate of 3.1% [38]. This study also reported a reduction in medication administration errors to 0.5% following the introduction of a set of warning labels printed on each patient's unit dose packaging indicating whether a medication could be crushed, as well as education sessions for staff.

4.1. Implications for Practice

This study reports that a minimum of one in every seven adult acute hospital inpatients have difficulties in swallowing SODFs, with approximately one third of those having an enteral feeding tube for medicines administration. Whether SODFs are administered via an enteral feeding tube or not, swallowing difficulties lead to SODF modification, most often by crushing tablets or opening capsules [13]. Medication administration errors occur when SODFs are manipulated to facilitate oral administration in patients with swallowing difficulties [39]. This can have catastrophic consequences for individual patients [40]. Studies have shown that the inappropriate manipulation of SODFs, such as crushing sustained release tablets, decreases when guidelines on administration are available and followed [12] and when advice labels are used [38].

4.2. Strengths and Limitations

This study was completed at three different time points, with consistent findings in relation to study outcomes enhancing confidence in the results. However, all data were collected from the acute inpatient population of a single hospital. The study results would have been strengthened if multiple hospitals had been included in the PPS.

4.3. Recommendations

All acute hospitals should screen patients for difficulties in swallowing SODFs at the point of admission and have administration guidelines available to those who administer medicines to inpatients with difficulties in swallowing. Practice with regard to the manipulation of medicines to facilitate SODF administration to patients with swallowing difficulties should be audited to ensure that practices are safe for the patient. Training should be offered to staff in relation to prescribing and administering SODFs to adult acute hospital inpatients with swallowing difficulties, and, considering the risks associated with medication administration errors, a multidisciplinary approach is warranted [41]. It has been shown that administration errors due to inappropriately crushing tablets can be significantly reduced by using warning symbols as part of the labelling system in conjunction with education [38]. Additionally, it has been reported that significant and sustainable quality improvement in medication administration in nursing home residents with swallowing difficulties can be achieved following the implementation of a programme that includes education, the introduction of a protocol and pocket cards, the screening of medicines by pharmacy technicians, and the annotation of charts with advice on crushing [33]. Additionally, some medicines, including those with antimuscarinic activity and calcium channel blockers, are considered to potentially induce dysphagia, something that also needs to be recognized at patient reviews [26].

5. Conclusions

The results of this point prevalence show that at least one in seven adult inpatients in acute hospitals may have difficulties in swallowing medicines. Systems in acute hospitals need to be aware of this prevalence in order to identify these patients, to allow swallowing difficulties to be considered when prescribing, dispensing, and administering SODFs. To allow a proactive pragmatic approach to medicine administration in these patients, we suggest the use of a screening tool to identify them at the point of admission, allowing targeted advice regarding the administration of their medications. This will ensure that the risk of medication administration error is minimised and patient adherence is maximised.

Author Contributions: Conceptualization, A.H., S.B. and L.J.S.; methodology, A.H., L.J.S., S.B., J.O., E.B., L.S. and D.L.; software, A.H. and L.J.S.; writing—original draft preparation, A.H., J.O. and E.B.; writing—review and editing, A.H., L.J.S., S.B., J.O., E.B., D.L. and L.S.; supervision, L.J.S., S.B. and D.L. All authors have read and agreed to the published version of the manuscript.

Funding: This research received no external funding.

Institutional Review Board Statement: The study was conducted in accordance with the Declaration of Helsinki and approved by the Research Ethics Committee of University Hospital Limerick (REC Ref: 084/2022, 16 June 2023, REC Ref: 056/2023, 30 May 2023, REC Ref: 057/2023, 30 May 2023).

Informed Consent Statement: Informed consent was obtained from all subjects involved in the study.

Data Availability Statement: The ethics application in this study neither sought nor received permission to share these data publicly.

Acknowledgments: The authors would like to acknowledge the contribution of patients who took part in these studies and the nursing staff who supported data collection.

Conflicts of Interest: The authors declare no conflicts of interest.

References

1. Kim, J.; De Jesus, O. Medication Routes of Administration. In *StatPearls*; StatPearls Publishing: Treasure Island, FL, USA, 2023. Available online: http://www.ncbi.nlm.nih.gov/books/NBK568677/ (accessed on 9 December 2023).
2. Richey, R.H.; Craig, J.V.; Shah, U.U.; Ford, J.L.; Barker, C.E.; Peak, M.; Nunn, A.; Turner, M.A. The manipulation of drugs to obtain the required dose: Systematic review. *J. Adv. Nurs.* **2012**, *68*, 2103–2112. [CrossRef] [PubMed]
3. Speyer, R.; Cordier, R.; Farneti, D.; Nascimento, W.; Pilz, W.; Verin, E.; Walshe, M.; Woisard, V. White Paper by the European Society for Swallowing Disorders: Screening and Non-instrumental Assessment for Dysphagia in Adults. *Dysphagia* **2022**, *37*, 333–349. [CrossRef] [PubMed]
4. McCloskey, A.P.; Penson, P.E.; Tse, Y.; Abdelhafiz, M.A.; Ahmed, S.N.; Lim, E.J. Identifying and addressing pill aversion in adults without physiological-related dysphagia: A narrative review. *Br. J. Clin. Pharmacol.* **2022**, *88*, 5128–5148. [CrossRef]
5. Royal Pharmaceutical Society. *Pharmaceutical Issues When Crushing, Opening or Splitting Oral Dose Forms*; Royal Pharmaceutical Society: London, UK, 2011. Available online: https://www.rpharms.com/Portals/0/RPS%20document%20library/Open%20access/Support/toolkit/pharmaceuticalissuesdosageforms-(2).pdf (accessed on 5 December 2022).
6. Mc Gillicuddy, A.; Kelly, M.; Crean, A.M.; Sahm, L.J. The knowledge, attitudes and beliefs of patients and their healthcare professionals around oral dosage form modification: A systematic review of the qualitative literature. *Res. Soc. Adm. Pharm.* **2017**, *13*, 717–726. [CrossRef] [PubMed]
7. Mc Gillicuddy, A.; Crean, A.M.; Sahm, L.J. Older adults with difficulty swallowing oral medicines: A systematic review of the literature. *Eur. J. Clin. Pharmacol.* **2016**, *72*, 141–151. [CrossRef] [PubMed]
8. Duncan, S.; Blackwood, B.; McAuley, D.F.; Walshe, M. Prevalence, pathophysiology and treatment of dysphagia in cardiac surgical intensive care patients following tracheostomy and/or prolonged intubation: A case series. In *Poster Session 5J*; Trinity College Dublin: Dublin, Ireland, 2018. Available online: https://www.tcd.ie/slscs/clinical-speech-language/dysphagia/assets/Duncan.pdf (accessed on 5 December 2022).
9. Kenny, C.; Regan, J.; Balding, L.; Higgins, S.; O'Leary, N.; Kelleher, F.; McDermott, R.; Armstrong, J.; Mihai, A.; Tiernan, E.; et al. Dysphagia Prevalence and Predictors in Cancers Outside the Head, Neck, and Upper Gastrointestinal Tract. *J. Pain Symptom Manag.* **2019**, *58*, 949–958.e2. [CrossRef] [PubMed]
10. Gilheaney, Ó.; Béchet, S.; Kerr, P.; Kenny, C.; Smith, S.; Kouider, R.; Kidd, R.; Walshe, M. The prevalence of oral stage dysphagia in adults presenting with temporomandibular disorders: A systematic review and meta-analysis. *Acta Odontol. Scand.* **2018**, *76*, 448–458. [CrossRef] [PubMed]
11. Fodil, M.; Nghiem, D.; Colas, M.; Bourry, S.; Poisson-Salomon, A.-S.; Rezigue, H.; Trivalle, C. Assessment of Clinical Practices for Crushing Medication in Geriatric Units. *J. Nutr. Heal. Aging* **2017**, *21*, 904–908. [CrossRef]
12. Bourdenet, G.; Giraud, S.; Artur, M.; Dutertre, S.; Dufour, M.; Lefèbvre-Caussin, M.; Proux, A.; Philippe, S.; Capet, C.; Fontaine-Adam, M.; et al. Impact of recommendations on crushing medications in geriatrics: From prescription to administration. *Fundam. Clin. Pharmacol.* **2015**, *29*, 316–320. [CrossRef] [PubMed]
13. Kelly, J.; Wright, D.; Wood, J. Medicine administration errors in patients with dysphagia in secondary care: A multi-centre observational study. *J. Adv. Nurs.* **2011**, *67*, 2615–2627. [CrossRef]
14. Belissa, E.; Vallet, T.; Laribe-Caget, S.; Chevallier, A.; Chedhomme, F.-X.; Abdallah, F.; Bachalat, N.; Belbachir, S.-A.; Boulaich, I.; Bloch, V.; et al. Acceptability of oral liquid pharmaceutical products in older adults: Palatability and swallowability issues. *BMC Geriatr.* **2019**, *19*, 344. [CrossRef] [PubMed]
15. A Patel, D.; Krishnaswami, S.; Steger, E.; Conover, E.; Vaezi, M.F.; Ciucci, M.R.; O Francis, D. Economic and survival burden of dysphagia among inpatients in the United States. *Dis. Esophagus* **2018**, *31*, dox131. [CrossRef] [PubMed]
16. Harnett, A.; Byrne, S.; O'Connor, J.; Lyons, D.; Sahm, L.J. Adult Patients with Difficulty Swallowing Oral Dosage Forms: A Systematic Review of the Quantitative Literature. *Pharmacy* **2023**, *11*, 167. [CrossRef] [PubMed]
17. Health Service Executive. *UL Hospitals Group Strategic Plan 2023–2027*; Health Service Executive: Limerick, Ireland, 2023. Available online: https://healthservice.hse.ie/filelibrary/ul-hospitals-group-strategic-plan-2023-2027.pdf (accessed on 28 December 2023).
18. Health Service Executive. UL Hospitals Operational Plan 2014. 2014. Available online: https://www.hse.ie/eng/services/list/3/acutehospitals/hospitals/ulh/staff/resources/library/testdoc.pdf (accessed on 28 December 2023).

19. World Health Organisation. *WHO Methodology for Point Prevalence Survey on Antibiotic Use in Hospitals*; World Health Organisation: Geneva, Switzerland, 2018. Available online: https://iris.who.int/bitstream/handle/10665/280063/WHO-EMP-IAU-2018.01-eng.pdf?sequence=1 (accessed on 3 June 2022).
20. Dean, A.G.; Sullivan, K.M.; Soe, M.M. Open Epi: Open Source Epidemiologic Statistics for Public Health. 2013. Available online: https://www.openepi.com/Menu/OE_Menu.htm (accessed on 9 April 2024).
21. White, R.; Bradnam, V. *Drug Administration via Enteral Feeding Tubes*; Pharmaceutical Press: London, UK. Available online: https://www.pharmaceuticalpress.com/products/drug-administration-via-enteral-feeding-tubes/ (accessed on 26 April 2023).
22. Wrexham Maelor Hospital Pharmacy Department. The NEWT Guidelines for Administration of Medications to Patients with Enteral Feeding Tubes or Swallowing Difficulties. Wrexham. Available online: https://www.newtguidelines.com/index.html (accessed on 26 April 2023).
23. World Health Organisation. International Statistical Classification of Diseases and Related Health Problems (10th ed.). 2019. Available online: https://www.google.ie/url?sa=t&rct=j&q=&esrc=s&source=web&cd=&cad=rja&uact=8&ved=2ahUKEwjrjeTOkMyDAxXNSUEAHVpUDg8QFnoECBsQAQ&url=https://icd.who.int/browse10/2019/en&usg=AOvVaw3IW_-42aAndAuKbwlieCVZ&opi=89978449 (accessed on 12 July 2023).
24. Cohen, J. *Statistical Power Analysis for the Behavioural Sciences*, 2nd ed.; Erlbaum Associates: Hillside NJ, USA, 1988.
25. Christmas, C.; Rogus-Pulia, N. Swallowing Disorders in the Older Population. *J. Am. Geriatr. Soc.* **2019**, *67*, 2643–2649. [CrossRef] [PubMed]
26. Blaszczyk, A.; Brandt, N.; Ashley, J.; Tuders, N.; Doles, H.; Stefanacci, R.G. Crushed Tablet Administration for Patients with Dysphagia and Enteral Feeding: Challenges and Considerations. *Drugs Aging.* **2023**, *40*, 895–907. [CrossRef] [PubMed]
27. Fields, J.; Go, J.T.; Schulze, K.S. Pill Properties that Cause Dysphagia and Treatment Failure. *Curr. Ther. Res. Clin. Exp.* **2015**, *77*, 79–82. [CrossRef] [PubMed]
28. Hummler, H.; Stillhart, C.; Meilicke, L.; Grimm, M.; Krause, E.; Mannaa, M.; Gollasch, M.; Weitschies, W.; Page, S. Impact of Tablet Size and Shape on the Swallowability in Older Adults. *Pharmaceutics* **2023**, *15*, 1042. [CrossRef]
29. Stegemann, S.; Gosch, M.; Breitkreutz, J. Swallowing dysfunction and dysphagia is an unrecognized challenge for oral drug therapy. *Int. J. Pharm.* **2012**, *430*, 197–206. [CrossRef]
30. Messerli, M.; Aschwanden, R.; Buslau, M.; Hersberger, K.E.; Arnet, I. Swallowing difficulties with medication intake assessed with a novel self-report questionnaire in patients with systemic sclerosis—A cross-sectional population study. *Patient Prefer. Adherence* **2017**, *11*, 1687–1699. [CrossRef]
31. Arnet, I.; Messerli, M.; Oezvegyi, J.; Hersberger, K.; Sahm, L. Translation to English, cross-cultural adaptation, and pilot testing of the self-report questionnaire on swallowing difficulties with medication intake and coping strategies (SWAMECO) for adults with polypharmacy. *BMJ Open* **2020**, *10*, e036761. [CrossRef]
32. Mercovich, N.; Kyle, G.J.; Naunton, M. Safe to crush? A pilot study into solid dosage form modification in aged care. *Australas. J. Ageing* **2014**, *33*, 180–184. [CrossRef] [PubMed]
33. Stuijt, C.C.M.; Klopotowska, J.E.; van Driel, C.K.; Le, N.; Binnekade, J.; van der Kleij, B.; van der Schors, T.; Bemt, P.v.D.; Lie-A-Huen, L. Improving medication administration in nursing home residents with swallowing difficulties: Sustainability of the effect of a multifaceted medication safety programme. *Pharmacoepidemiol. Drug Saf.* **2013**, *22*, 423–429. [CrossRef] [PubMed]
34. Solberg, H.; Devik, S.A.; Bell, H.T.; Zeiss, D.H.; Olsen, R.M. Drug modification by nurses in Norwegian nursing homes: A cross-sectional study. *Geriatr. Nur.* **2021**, *42*, 351–357. [CrossRef] [PubMed]
35. Kirkevold, Ø.; Engedal, K. What is the matter with crushing pills and opening capsules? *Int. J. Nurs. Pract.* **2010**, *16*, 81–85. [CrossRef] [PubMed]
36. Santos, J.M.S.; Poland, F.; Wright, D.; Longmore, T. Medicines administration for residents with dysphagia in care homes: A small scale observational study to improve practice. *Int. J. Pharm.* **2016**, *512*, 416–421. [CrossRef] [PubMed]
37. Drumond, N.; Stegemann, S. Better Medicines for Older Patients: Considerations between Patient Characteristics and Solid Oral Dosage Form Designs to Improve Swallowing Experience. *Pharmaceutics* **2020**, *13*, 32. [CrossRef] [PubMed]
38. van Welie, S.; Wijma, L.; Beerden, T.; van Doormaal, J.; Taxis, K. Effect of warning symbols in combination with education on the frequency of erroneously crushing medication in nursing homes: An uncontrolled before and after study. *BMJ Open* **2016**, *6*, e012286. [CrossRef]
39. Apolo Carvajal, F.; González Martínez, M.; Capilla Santamaría, E.; Cáliz Hernández, B.; Cañamares Orbis, I.; Martínez Ca-sanova, N.; Martínez Sánchez, E.; Aranguren Oyarzábal, A.; Calvo Alcántara, M.J.; Cruz Martos, E. Adaptation of oral medication in people institutionalized in nursing homes for whom medication is crushed: The ADECUA Study. *Farm Hosp.* **2016**, *40*, 514–528. [CrossRef]
40. Schier, J.G.; Howland, M.A.; Hoffman, R.S.; Nelson, L.S. Fatality from Administration of Labetalol and Crushed Extended-Release Nifedipine. *Ann. Pharmacother.* **2003**, *37*, 1420–1423. [CrossRef]
41. Sestili, M.; Logrippo, S.; Cespi, M.; Bonacucina, G.; Ferrara, L.; Busco, S.; Grappasonni, I.; Palmieri, G.F.; Ganzetti, R.; Blasi, P. Potentially Inappropriate Prescribing of Oral Solid Medications in Elderly Dysphagic Patients. *Pharmaceutics* **2018**, *10*, 280. [CrossRef]

Disclaimer/Publisher's Note: The statements, opinions and data contained in all publications are solely those of the individual author(s) and contributor(s) and not of MDPI and/or the editor(s). MDPI and/or the editor(s) disclaim responsibility for any injury to people or property resulting from any ideas, methods, instructions or products referred to in the content.

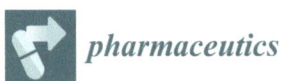

Review

Advancing Precision Medicine: A Review of Innovative In Silico Approaches for Drug Development, Clinical Pharmacology and Personalized Healthcare

Lara Marques [1,2,3], Bárbara Costa [1,2,3], Mariana Pereira [1,2,4], Abigail Silva [1,2,5], Joana Santos [1,2,3], Leonor Saldanha [1,2,3], Isabel Silva [1,2,3], Paulo Magalhães [6], Stephan Schmidt [7] and Nuno Vale [1,2,3,*]

1. PerMed Research Group, Center for Health Technology and Services Research (CINTESIS), Rua Doutor Plácido da Costa, 4200-450 Porto, Portugal; lara.marques2010@hotmail.com (L.M.); b.c.211297@gmail.com (B.C.); mariana.m.pereira2097@gmail.com (M.P.); abigailsilva@outlook.pt (A.S.); jmdmsantos@hotmail.com (J.S.); leonorpessanha@gmail.com (L.S.); iumsmed@gmail.com (I.S.)
2. CINTESIS@RISE, Faculty of Medicine, University of Porto, Alameda Professor Hernâni Monteiro, 4200-319 Porto, Portugal
3. Department of Community Medicine, Health Information and Decision (MEDCIDS), Faculty of Medicine, University of Porto, Rua Doutor Plácido da Costa, 4200-450 Porto, Portugal
4. ICBAS—School of Medicine and Biomedical Sciences, University of Porto, Rua de Jorge Viterbo Ferreira 228, 4050-313 Porto, Portugal
5. Department of Biomedicine, Faculty of Medicine, University of Porto, Rua Doutor Plácido da Costa, 4200-450 Porto, Portugal
6. Coimbra Institute for Biomedical Imaging and Translational Research, Edifício do ICNAS, Polo 3 Azinhaga de Santa Comba, 3000-548 Coimbra, Portugal; paulo.r.magalhaes1@gmail.com
7. Center for Pharmacometrics and Systems Pharmacology, Department of Pharmaceutics, College of Pharmacy, University of Florida, 6550 Sanger Road, Office 465, Orlando, FL 328227-7400, USA; sschmidt@cop.ufl.edu
* Correspondence: nunovale@med.up.pt; Tel.: +351-220426537

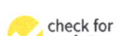

Citation: Marques, L.; Costa, B.; Pereira, M.; Silva, A.; Santos, J.; Saldanha, L.; Silva, I.; Magalhães, P.; Schmidt, S.; Vale, N. Advancing Precision Medicine: A Review of Innovative In Silico Approaches for Drug Development, Clinical Pharmacology and Personalized Healthcare. *Pharmaceutics* **2024**, *16*, 332. https://doi.org/10.3390/pharmaceutics16030332

Academic Editors: Cristina Manuela Drăgoi, Alina Crenguța Nicolae, Ion-Bogdan Dumitrescu and Pedro Dorado

Received: 1 November 2023
Revised: 21 February 2024
Accepted: 25 February 2024
Published: 27 February 2024

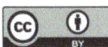

Copyright: © 2024 by the authors. Licensee MDPI, Basel, Switzerland. This article is an open access article distributed under the terms and conditions of the Creative Commons Attribution (CC BY) license (https://creativecommons.org/licenses/by/4.0/).

Abstract: The landscape of medical treatments is undergoing a transformative shift. Precision medicine has ushered in a revolutionary era in healthcare by individualizing diagnostics and treatments according to each patient's uniquely evolving health status. This groundbreaking method of tailoring disease prevention and treatment considers individual variations in genes, environments, and lifestyles. The goal of precision medicine is to target the "five rights": the right patient, the right drug, the right time, the right dose, and the right route. In this pursuit, in silico techniques have emerged as an anchor, driving precision medicine forward and making this a realistic and promising avenue for personalized therapies. With the advancements in high-throughput DNA sequencing technologies, genomic data, including genetic variants and their interactions with each other and the environment, can be incorporated into clinical decision-making. Pharmacometrics, gathering pharmacokinetic (PK) and pharmacodynamic (PD) data, and mathematical models further contribute to drug optimization, drug behavior prediction, and drug–drug interaction identification. Digital health, wearables, and computational tools offer continuous monitoring and real-time data collection, enabling treatment adjustments. Furthermore, the incorporation of extensive datasets in computational tools, such as electronic health records (EHRs) and omics data, is also another pathway to acquire meaningful information in this field. Although they are fairly new, machine learning (ML) algorithms and artificial intelligence (AI) techniques are also resources researchers use to analyze big data and develop predictive models. This review explores the interplay of these multiple in silico approaches in advancing precision medicine and fostering individual healthcare. Despite intrinsic challenges, such as ethical considerations, data protection, and the need for more comprehensive research, this marks a new era of patient-centered healthcare. Innovative in silico techniques hold the potential to reshape the future of medicine for generations to come.

Keywords: precision medicine; in silico; clinical pharmacology; computational tools; patient-centered healthcare

1. Introduction

The concept of tailoring medical treatments to a patient's characteristics based on modern tools is relatively recent. About three decades ago, many scientists thought such an idea was utopian [1,2]. Historically, clinical decision-making relied on clinical experience and pathophysiology knowledge, following a "one size fits all" approach [1,3]. The Human Genome Project accelerated this paradigm shift, as the rapid development of affordable DNA sequencing methods facilitated targeted therapies, revolutionizing healthcare [2–5].

Modern medicine now integrates several technologies for precise identification and treatment The framework for successful clinical outcomes revolves around the "five rights": administration of the right drug to the right patient at the right time, in the right dose, and through the right route of administration [6]. This approach, considering the patient's medical history, genes, environment, and lifestyle, defines precision medicine. In 2011, the United States National Research Council's *Toward Precision Medicine* defined precision medicine as the "tailoring of medical treatment to the individual characteristics of each patient (. . .) to classify individuals into subpopulations that differ in their susceptibility to a particular disease or their response to a specific treatment" [7]. This trending field is based on a healthcare model grounded on data, analytics, and information, yet it is often confused with personalized medicine due to their similar meanings. Personalized medicine, an older concept, considers the patient's genetic makeup, beliefs, preferences, knowledge, and social context. However, the term "personalized" could be misinterpreted as implying the development of treatments uniquely tailored to each individual [8], leading to the preference for the term "precision medicine" by the US National Research Council. Many authors still question this definition, and it remains a subject of ongoing debate.

Therefore, precision medicine addresses the growing need for precise and effective treatments, aligning with the cornerstones of the clinical medicine model, the four Ps: predictive, preventive, personalized, and participative [9]. This shift toward a patient-centered clinical decision-making system marks a transition from reactive medicine based on gold standards to patient-specific diagnostics and therapeutics [4]. In pursuit of robust precision medicine, in silico approaches have gained prominence, using computational methods to tailor therapies to individual patient characteristics (Figure 1). In this article, we aimed to present an updated review of in silico approaches, highlighting their impact on advancing precision medicine while spotlighting notable gaps and challenges within this field.

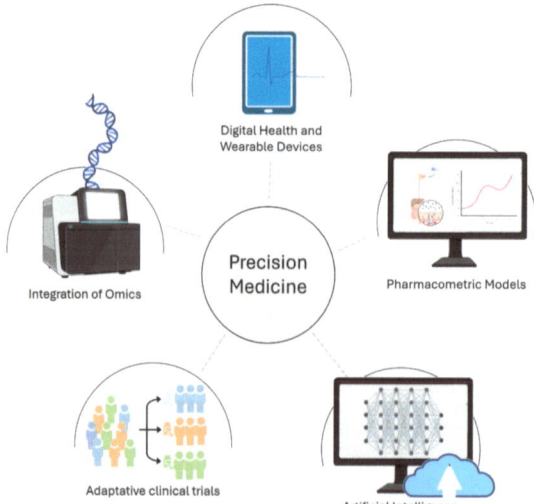

Figure 1. Key elements of in silico approaches in precision medicine. Created with Biorender.com. Available online: http://biorender.com/ (accessed on 12 October 2023).

2. OMICS in Advancing Clinical Decision-Making

Advances in omics technologies since the discovery of the DNA structure have transformed precision medicine, offering unprecedented insights into the complex biological systems that underpin human health and disease. Omics, an umbrella term encompassing a set of biological fields such as genomics, proteomics, metabolomics, and other omics, which analyze the "omes" (the suffix comes from "chromosome"), refers to the collective technologies used to explore the roles, relationships, and actions of various molecules in an organism's cells, significantly improving clinical decision-making, as they provide comprehensive insights into patient-specific molecular profiles, opening up new avenues for more precise prevention, diagnosis, and treatments [10–12]. While standard methods to study molecular mechanisms are time-consuming and proven to be inefficient, omics are structured on high-throughput analytical methods and have proven records of greater efficiency [13].

Drawing from our current understanding, precision medicine strives to deliver treatment to patients according to their own molecular characteristics (individual level) but also considers data related to the remaining population [14]. Its focus is on combining individualized data from patient-specific multi-omics with collective data in order to target the most suitable therapeutic strategy and founding structure for precision medicine in diverse populations [15]. Factors beyond genetic makeup, such as environmental influences and lifestyle, can also contribute to the complexity of predicting drug responses accurately.

The decision-making process related to precision medicine is usually driven by biomarkers as they may serve as indicators of a disease or a certain physiological state. In fact, research development of biomarkers is a current trend for pharmaceutical industries. As an example, the proteomics study of cancer is capable of revealing crucial information about the growth of the tumor and metastasis, leading to the identification of biomarkers and therapeutic targets [16]. The omics-based personalized medicine approach aims to discover biomarkers that provide highly detailed information about the pathology of the disease and therefore contribute to the decision-making process [17].

Considering the above, it means that clinicians should know how to interpret genomic data and biomarker results and apply them in current practice. Computer-based decision support (CBDDS) tools are able to offer support by listing the latest research and guidance and are required in order to aid clinicians through this process [18]. However, not all health care systems or clinicians are ready for this. A commitment to train personnel and to change the healthcare structure should be put in place to encourage precision medicine.

Indeed, there is a high hope within the scientific community regarding precision medicine and its power to improve the effectiveness of treatment and tolerability. However, before being applied in clinical practice, these studies typically undergo a complex process known as multi-omics. For example, the progression of a study involving multi-omics in metabolic diseases is usually followed by: (1) genomics for determining an individual's complete genome and developing biomarkers; (2) pharmacogenomics to predict the treatment efficacy by analyzing genetic variants; (3) transcriptomics, studying external factors that influence gene expression and affect the patient's phenotype; (4) epigenomics, to examine mechanisms that regulate gene expression; (5) proteomics, which focuses on studying protein function; (6) pharmacoproteomics, applying proteomics to pharmacology; (7) metabolomics, to identify metabolism variants; (8) pharmacometabolomics, applying metabolomics to pharmacology in order to support the development of personalized medicine by measuring metabolic phenotypes and drug metabolism; and finally, (9) integrating multi-omics, the integration and interpretation of the diverse omics, a complex exercise to apply in clinical routine [19].

2.1. Pharmacogenomics: Tailoring Treatment to Genetic Profiles

Pharmacogenomics stands at the forefront of precision medicine, integrating pharmacology and genomics to align medical treatments with the unique genetic makeup of each individual. The promise of pharmacogenomics lies in its potential to optimize drug therapy, minimize adverse drug reactions, and enhance treatment efficacy. By understanding the genetic variations that influence drug metabolism, transport, and mechanisms of action, healthcare providers can select medications and dosages that are best suited to an individual's genetic profile [20]. Some examples include treatments for viral infections [21], oncology [22], and the choice of antidepressants [23] and heart disease medications [24]. For instance, pharmacogenomic testing for the HLA-B*5701 allele aids in identifying individuals at risk of hypersensitivity reactions to abacavir, improving treatment efficacy and safety [25]. In cancer patients, the testing for the thymidine synthase (TS) gene can help identify patients who may experience diarrhoea as a side effect of 5-fluorouracil (5-FU) chemotherapy. By adjusting the treatment plan based on the pharmacogenomic test results, healthcare providers can improve patient outcomes and reduce the risk of adverse effects [26].

Some common medications that require pharmacogenomic testing include: warfarin, because genes such as CYP2C9 and VKORC1 can help determine the most effective and safe dosage for an individual, reducing bleeding risks [27]; carbamazepine, because genetic testing for the HLA-B*1502 allele identifies those at higher risk of severe skin reactions, such as Stevens–Johnson syndrome [28]; and tamoxifen, because testing for the CYP2D6 gene can help identify individuals who may have a reduced ability to metabolize tamoxifen into its active form, allowing for personalized treatment plans to improve efficacy [29]. These examples illustrate how pharmacogenomic testing has been integrated into clinical decision-making to personalize medication choices and dosing, ultimately improving patient care and safety. As the field of pharmacogenomics continues to advance, it is expected that more medications and health conditions will benefit from personalized care guided by genetic testing.

Pharmacogenomics is an emerging and challenging field with limited clinical utility and applicability currently, but its impact is growing rapidly, with US Food and Drug Administration (FDA) approvals of personalized therapeutics involving biomarkers. Nonetheless, the clinical application of pharmacogenomics encounters substantial hurdles such as unknown validity across ethnic groups, underlying bias in healthcare, and real-world validation. Recent developments in the implementation of pharmacogenomics in personalized care include the Pharmacogenomic Clinical Decision Support System (PGx-CDS), which has been crucial in minimizing complexity and enabling clinicians to make informed medication decisions based on patients' genetic profiles. There is a growing emphasis on the clinical implementation of pharmacogenomics, with proposed drug–gene pairs for implementation and the development of guidelines to integrate pharmacogenomic information into electronic health records (EHRs) and clinical decision support (CDS) systems.

2.2. Challenges and Considerations in Integrating OMICS: Navigating the Road to Precision Medicine

Progress in laboratory-based protocols, data storage, and bioinformatic capabilities has enabled the efficient generation of huge amounts of omics data in terms of both cost and time. This has been exemplified by the extensive COVID-19 research data generated within a few months [14]. However, omics methods, though widely employed in biomedical research, with several scientific studies being published in recent years, are still far from clinical reality. There are still many obstacles preventing translational-omics, a term that refers to the utilization of these new technologies in the clinical decision-making process [18]. Among these, maybe due to a lack of clinicians' knowledge on this topic, there is a willingness of physicians to accept findings that primarily convey probabilities, such as the likelihood of disease presence or prognosis [14,30,31]. Furthermore, the large amounts of acquired data raise complex challenges, including the lack of technical knowledge to collect, handle, store, and transport samples, and limitations regarding multi-omics integration techniques. New creative approaches have been applied in this field. Machine learning (ML) and big data have been integrated with omics, leading to an improvement in the rapid and efficient collection, processing, and integration of vast amounts of data [30].

However, not all regions and healthcare settings have access to these advanced testing and interpretation tools.

Furthermore, the integration of pharmacogenomics and omics raises regulatory challenges, including standardization of testing methodologies and ensuring ethical use of genetic information. Navigating these regulatory landscapes is crucial for widespread adoption. Addressing these challenges requires ongoing research, technological advancements, and collaboration among researchers, clinicians, and policymakers.

The complexity of genomic medicine requires the development of guidelines and strategies for the integration of genomics into precision medicine. A structured clinical decision support system, combining clinical data and bioinformatics, is fundamental for this purpose [32]. Although CDS tools were created to guide clinicians to better integrate, use, and interpret genomic data, a recent study has shown that is still not clear what would be the best strategy [33]. Not only it is important to bring standard guidelines and strategies that can provide consistency in order to better train clinicians, but it is also important to promote an environment among different stakeholders (academics, clinicians, patients, government) to raise scientific awareness of the need and importance of creating more knowledge in precision medicine. Clinicians must be able to interpret this data for strong and effective decision-making; patients must be aware and well-informed to accept the treatment regimen they are prescribed; and the government must restructure the healthcare system, providing the necessary tools for this to become a reality in clinical practice. In fact, some of these measures are already implemented by regulatory agencies.

Until now, there has been a proven record that reflects the advances of omics in precision medicine which contributed to relevant discoveries. Several FDA-approved treatments now target individual characteristics of patients [34,35]. Among these, most are for the treatment of cancer (47%), rare diseases (37%), and other diseases (16%). The table below outlines some of the approved treatments for these therapeutic indications (Table 1).

Table 1. Some new therapeutic molecular personalized medicines approved by the FDA [34,35].

	Therapeutic Indication
	Cancer
Products	Abecma (multiple myeloma) Exkivity (lung cancer) Lumakras (lung cancer) Jemperli (endometrial cancer) Rybrevant (lung cancer) Scemblix (myeloid leukaemia) Tepmetko (lung cancer) Truseltiq (cholangiocarcinoma)
	Rare Diseases
	Amondys (muscular dystrophy) Evkeeza (homozygous familial hypercholesterolaemia) Nexviazyme (Pompe disease) Nulibry (molybdenum cofactor deficiency) Vyvgart (Myasthenia Gravis) Welireg (von Hippel–Lindau)
	Other Diseases
	Bylvay (progressive familial intrahepatic cholestasis) Cabenuva (HIV-1) Leqvio (hypercholesterolaemia)

According to the FDA, effective precision medicines require efficient tests able to aid diagnosis and a suitable treatment. These tests, or companion diagnostics, are named next generation sequencing (NGS) and are able to identify or sequence huge sections of patients' genomes; therefore, they are considered a key advanced tool to be used in clinical practice [36]. The International Consortium for Personalized Medicine (ICPerMed) is another important international initiative to support precision medicine research [37]. Launched in 2016, it involves the European Commission and around 30 European and international members, including funders and policy-making organizations. ICPerMed, by conducting workshops and debates and providing reports on precision medicine implementation, aims to position Europe as a global leader in precision medicine research, actively promoting the science and demonstrating its societal benefits.

While omics technologies have significantly advanced the field of pharmacometrics, their contribution to precision medicine is not direct, but rather via the identification of relevant biomarkers. The high-throughput nature of omics technologies enables the fast discovery of candidate biomarkers, but their clinical validation and integration into precision medicine approaches require careful consideration of analytical development, computational modeling of the predictor, and clinical utility assessment.

3. Biomarkers and Molecular Diagnostics

Having explored the transformative role of omics in advancing clinical decision-making, a pivotal component in this journey is the identification and utilization of biomarkers through molecular diagnostics. Biomarkers are biological observations, such as small molecules or clinical points, which are applied in drug discovery and used extensively in medical practice for screening, diagnosing, and characterizing diseases, as well as informing prognosis or therapy effects [38]. Biomarker analysis has started the shift toward an individualized treatment for each patient, and, as such, biomarker discovery is of high importance in this approach (Figure 2). New methods and techniques for efficient and quick analysis of biomarkers, surpassing the need for conventional monitoring, usually involve blood draws for imaging techniques [39].

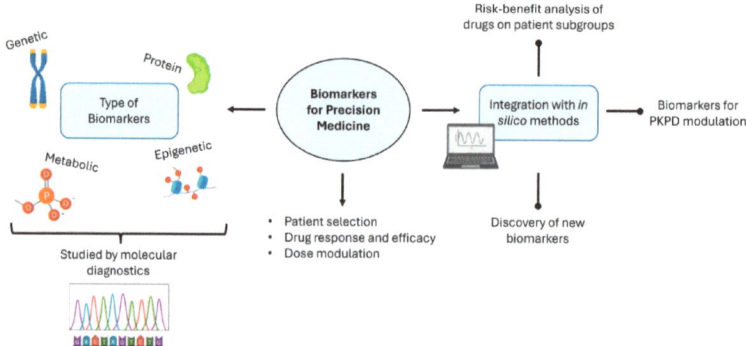

Figure 2. Biomarker integration in precision medicine and in silico approaches. Created with Biorender.com. Available online: http://biorender.com (accessed on 16 October 2023).

The use of biomarkers in physiologically based pharmacokinetic (PBPK) modeling has shown promising potential in predicting drug responses and optimizing therapeutic strategies across diverse populations. These biomarkers offer valuable information about drug absorption, distribution, metabolism, and elimination (ADME) within an individual's body, allowing for more precise drug exposure and response modeling. Additionally, biomarkers can help identify patient subgroups that are more likely to respond positively to drug therapy or those at higher risk of experiencing adverse events [40]. Incorporating pharmacokinetic (PK) biomarkers, such as drug concentrations, into research can enhance the accuracy and efficacy of drug development and personalized medicine.

Biomarkers are categorized based on their research and clinical practice roles. Genetic biomarkers, identifying genetic variations, play a crucial role in assessing disease risk and predicting treatment responses [41,42]. Protein biomarkers, such as enzymes, receptors, and cytokines, can indicate organ damage or dysfunction, abnormal cellular processes, or inflammation processes [43–46]. Metabolic biomarkers, derived from the analysis of metabolites and small molecules in various biological samples, provide valuable insights into metabolic pathways and can be used to identify markers of disease progression or treatment response [47]. Epigenetic markers, in turn, analyze alterations in DNA methylation, non-coding RNAs, or histone modifications, and samples can be obtained through either noninvasive or minimally invasive procedures, making these markers accessible, stable, and frequently chosen. They have been found to be very useful for cancer, as there are known epigenetic changes in the shift from somatic to cancerous cells [48]. One such example is the panel of promoter hypermethylation of the RASSF1A, RARβ2, and APC genes in serum and urine, which has a 94% specificity and sensitivity in detecting renal cell carcinoma [49].

The analysis of these biomarkers can be performed through molecular diagnostics, which encompasses several technologies that allow the study of genomic and proteomic biomarkers [50]. Essential assays include sequencing-based and non-sequencing methods, like immunohistochemistry (IHC), microsatellite instability testing (MSI), and chromosomal microarray analysis (CMA). Beyond those important tools for molecular diagnostics and biomarker analysis, they also include polymerase chain reaction (PCR), Sanger and NGS, and emerging techniques like liquid biopsies, RNA sequencing, and long-read sequencing [51].

Human PK investigations and clinical trials are the mainstays of conventional drug development procedures. However, these traditional methods frequently fall short of accurately portraying the wide variety of patient groups found in real-world situations. This restriction is particularly important since drug reactions might differ significantly between people due to their specific demographic, genetic, and environmental characteristics [52]. Generalized pharmacometric modeling (GPM) stands out as an effective remedy to these problems by integrating ML approaches with sizable, diverse datasets into the renowned framework of pharmacometrics methods, improving our understanding of drug disposition and its effects across a wide range of distinct patient groups. GPM might revolutionize the individualization of drug therapy by finding instructive and pertinent patient-specific variables, with a strong focus on biomarkers that affect drug dynamics [53]. Treatment plans that are customized for certain patient populations may result in safer and more efficient drug regimens [54]. GPM makes use of the capabilities of ML algorithms, particularly random forest regression [55] and Bayesian networks [56], to handle and comprehend vast and complex datasets, which traditional models sometimes find difficult to process, and unveil intricate connections and interactions between variables that could not have been seen otherwise. The biological and therapeutic significance of the GPM-identified biomarkers is an important topic for debate. Surprisingly, GPM occasionally reveals unanticipated biomarkers that appear to have no connection to drug dynamics but that are strongly grounded in the current scientific literature and can actually affect certain dynamics. The identification of biomarkers influencing the inter-individual variability in drug pharmacokinetics/pharmacodynamics (PK/PD) may be made easier with the use of this new knowledge, which will eventually lead to the development of more individualized and successful pharmacological regimens [53].

3.1. Harnessing Biomarkers for Precision Drug Development and Treatment Optimization

Biomarkers can be used for the development of in silico PKPD models of enzymatic activity. For example, a study aimed to assess the induction or inhibition of the cytochrome P450 (CYP450) enzyme CYP3A4 by using the biomarker 4β-hydroxycholesterol (4βHC) [57], which is directly associated with CYP3A4 activity [58]. The researchers applied a Bayesian technique for parameter estimation to develop the PKPD model [59,60], which predicts a differential impact of rifampin and ketoconazole on 4βHC and midazolam (MDZ), the industry standard CYP3A4 inhibitor detectors. Despite limitations, the PKPD model holds promise for precision medicine, allowing tailored prescription regimens, predicting drug–drug interactions (DDIs), and reducing negative consequences through early identification of CYP3A4-related dynamics [57].

The study of biomarkers using ML can allow benefit–risk analysis of drugs in various patient subgroups, enabling predictions of efficacy and adverse effects [61]. A study exemplified this approach by utilizing the random forest algorithm to analyze clinical trial results of acute melanoma patients treated with nivolumab to establish a relation between nivolumab clearance and several cytokines [62]. The researchers were able to establish a panel of biomarkers using the 16 top inflammatory cytokines that, even without the use of the drug, could be related with clinical benefit. Moreover, these biomarkers were able to predict nivolumab clearance, which is related to overall survival (OS) [63]. Effectively, this algorithm could predict OS by the clearance, in which patients with high clearance have decreased OS. This allows the stratification of patients in high and low clearance groups, enabling the prediction of treatment outcomes and an informed choice of treatment [64].

New biomarkers can also be discovered using in silico techniques. Radiomics collects digital medical images from magnetic resonance (MR), computed tomography (CT), positron emission tomography (PET), and other imaging techniques and transforms them into mineable data that can be quantitatively linked with pathophysiology. This effectively creates new imaging biomarkers that, when combined with patient characteristics and even genomic data, can help inform diagnostics, prognosis, and response to therapy, the basis of precision medicine [64]. Radiomics information can fundamentally reshape the development of pharmacometrics models, particularly in understanding the dynamics of tumor size. These cutting-edge pharmacometrics models shed light on the complicated interplay within a tumor ecosystem by accounting for the numerous characteristics of tumor heterogeneity both within and between lesions, and an example of such a model is the classification clustering of individual lesions (CICIL) methodology [65]. Still in the oncologic area, by drawing conclusions from radiomic data, this method can also be useful in understanding resistance mechanisms and identifying new biomarkers for drug resistance [66]. In a recent study, pharmacometric models were employed to explore the potential of biomarkers in predicting the efficacy of brazikumab, an anti-interleukin 23 monoclonal antibody [67], in the treatment of Crohn's disease (CD). Two predictive biomarkers emerged from this study, baseline IL-22 (BIL22) and baseline C-reactive protein (BCRP), whose higher baseline levels represent a notably enhanced response to the drug [68]. Moreover, the study unveiled a strong negative correlation between the placebo effect and the baseline Crohn's Disease Activity Index (BCDAI) [69], serving as a prognostic biomarker. Recognizing that the impact of the placebo effect is vital for interpreting clinical trial results accurately and refining treatment strategies accordingly, a correlation between high BCDAI and low clinical response to drugs has been found previously in the literature [70]. The pharmacometrics analysis also established quantitative cutoff values for BIL22 and BCRP, offering precise thresholds for patient stratification, a significant departure from traditional median-based cutoffs. Such precision in patient selection can pave the way for more effective clinical trial designs and enhance the likelihood of success in future studies. Furthermore, the study highlighted the superiority of pharmacometrics modeling over conventional statistical analysis. Its capacity to integrate longitudinal data while considering various sources of variability, including drug PK and placebo effects, proved to be a powerful tool for elucidating biomarker-dependent responses in biologic therapies [68].

3.2. Challenges in Implementing Biomarkers and Molecular Diagnostics in Precision Medicine

Thus, biomarkers and molecular diagnostics offer significant promise in healthcare, enabling early disease detection and personalized treatment. However, their effective implementation faces challenges that warrant attention. These include ensuring the accuracy and reliability of biomarker tests, which often require complex validation processes; standardization, as variations in measurement and interpretation can lead to inconsistent results across different laboratories; time related to regulatory approval; and ethical concerns surrounding informed consent, data privacy, and genetic discrimination, which require careful consideration. Clear guidelines for interpretation, addressing limited biomarkers, and integrating data effectively are crucial.

There have been some collaborations between academia, industry, and regulatory bodies to accelerate biomarker discovery and establish standardized approaches for biomarker validation for precision medicine. The European Medicines Agency (EMA) emphasizes early engagement with biomarker developers through various platforms like the Innovation Task Force, the Qualification of Novel Methodologies procedure, and the Scientific Advice procedure [71]. The EMA's Regulatory Science Strategy includes measures to facilitate regulatory qualification for biomarkers. The FDA has a Biomarker Qualification Program (BQP), which is a voluntary process that allows biomarker developers to submit their data and information for FDA review and qualification as drug development or regulatory tools. The FDA also collaborates with other stakeholders through consortia, such as the Biomarkers Consortium and the Critical Path Institute [72].

The Innovative Medicines Initiative (IMI), a public–private partnership between the European Union and the European Federation of Pharmaceutical Industries and Associations (EFPIA), supports several projects such as PRECISESADS, AETIONOMY, RHAPSODY, and CANCER-ID [73], focusing on biomarker discovery, molecular mechanisms of non-response to treatments, and the development of tools, standards, and approaches to address unmet medical needs for effective disease-modifying treatments.

4. Pharmacometrics Tools: Significance and Challenges in Precision Medicine

Pharmacometrics is a critical tool in the field of clinical pharmacology, providing a quantitative framework for understanding, characterizing, and predicting drug exposure and response. The integration of omics and biomarkers is fundamental to pharmacometrics, providing vital quantitative data for characterizing and predicting drug behavior, ultimately enabling the optimization of therapeutic strategies and the development of precision medicine approaches. Therefore, drug development and optimization have become increasingly challenging over the years due to the diversity of compounds and therapeutic targets, the inherent variability in patient responses, and the evolving landscape of regulatory agencies in the drug approval process. Pharmacometrics has emerged as a multidisciplinary scientific discipline to address all these challenges, employing advanced mathematical and statistical methods based on biology, pharmacology, and physiology to quantify the interaction between the drug and the patient [74–78].

The introduction of the concept of pharmacometrics dates back to the 1960s, with the quantification of PK data in laboratory experiments and the development of methods to connect to pharmacodynamics (PD) [79–81]. Sheiner and Stuart Beal are the pioneers in this field, having created the Nonlinear Mixed Effects Modeling (NONMEM) software system in the 1970s, particularly well-known for its applications in population pharmacokinetic (popPK) studies [82], allowing the characterization of individual PK profiles and sources of variability in a population. From 1980 onwards, drug regulatory authorities, namely, the FDA, began to endorse the practice of pharmacometrics and, since then, this area has had a high impact on decisions related to clinical trial design, drug development, approval, and therapeutic regimen optimization [83]. Indeed, the pharmacometrics resources enable tailoring the therapeutic plan—the most appropriate drug dose and dosing schedule—for an individual patient based on factors such as genetics, age, weight, and underlying health conditions. In the preclinical phase, modeling and simulating the drug's behavior in different patient populations allow for the design of clinical trials more efficiently, reducing costs and the time required in the drug development process [83]. Pharmacometrics tools also empower the prediction of different patient responses to a drug based on their unique characteristics, thus enabling the identification of biomarkers and patient subgroups that may benefit more or less from a specific drug [84–86]. Consequently, this allows for quicker decision-making regarding safety and efficacy, streamlining the evaluation and approval process of new drugs. Additionally, therapeutic regimen optimization also relies on modeling. This field has been supported by increasingly complex mathematical models, assuming a pivotal role in the era of precision medicine [87,88].

Initially met with skepticism, pharmacometrics faced challenges in integrating diverse data types for precision medicine research, slow adoption due to limited understanding, regulatory hurdles aligning with FDA requirements, and computational challenges in developing advanced models. Overcoming these required collaboration among clinicians, researchers, bioinformatics specialists, and biostatisticians. As the field has evolved, researchers, regulatory authorities, and funding bodies have recognized the power of pharmacometric analyses in improving pharmacotherapeutic use, drug development, and regulatory decisions. As the field continues to advance, it is essential to address these challenges and solidify pharmacometrics' role in the era of precision medicine.

4.1. A Triad of Precision: PKPD, PBPK, and Population PK Models in Pharmacological Insights

PK and PD modelling, PBPK modelling, and popPK modelling are all tools used in pharmacometrics to understand drug behavior and optimize therapeutic strategies. PKPD modelling interrelates PK (ADME) and PD (effect on patients). PD models focus on concentration–effect relationships and are often integrated with PK modelling to optimize drug efficacy and minimize adverse effects [89,90].

The primary basis for PD models is concentration–effect relationships [91]. To our knowledge, there is a limited body of research exclusively focused on PD modelling, although some approaches may be outlined: simple direct effect models, biophase distribution, indirect response models, signal transduction models, and irreversible effect models [92,93]. Typically, these techniques are integrated with PK modelling, allowing for the characterization of the dose–exposure–response relationship, which is a crucial step in optimizing the drug efficacy and minimizing adverse effects, ultimately leading to improved therapeutic outcomes. Lin et al. [94] developed a population-based PKPD model for carfilzomib in adult patients with relapsed/refractory diffuse large B-cell lymphoma using the NONMEM® software (version 7.4.1). Such studies contribute to ongoing research aiming to identify characteristics of patients who benefit from this specific treatment. Additionally, the relevance of PKPD model integration in drug development has also been stated. For instance, Palmer et al. [95] reviewed the implementation of PK and PD studies in antimicrobial drug development. Derendorf et al. [96] have also demonstrated that corticosteroids represent a class of drugs suitable for PKPD modelling studies, allowing the prediction of the systemic activity of novel corticosteroids based on their PK profiles. According to Zou et al. [89], this model technique also finds extensive application in drug delivery systems and the modification of large molecules, both in preclinical and clinical trials, providing essential insights for animal-to-human translation and facilitating the selection of therapeutic regimens. Even at the initial stages, during the discovery of novel compounds phase, these strategies can be effectively implemented [97]. PKPD model-based analysis enables a faster in vitro to in vivo translation, reduces the number of animal studies, and improves bench-to-bed translation. As evident, PKPD models offer a broad spectrum of applications, spanning from preclinical drug assessment to drug optimization, maximizing the patient's therapeutic response.

PK itself represents a powerful tool to characterize the kinetic profile of several drugs. To explore the effects of the human body on a drug, specifically, to analyse its PK data, there are two common approaches: compartmental PK analysis and noncompartmental PK analysis (NCA) [98–101]. In the first method, the human body is conceptualized as a finite number of interconnected and kinetically homogenous compartments (representing various parts of the body, such as blood, organs, and other tissues), assuming that the rate of transfer between compartments and the rate of drug elimination from compartments follow first-order or linear kinetics. In turn, NCA is a simpler method that does not rely on specific compartmental models. Instead, it estimates PK parameters directly from the observed concentration–time data through algebraic equations. These analytical approaches have proved specific utility in advancing the development of complex drug delivery systems, namely, nanoparticles. Recently, Osipova et al. [102] compared two nanoparticle formulations using both NCA and compartmental analysis. Their findings underscored the potential of compartmental analysis to provide valuable insights into a crucial step in drug development, such as drug delivery.

Among the various PK modeling approaches, the most common mathematical models are popPK models and PBPK models. They are complementary techniques that scientists often use and are instrumental in the era of precision medicine [81]. There are a variety of software packages available to analyze, model, and simulate pharmacological data, including NONMEM®, Phoenix® WinNonlin®, Simcyp, MATLAB®, GastroPlus, and Monolix. Most of these programs are user-friendly for scientists from diverse disciplines, but they are mainly used by experts in the field [103]. Based on evidence that concentrations of chemical substances within target tissues hold greater predictability for biological responses than external doses, the pre-eminence of PBPK modelling has increased significantly [104,105]. The concept of employing multicompartmental models that incorporate biological and physiological components to simulate PK data was originally introduced by Teorell in the 1930s [106]. Over subsequent decades, the number of publications involving PBPK models has increased significantly, demonstrating the growing interest in the implementation of this approach in the pharmaceutical industry, from the drug discovery and development process to post-market drug optimization [107,108].

PBPK models, which mechanistically describe drug disposition within the body by simulating ADME processes, have a huge focus on DDI. In a study conducted by Umehara et al. [109], the efficacy of a robust PBPK model in accurately predicting DDI was demonstrated. It can help reduce the number of DDI clinical trials. Previously, we have also highlighted the valuable utility of this tool within this field [110]. Specifically, we have developed a PBPK model of salbutamol and fluvoxamine to simulate the interaction between both drugs in different regimens and under diverse patient profiles.

Furthermore, the prediction of drug behavior in different populations and under varying physiological conditions, namely, age, ethnicity, or disease status, is easily conducted with PBPK models. Zamir et al. [111] assessed the PK of metoprolol in distinct cohorts comprising healthy, chronic kidney disease (CKD), and acute myocardial infarction (AMI) patients through PBPK modelling. Their findings led to the recommendation of metoprolol dosage adjustments at various CKD stages, along with the elucidations of PK differences in this β-blocker between the different subgroups. PBPK modelling can also predict drug disposition during pregnancy. For instance, Amaeze et al. [112] developed a PBPK model to evaluate N-acetyltransferase 2 phenotype-specific effects of pregnancy on isoniazid disposition. Hence, tailoring dosage strategies for vulnerable groups is increasingly becoming a reality.

PopPK modelling involves examining PK on a broader scale, where data from all individuals in a population are simultaneously analyzed using a NONMEM. The development of a popPK model encompasses five key elements: the data, structural model, statistical model, covariate model, and modeling software. Mould et al. detail all these aspects [113]. Similar to all the aforementioned approaches, popPK models have wide applicability in the pharmaceutical industry, and an increasing number of studies are being conducted. In particular, the optimization of therapeutic regimens along with the identification of patient characteristics (also referred to as covariates) with an impact on drug kinetics has been the core of this area. There has been a growing use of popPK models to study various diseases across diverse areas. Researchers are now employing retrospective studies using real-world data to examine relationships between covariates and drug PK parameters [114]. Other studies are being developed within clinical trials. For instance, a study used PK data from an open-label, randomized, two-treatment, two-period, two-sequence, single oral dose, crossover, bioequivalence study to develop a popPK model for simulating various doses of a recently produced drug for acute lymphoblastic leukemia (ALL), aiding in selecting the bioequivalence dose. Some authors also focus on addressing significant gaps in clinical knowledge. For example, the impact of renal function on amisulpride PK was examined using popPK modeling by Li et al. [114]. A popPK model of dasatinib developed by He et al. [115] evidenced that low doses should be recommended for Chinese patients.

Currently, researchers have at their disposal a modelling continuum, ranging from popPK to quantitative systems pharmacology (QSP) models. QSP models integrate complex biological pathways and drug interactions to predict responses to drug interventions. For example, a QSP model might be used to understand the impact of a new cancer drug on various signalling pathways involved in tumor growth. A recent study aimed to assess if targeting regulatory T cells (Treg) could enhance the efficacy of a checkpoint inhibitor (anti-PD1) in inhibiting tumor growth. Mice experiments alone were insufficient in providing insights into longitudinal changes in biomarkers. QSP modelling was employed to elucidate the mechanistic interplay of anti-PD1 and anti-Treg on Treg and effector T cell (Teff) longitudinal changes. The QSP model focused on essential components characterizing major pathways in the immune system. It represented the dynamics through Teff (cytotoxic effector T cells), Treg, and PD1/PDL1, linking these components to tumor growth modulation. The findings suggest that Teff profiles may be more predictive of pharmacological responses than Treg profiles, which provides valuable insights for drug development decisions in immuno-oncology [116].

The decision of which modeling approach to use should be based on the specific goals of the research or application, considering factors like data availability and system complexity.

4.2. Challenges of Quantitative Drug Modeling

Pharmacometrics mainly relies on data, and the quality and quantity of available data can vary significantly. Poor quality data collection compromises model development and validation, leading to less accurate predictions. For example, popPK models may not be well supported by commonly used sparse sampling because of the slow absorption and long half-life of some drugs [117]. In fact, scientists with training and expertise in quantitative drug modelling may face some concerns when it comes to collecting PK data. While PK data is typically gathered during early clinical trials, the number of data points collected per subject is quite limited in phase II and III studies due to ethical and medical considerations, resulting in sparse PK sampling [118]. This constraint also applies to pediatric studies, where efforts are made to minimize the volume of blood sampled. In addition, data collection often lacks accurate time information, leading to measurement errors (ME). Choi et al. [119] have highlighted that time ME can lead to bias in parameter estimators since the time variable used in PK modelling differs from the actual collection time. To address this, the authors have proposed two methods for correcting time ME: in cases where the PK profile exhibits minor curvature, conventional population PK modeling can be employed; however, in scenarios where the curvature is moderate or large, the most reliable approach is the transform both sides (TBS) model, which preserves a nonlinear relationship between response and structural variables such as time, ensuring that PK parameters maintain their original interpretation. Another innovative approach involves the use of dried blood samples through wearable automatic sampling systems rather than conventional blood sampling techniques. In a study conducted using blood samples from Beagle dogs [120], these novel systems demonstrated the capability to yield a higher number of samples, allowing the collection of more PK data, representing a promising alternative to established methods.

Traditionally, parameter estimation in PK modelling relied heavily on mathematical equations and assumptions about physiological processes. However, these classical methods often struggled to capture the complexities and inter-individual variations in drug PK. Data-driven approaches offer a paradigm shift by leveraging vast datasets, advanced computational techniques, and ML algorithms to improve parameter estimation. Traditional parameter estimation methods in PK can include the standard two-stage (STS) approach, which involves fitting a PK model to individual data, estimating individual PK separately for each individual, and then combining the individual parameter estimates [121]. The naive pooled data (NPD) approach involves fitting all individuals' data together as though there were no individual kinetic differences [122]. Furthermore, the Bayesian estimation method provides a powerful approach to individualizing dosing regimens. It incorporates elements of variability in previously known population estimates and variability in the PK parameters and known errors intrinsic to the assay method used to estimate the blood fluid drug concentrations [123]. However, these traditional methods have some limitations. They often require distributional assumptions and model linearization. They may encounter issues with local minima and underdetermined problems [124]. They are based solely on the plasma concentrations obtained from individual patients and applied directly to PK equations [123].

In addition, model evaluation represents a significant hurdle in pharmacometrics. Generally, models can be evaluated internally or externally [125]. Internal evaluation involves basic methods such as analyzing goodness-of-fit (GOF) graphs to detect potential biases or problems in the structural model, as well as the evaluation of the accuracy of parameter estimates from standard errors or confidence intervals. Advanced methods include data splitting, resampling techniques, or Monte Carlo simulations (visual predictive check). External evaluation, which is not very common, involves comparing a validated dataset with the predictions obtained from the built model. For this reason, ensuring an accurate predictive model is challenging.

Nonetheless, we also face ethical issues since dose-finding PK studies may not provide direct participant benefit, posing the dilemma of balancing individual research-associated burdens with intended long-term benefits [126,127]. There are also difficulties in recruiting peer-reviewers with appropriate modelling expertise and experience, lack of confidence in PBPK models for which no tissue/plasma concentration data exist for model evaluation, lack of transferability across modelling platforms, poor in vitro–in vivo correlations, and knowledge gaps in system parameters [128,129].

5. Data Integration and Analytics: Data-Driven Approaches in Pharmacokinetic Modeling

The demand for precision dosing of established medications post-approval has become routine in the evolving healthcare landscape. As aforementioned, mathematical modelling is a valuable tool that extends its utility beyond late-stage clinical development [130,131]. Healthcare professionals, including clinicians and providers, increasingly recognize the significance of patient-specific responses to standardized dosing protocols [132,133]. This awareness holds particular importance in the context of diseases such as cancer [134], human immunodeficiency virus (HIV) [135], and tuberculosis (TB) [136], where drug PK variability can profoundly influence treatment outcomes.

5.1. Unraveling Complexity: Data-Driven Pharmacokinetic Modeling in Combination Therapy

In the context of data integration and analytics, these diseases benefit from the ability to gather and analyze vast amounts of data. When modelling monotherapy, the focus is primarily on understanding the PK and PD of a single drug to predict its behavior and efficacy. In contrast, modelling combination therapy involves the complex interplay of multiple drugs, each with its own PK properties, mechanisms of action, and potential for DDIs. Data integration and analytics became crucial for assessing how these drugs work together. In data-driven PL modelling for combination therapy, researchers and healthcare professionals need to consider the additional layers of complexity introduced by multiple drugs. This complexity underscores the importance of data integration and analytics in tailoring treatment regimens to individual patients effectively. The goal is to achieve the best possible therapeutic outcomes while addressing the unique challenges posed by these complex interactions (Figure 3).

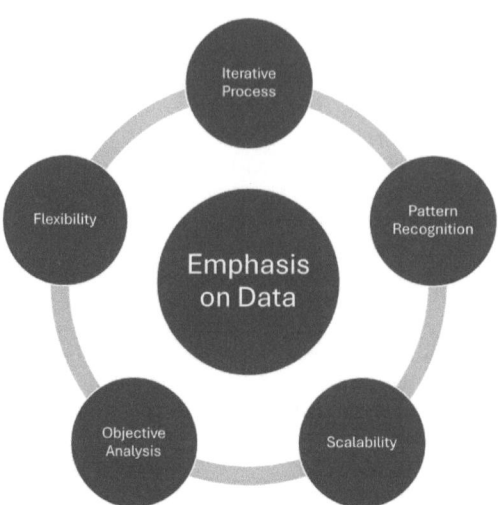

Figure 3. Key characteristics of data-driven approaches.

Access to a growing volume of patient-specific digital health data and an expanding pharmacological and disease-specific pathophysiological knowledge presents new opportunities. This data, often beyond the scope of traditional clinical trials, can be used to create models that support clinical decision-making, leading to enhanced patient care and improved treatment outcomes [137]. As previously stated, precision medicine relies on integrating and analyzing diverse datasets to understand individual patient profiles, identify biomarkers, and tailor treatments. This step involves merging datasets from various sources, including EHRs, genomic data, proteomic data, and other "omics" data (e.g., metabolomics), to derive meaningful insights that guide personalized healthcare decisions. The integration of omics and EHR data is particularly important, as it allows for a more comprehensive understanding of a patient's health status and treatment history. For example, EHR data can provide information on a patient's medical history, medication use, and clinical outcomes, while omics data can provide information on genetic variations, protein expression, and metabolic profiles. Nevertheless, standardized data formats and interoperability between different data sources (as EHR data is often stored in different formats and systems) and privacy concerns and regulatory requirements represent some of the challenges encountered. Despite this, the integration of omics and EHR data holds great promise for advancing precision medicine [138,139].

Advanced analytics methodologies, including ML and artificial intelligence (AI), are pivotal in making sense of integrated datasets [140]. These technologies can identify patterns, correlations, and predictive insights that might be challenging to uncover through traditional methods. Predictive models can be developed to forecast disease risk, treatment response, and patient outcomes [141]. ML algorithms can adapt and improve these models as new data becomes available. As previously discussed, data integration and analytics help discover biomarkers that can guide the development of targeted therapies [142,143]. Precision medicine acknowledges the heterogeneity in patient populations [3], and data-driven methods can account for this variability by estimating inter-individual differences in drug disposition, enabling tailored dosing regimens for diverse patient groups and helping to identify relevant biomarkers or patient characteristics significantly impacting drug PK [144,145].

Integrated data empowers CDS systems, aiding healthcare providers in personalized treatment decisions based on individual patient data and the latest research [146]. This approach enhances early disease detection, tailors treatments, and deepens the understanding of factors influencing health. In PK modeling, data-driven approaches utilize observed data, often from clinical trials or real-world settings, to estimate model parameters governing drug behavior [146]. Unlike theory-driven methods, these approaches prioritize empirical relationships and statistical methods, enabling pharmacometricians to capture complex interactions between drug concentrations and patient-specific factors for more accurate parameter estimates [147]. Nevertheless, there is a symbiotic relationship among data-driven, theory-driven, and hypothesis-driven strategies in scientific research. Data-driven methods offer the advantage of uncovering unexpected insights and patterns that might not be apparent through preconceived theories. Theory-driven approaches provide a theoretical framework that guides research design and interpretation. Hypothesis-driven strategies, in turn, enable researchers to test specific predictions and refine theories. An integrated use of these methodologies enhances the rigor and depth of scientific investigations.

Optimizing clinical trial designs by identifying relevant covariates that influence drug PK streamlines trial enrollment, ensuring the inclusion of precisely the right patients [148], and enhances the accuracy and efficiency of clinical investigations, allowing advances in accurate parameter estimation for drug safety and efficacy [149]. Data-driven methods excel in predicting adverse events, guiding dose adjustments, and minimizing side effects. Rigorous validation and refinement using real-world data reinforces their applicability across diverse clinical settings and patient populations. Their adaptability to changing patient data aligns with the dynamic nature of precision medicine applications [150], optimizing treatment plans and clinical trial designs and leading to cost savings in drug development and healthcare services.

Data-driven approaches involve statistical and computational techniques to collect, analyze, and interpret data, prioritizing the identification of patterns, correlations, trends, and relationships [151]. They are well-suited for handling large datasets, making them valuable in ML, AI, and big data analytics. They can adapt to changing data and evolving insights, allowing dynamic decision-making and the extraction of complex patterns and relationships within PK data. Their strength lies in multivariate analysis, effectively considering numerous variables simultaneously to uncover hidden correlations that classical methods might miss. One real-life example of a hidden correlation that data-driven approaches can identify is the relationship between certain genetic markers and drug efficacy. Classical methods might not detect this correlation due to the complex interplay of genetic factors. These examples illustrate how data-driven approaches can reveal insights that are not immediately obvious, leading to a deeper understanding of complex phenomena and informing more effective decision-making.

By considering individual patient characteristics, data-driven approaches enable the tailoring of drug dosages to maximize therapeutic benefits while minimizing side effects [152,153]. In contrast to traditional approaches, which often require extensive trial-and-error adjustments to find optimal dosages [154,155], these methods accelerate this process, reducing costs and risks, and can be used in early drug development stages to predict PK parameters, facilitating decision-making and dose selection [156,157]. These approaches support adaptive dosing strategies that can be modified in real time based on a patient's response and changing clinical conditions [158,159].

5.2. Challenges and Regulatory Considerations in Data-Driven Pharmacokinetic Modeling

While data-driven approaches offer substantial advantages, they face challenges, such as ensuring data quality, addressing bias in datasets, and interpreting complex ML models. Strategies to mitigate these concerns include: (a) Data preprocessing, which involves cleaning, normalizing, and handling missing values to ensure consistency and quality, removing outliers, addressing imbalanced classes, and ensuring data representativeness; (b) Feature selection, identifying the most relevant features for the model using techniques such as principal component analysis or correlation analysis to reduce the impact of noise and improve the model's performance; (c) Model evaluation, employing appropriate metrics, such as accuracy, precision, recall, and F1-score to assess the performance of the model on a validation set or cross-validation techniques, preventing overfitting and ensuring effectiveness on unseen data; (d) Hyperparameter tuning, optimizing the hyperparameters of the ML models through techniques like grid searching or random searching to find the best combination of hyperparameters for optimal performance; (e) Ensemble methods, combining multiple ML models to make predictions by aggregating their individual predictions, which can help to reduce the impact of any single model's errors and improve the overall accuracy; (f) Regulatory guidelines, adhering to regulatory guidelines, such as those set by the FDA, to ensure responsible and compliant use of AI and ML in PK modelling.

The current state of regulatory guidelines for incorporating data-driven models into drug development and clinical practice is still evolving. Regulatory agencies like the FDA have released guidance documents on the use of AI and ML in drug and biological product development, providing recommendations on data quality, algorithm development, and validation. The use of ML/AI-based modeling approaches in PBPK modeling can help support dose selection for future clinical trials or guide drug development strategies. Collaborations between researchers, regulatory agencies, and industry partners can help to advance the understanding of AI and ML applications in PK modelling and address the challenges associated with their implementation. Key challenges and opportunities include: (1) Ensuring data quality and diversity for robust ML model training; (2) Addressing model interpretability to understand the underlying mechanisms and reasoning behind the model's outputs, especially in the context of drug development and clinical practice; (3) Securing regulatory acceptance by transparently communicating the model's performance, data quality, and potential limitations; (4) Integrating traditional pharmacometric methods into data-driven models, such as popPK and PD models, to improve overall model performance.

6. Artificial Intelligence: Integration of Machine Learning in Pharmacometrics

The introduction of AI to healthcare coincided with the emergence of PK modelling and simulation techniques [160,161]. Since then, AI has played a crucial role in the medical field, particularly in the analysis and processing of complex and diverse healthcare data, such as EHRs. Within AI, ML is a subgroup that has contributed to advancing mathematical and statistical algorithms capable of effectively learning from data to generate predictions and insights [162].

Pharmacometrics and ML are distinct yet complementary approaches to enhance drug therapy and disease management. As previously stated, pharmacometrics utilizes mathematical models to describe the behavior of drugs in the body, the effects of drugs over time, and the variability among individuals and to optimize and predict dosing and outcomes. ML, in turn, is a subset of artificial intelligence that focuses on building systems that learn from data, identify patterns, and make decisions with minimal human intervention. In healthcare, ML algorithms analyzes large datasets to predict disease progression, identify potential drug targets, and personalize treatment plans based on patient characteristics. Pharmacometrics quantitatively describe and predict drug and disease behavior, enabling the optimization of therapeutic strategies. In contrast, ML prioritizes the accuracy of outcome predictions [163]. As Poweleit et al. note, popPK modelling differs from ML in the kinds of models it uses, despite being considered a subset of ML. To ensure the physiological and pharmacological relevance of parameter estimations, popPK modeling depends on structurally grounded models founded in pharmacokinetic and pharmacodynamic concepts [164]. On the other hand, ML is focused on minimizing prediction errors by selecting the most appropriate model from a range of possibilities.

The convergence of pharmacometrics and AI approaches, rooted in the 1990s, when neural networks were first applied to PK/PD analyses [165,166], is gaining momentum. However, the success of both pharmacometrics and ML fundamentally depends on the quality of analysis datasets, which, in turn, hinges on the calibre of reference data sources and the meticulousness of data preparation processes [162]. Pharmacometrics datasets, frequently developed for specific analysis, face challenges in review and exchange due to their unique construction and lack of standardization [167]. By serving as a computational link and enabling the integration of massive data sources into pharmacometrics analysis, ML can overcome these problems.

Integrating ML into pharmacometrics enhances precision dosing for precision medicine, emphasizing synergy rather than the replacement of conventional methods. ML-driven PBPK/popPK models, considering genetics and patient-specific data, enable precise dosing regimens tailored to individual physiology. Thus, this approach improves drug exposure, efficacy, and disease control, improving therapeutic success [168]. ML's impact on drug development includes predicting metabolism, identifying safety concerns, and reducing side effects [169]. Tailored dosing considering patient variability ensures individualized treatment recommendations, crucial in diverse populations [170]. Personalized models improve the allocation of healthcare resources [132], reduce overmedication risks, and cut costs. These models can also aid in the early stages of drug development by identifying patient subgroups that may benefit most from a new drug. Again, this can streamline clinical trials, improve patient recruitment, and increase the chances of successful drug development [171]. Ultimately, personalized dosing and treatment regimens are aligned with the goal of patient-centered care, fostering satisfaction and adherence to therapies [172].

Traditional PBPK and popPK models often rely on static datasets that may not reflect the latest patient information or trends in health data. ML-driven dynamic data integration enables the continuous flow of real-time patient data into these models. This ensures that the models remain up-to-date and relevant, reflecting changes in patient health status, treatment responses, and demographics as they occur. This timeliness is crucial for optimizing treatment decisions [147,173]. This influx of data can lead to more accurate and comprehensive models and identify subtle patterns and associations that may not be apparent in smaller or less diverse datasets. As a result, ML-driven PBPK and popPK models can be continuously validated against real-world patient data [174]. This validation process ensures that the models are not only accurate in controlled clinical settings but also in the messy and complex environment of real-world healthcare, which enhances confidence in model predictions and their utility in clinical practice [169].

Additionally, ML-based models support adaptive CDS systems, providing real-time recommendations for drug dosing, treatment adjustments, and monitoring based on the latest patient data. The real-time integration of data sources also benefits research and drug development. Researchers can access a wealth of real-world data to study drug responses, patient outcomes, and the impact of treatments on diverse populations. ML-driven data integration can also reduce the administrative burden on healthcare providers due to the automated data processing and model updates [175].

Additionally, ML-driven PBPK models offer a cost-effective alternative to traditional drug development, which involves a substantial amount of experimentation and data collection to understand a drug's PK [176,177]. They significantly reduce the need for expensive and time-consuming experiments, especially in the early stages. This cost-saving aspect is highly advantageous for pharmaceutical companies and researchers. ML-driven models can uncover complex relationships between drug PK and patient characteristics, such as genetics, demographics, and comorbidities [178]. Moreover, traditional methods for selecting relevant covariates in popPK models often involve manual and time-consuming processes, with pharmacometricians performing stepwise covariate modelling, which entails sequentially testing and adding covariates, leading to an iterative and time-intensive procedure [177]. ML frameworks, on the other hand, can automate and expedite this procedure by simultaneously analyzing a broad range of potential covariates. This not only reduces the time required for model development and refinement, but also handles large datasets and a multitude of potential covariates more comprehensively than manual methods [168]. In fact, this comprehensive exploration increases the likelihood of identifying important covariates that may have been overlooked in a manual approach, since manual stepwise covariate modelling can introduce bias due to the subjective decisions made by modelers during the process [178]. ML frameworks, in contrast, rely on data-driven algorithms that are less prone to these types of biases, resulting in more objective and data-supported covariate selection. Moreover, they can capture nonlinear associations and synergistic effects that may be challenging to detect manually. This enhanced predictive accuracy can lead to better individualized dosing recommendations and improved clinical outcomes. For example, Zhu et al. [179] discuss how ML serves as a rapid screening tool for covariates in popPK models.

ML-driven PBPK models offer a versatile solution to address the variability in clinical practice, demonstrating robust performance across diverse patient populations and medical conditions. As these models learn effectively from extensive patient data, they provide reliable predictions for various groups, from pediatrics to geriatrics, and across different demographics. In addition, the ability to adapt predictions according to new PK data [169] due to changes in physiology and organ function resulting from different diseases and medical conditions is crucial for optimizing drug therapy in patients with various medical conditions, including chronic diseases or infections.

ML-driven PBPK models can account for demographic factors, which are essential for individualizing drug dosages based on patient-specific characteristics, highlighting robust performance across various patient subgroups [180]. This consistent accuracy in predictions for different populations and clinical scenarios, ensuring generalization across diverse contexts, enhances trust and acceptance among healthcare providers and regulators. Therefore, the fact that decision-making on treatment strategies may be supported by this type of model also enables questions related to complex medical cases or rare diseases to be addressed [85], where available clinical data is limited [181].

ML-PBPK/popPK models can also predict drug toxicity and safety profiles more accurately, aiding in the early identification of potential adverse effects during drug development [182,183]. Pharmaceutical companies can decide whether to continue development, modify the drug's formulation, or explore alternative compounds. Once more, this early detection can save substantial time and resources that might have been invested in less promising candidates, and avoiding late-stage safety issues can significantly reduce the costs of drug development [184]. Identifying safety concerns early can prevent costly clinical trial failures or regulatory setbacks, leading to extensive delays and financial losses [185]. Regulatory agencies, such as the FDA, require thorough safety assessments during drug approval processes [186,187], and ML-PBPK/popPK models can provide valuable insights and data to support these assessments, helping pharmaceutical companies meet regulatory requirements more effectively. The following table (Table 2) summarizes the integration points of ML and phamacometrics.

Table 2. Integration points between ML and pharmacometrics.

Integration Points	Details
Data analysis	ML processes big data efficiently, improving patient outcomes in drug therapy. It identifies salient variables and delineates their interdependencies.
Predictive capabilities	ML algorithms excel in predictive capabilities, aiding pharmacometrics in understanding dose–exposure relationships (pharmacokinetics) and exposure marker effects (pharmacodynamics).
Complementing pharmacometric modelling	ML acts as a computational bridge, leveraging its flexibility to complement the complexity of principled pharmacometric modelling, resulting in synergistic effects in pharmacological applications.
Robustness of datasets	ML implementation in pharmacometrics requires robust datasets for training and testing, capturing the distribution of intrinsic and extrinsic factors of interest.
Overfitting	Evaluation data should not be used for training to prevent overfitting, ensuring the model generalizes well to unseen observations and doesn't fit the training data perfectly.

6.1. Examples of ML Approaches That Can Address Unique Challenges and Opportunities within Pharmacometrics

ML empowers PBPK and popPK models with notable benefits. Pioneering work by Woillard et al. utilized extreme gradient boosting (XGBoost) models to predict the exposure of drugs like tacrolimus and mycophenolic acid [188–190]. ML algorithms, including classification and regression trees, excel in optimizing doses, especially for drugs with a narrow therapeutic index like vancomycin [191,192]. Applications extend to predicting optimal doses for medications like lamotrigine and warfarin, demonstrating moderate to good accuracy and target attainment rates [193,194]. ML's pivotal role in enhancing Bayesian approaches within model-informed precision dosing (MIPD) systems is noteworthy.

Gill et al. used regression-based ML to predict drug exposure changes due to interactions [195]. The model, with 78% accuracy within twofold observed changes, highlighted early drug-discovery features for risk assessment. Despite potential biases, it showcased ML's power in capturing relationships, aiding decision-making in drug discovery [195]. Song et al. focused on DDI prediction using similarity-based ML, achieving an AUROC exceeding 0.97 [196]. Additionally, Minerali et al. compared ML algorithms, with the best Bayesian model, achieving a ROC of 0.814, illustrating ML's effectiveness in predicting DILI and identifying potential issues in clinical compounds and FDA-approved drugs. These studies collectively demonstrate ML's versatility and efficacy in pharmacology, advancing early risk assessment and safety evaluation in drug development.

A study developed an ML model predicting methicillin-resistant *Staphyloccocus aureus* (MRSA) infection likelihood in community-acquired pneumonia (CAP) patients within 72 h [197]. Using classification tree analysis, the model achieved high accuracy (ROC area: 0.775), aiding risk stratification for targeted interventions. Despite promising results, limitations include a small sample, lack of external validation, and interpretability concerns due to the "black box" nature of ML models. Further validation is crucial for real-world reliability and practicality.

Finally, Harun et al.'s study focuses on methodological considerations in ML-based exposure–response analysis [190]. The study underscores the importance of following proposed ML workflow practices, including SHAP analysis, hyperparameter tuning, and model reliability checks. Failure to adhere to these practices can lead to errors and confidence interval issues. The study showcases XGBoost's potential in accurately estimating exposure–response relationships. Exposure–response analysis in pharmacometrics is vital for drug development, optimizing therapeutic outcomes, and ensuring patient safety. Liu et al.'s study evaluates ML-based techniques in this type of analysis, highlighting their potential in handling complex datasets and identifying confounding factors [196,198]. The combination of ML and PK approaches has demonstrated reduced mean percentage errors and prediction errors compared to using only the maximum a posteriori method. ML frameworks have also facilitated efficient covariate modelling in popPK models, enabling faster and more streamlined selection of relevant covariates while maintaining computational efficiency. In supporting EHR systems and data collection, ML has proven useful in automating data extraction, processing, and preparation for PK analyses. ML-based systems have been developed to extract structured and unstructured EHR data, reducing the time and effort required for popPK analysis. These systems have efficiently formatted data for analysis using PK software like NONMEM. With the increasing availability of big data, there is a growing interest in leveraging ML (and AI) to enhance patient outcomes in drug therapy. Indeed, ML and AI are essential bridges between big data and pharmacometrics, facilitating efficient analysis and interpretation of vast information.

PBPK models are on the verge of expanding their capabilities to manage population-level data and create population-specific PBPK models routinely. Similarly, there are expectations for some level of automation in system pharmacology models. ML is expected to be central in bringing these subfields together, fostering smooth collaboration and integration. This paradigm shift in pharmacometrics reverberates across the broader pharmaceutical industry. Professionals in this sector are poised to transition into the role of model interpreters as ML algorithms progressively shoulder the computational workload [199]. Looking forward, the role of ML in this field is set for significant evolution. Prominent voices in the field have alluded to the transformation awaiting the landscape of pharmacometrics [200,201]. ML techniques are set to automate various facets of the process, such as popPK models, driven by methods like genetic algorithms [202,203]. However, it is imperative that a fundamental understanding of these algorithms and their limitations is retained. Interestingly, Kolluri et al. emphasize the importance of recognizing that the scientific method is not obsolete when making inferences about data and that informed decision-making on the optimal use of AI/ML in drug development is necessary [157]. A landscape analysis of regulatory submissions to the FDA reveals a rapid increase in AI and ML applications since 2016, with a particularly significant rise in 2021. This trend emphasizes the need for standards and best practices to guide and ensure the proper implementation of AI and ML applications in healthcare [204]. The International Coalition of Medicines Regulatory Authorities (ICMRA) has also published recommendations for stakeholders regarding the uses and challenges of AI in drug development, which the European Medicines Agency has endorsed [204]. As new applications and approaches emerge, the guidelines for AI and ML in healthcare will continue to evolve to address the specific needs and challenges of the field. However, limitations and challenges remain (Table 3).

Table 3. ML approaches that can address unique challenges and opportunities within pharmacometrics [157].

Opportunities	How to Address Them?
PKPD model personalization	Developing ML techniques for efficient personalization of PK/PD models to individual patients using sparse data. • Integrating patient-specific data, such as genetics, biomarkers, and historical treatment responses to improve model predictions and treatment optimization • Predicting the probability of a drug's success and identifying patient subgroups for maximum therapeutic benefit. **Challenges**: Determining appropriate endpoints and predicting success in pivotal trials. Unsupervised learning can be used for patient clustering to optimize clinical development.
Data integration for rare events	Designing models that integrate information from various sources (EHRs, social media, and wearable devices) to predict and manage rare adverse events not well-captured by traditional pharmacometrics models. **Challenges**: Scarcity of labeled data since rare events occur infrequently.
Adaptive clinical trials that can dynamically adjust treatment regimens based on real-time data analysis	Using ML as an assisted tool for clinical trial oversight, providing efficient ways to protect patient safety, reduce trial duration, and lower costs in clinical trial oversight. **Challenges**: Ensuring data quality and integrity when incorporating data from multiple sources.
Real-world evidence analysis	Using real-world evidence data to refine pharmacometrics models, accounting for patient heterogeneity, treatment variability, and long-term outcomes not adequately captured in controlled clinical trials. **Challenges**: Ensuring data quality and consistency.

Table 3. Cont.

Opportunities	How to Address Them?
Interpretable AI for decision Support	Developing interpretable ML models for transparent clinical decision-making. **Challenges**: Balancing model complexity and transparency; difficult interpretation potentially hindering their acceptance in clinical settings.
Uncertainty quantification	Enhancing pharmacometric models by incorporating uncertainty estimation techniques from ML, providing clinicians with confidence intervals for predictions and allowing for better risk assessment.
Multi-modal data fusion	Investigating methods to effectively fuse data from diverse modalities, such as genomics, proteomics, and imaging data, to create comprehensive patient profiles that can better inform treatment decisions. Breakdown of the multi-modal data fusion process: (1) data collection; (2) data preprocessing; (3) feature extraction and selection; (4) data fusion; (5) model development; (6) model validation; (7) clinical application; and (8) continuous learning (as new data becomes available, the models can be updated and refined, embodying the principles of continuous learning and improvement).
Longitudinal data analysis	Developing models for analyzing longitudinal data over extended periods to capture changes in patient response to treatments.
Ethical and regulatory Considerations	Addressing ethical implications and regulatory challenges of incorporating ML into pharmacometrics, including issues related to data privacy, bias, and validation.
Optimization of drug combination	Exploring ML algorithms to optimize drug combinations by predicting synergistic effects, potential adverse interactions, and tailoring treatments for individual patients.

6.2. Challenges and Future Directions

Navigating the intricate landscape of integrating ML with PBPK (ML-PBPK) and popPK (ML-PopPK) models presents many complex challenges and opportunities in pharmaceutical research and precision medicine. Concerning data integration and quality, pharmaceutical research relies on data from various sources, including clinical trials, EHRs, wearable devices, and omics data [205]. Each source may have different formats, standards, and levels of quality. Combining them into a cohesive dataset for ML modeling can be challenging. Thus, standardized data integration pipelines are required, addressing formats and maintaining compatibility. Implementing standard data formats, such as the CDISC (Clinical Data Interchange Standards Consortium), can facilitate this standardization process [206].

The accuracy and reliability of ML-driven models heavily depend on high-quality input data. To ensure this, preprocessing techniques are usually employed, particularly outlier detection, missing data imputations, and cleaning [207], as well as regular audits and validation checks to identify and rectify data quality issues without neglecting metadata management [208]. Establishing a robust metadata management system helps in tracking the lineage of data and assessing its reliability for modeling purposes.

Integrating data from various sources may involve sensitive patient information. Maintaining data privacy and complying with regulations like the General Data Protection Regulation (GDPR) and Health Insurance Portability and Accountability Act (HIPA) is essential. Anonymization and de-identification techniques can be employed to protect patient privacy while integrating data [205,209].

In addition to standardization, harmonizing data is a crucial step, particularly when dealing with patient-specific information. This involves reconciling differences in terminologies, units of measurement, and data collection methods to ensure the comparability and effective utilization of data. To ensure that different systems and platforms can interact and share data seamlessly, the development of application programming interfaces (APIs) and data exchange standards can facilitate interoperability [210]. Establishing clear data governance policies and practices is essential for managing data integration and quality. This includes defining roles and responsibilities, data stewardship, and data lifecycle management to maintain its integrity over time. ML models are dynamic and evolve with new data. Implementing data versioning protocols ensures that changes in data sources and quality are tracked and model updates can be managed effectively. For this reason, collaboration between data scientists, domain experts, clinicians, and information technology (IT) professionals is necessary to effectively address data integration challenges [211].

Moreover, patient data must be handled with utmost privacy and security. However, diversity, equity, and inclusion (DEI) and concern for bias are also critical considerations in the integration and analysis of diverse datasets in precision medicine. Biases can derail any attempt to improve the culture of DEI, and this is particularly relevant in healthcare. Human beings have inherent biases, and these biases can manifest in the collection, analysis, and interpretation of data, potentially culminating in disparities in healthcare access, treatment, and outcomes, particularly for underrepresented minority populations. Therefore, it is essential to consider DEI and bias in the integration and analysis of diverse datasets in precision medicine and to implement strategies to mitigate them, such as using diverse study populations, validating biomarkers across diverse populations, and using rigorous statistical methods to analyze data. Diversifying the composition of healthcare providers and research teams is one strategy to address DEI in precision medicine. Studies have demonstrated that underrepresented minority physicians and women are more likely to provide care to underserved populations and to address health disparities. Additionally, community engagement and education programs can help increase diversity in clinical trials and improve representation of underrepresented groups in research [212]. ML models can inadvertently perpetuate biases present in the training data. Mitigating bias and ensuring fairness in predictions, especially in healthcare decisions, is an ethical imperative [213]. For instance, Lee et al. demonstrated the significance of integrating ML techniques with robust de-identification methods to safeguard sensitive healthcare information. Advanced models can play a pivotal role in verifying the accurate application of de-identification techniques, thereby promoting both data confidentiality and usability while aligning with ethical and regulatory standards [214].

The opacity of ML models, that is, the fact that they are often considered "black boxes", can hinder their adoption in clinical practice [215]. Physicians and healthcare professionals need to understand the rationale behind a model's predictions to make informed decisions regarding patient care, and for this reason, a lack of interpretability can result in mistrust and reluctance to use ML-driven recommendations [216]. Therefore, transparent explanations for model predictions must be provided to solidify trust and empower patients to participate in their own care decisions [217,218]. Implementing model interpretability techniques like SHAP analysis can provide insights into model decision-making [219,220].

Patient-specific predictions should be actionable in a clinical setting, and this requires developing robust models [221,222] that align with clinical workflows and provide practical guidance to healthcare providers [223]. However, this exercise is quite complex due to substantial variability in response to drugs. Failing to account for such heterogeneity may lead to suboptimal treatment outcomes for specific patient groups, affecting its generalizability. Thus, ensuring that the model can handle healthy and diseased populations is essential for its clinical relevance [224,225]. One solution could be to continuously validate models across various patient subgroups and update them as needed.

Validation should encompass diverse datasets, including independent datasets not used during model training [226], to verify the reliability and robustness of ML-enhanced PBPK/popPK models. Models should be evaluated for their long-term predictive performance. This is particularly relevant in chronic diseases where treatment effects may evolve over time because it is crucial to ensure that the model remains accurate over extended periods. Therefore, rigorous validation approaches, including external validation using independent datasets can be helpful.

In addition, ML algorithms can be computationally demanding, particularly when dealing with large datasets or complex models. Efficient algorithm design, parallel computing, and graphics processing unit (GPU) acceleration can optimize resource usage [227]. ML models should be designed to scale with growing data volumes and computational demands, and therefore cloud computing resources are usually employed, which offer scalability and cost-effectiveness, especially for resource-intensive tasks like deep learning [228].

ML algorithms often require large sample sizes, which may exceed what is typically needed for the clinical application of AI and ML. Collaborative efforts are essential to develop comprehensive databases and enhance data quality. AI and ML should complement, not replace, traditional pharmacometrics. Ongoing advancements and collaborations are expected to drive the evolution of precision medicine, with a focus on research, validation, and integration into clinical practice. The future of ML-PBPK/popPK integration holds promise in various strategic directions:

- Expanded applications of PBPK models, informing clinical study design and predicting drug interactions.
- Pediatric dosing regimen prediction to ensure safer and more effective treatments for pediatric patients.
- Utilization of PBPK models for predicting drug exposure in patients with organ impairment.
- Estimation of maternal–fetal drug disposition during pregnancy.
- Prediction of pH-mediated drug interactions using PBPK models.
- Improved predictive performance of popPK models by focusing on data adequacy.
- Integration of generic PBPK models for extrapolations and continuous updates.

7. Digital Health and Wearable Technologies

As technology advances, digital health and wearable technologies have increasingly become integrated into patient care. Digital health has gained significant momentum due to several key factors and, besides improving access to healthcare, this discipline also mitigates any inefficiencies in the healthcare system, improves the quality of care, reduces the costs associated with healthcare, and offers more individualized care tailored to patients' needs [229].

Digital health, a term that refers to the application of information and communication technologies in the medical field and other health professions, plays a major role in precision medicine. It provides the essential tools and technologies for the collection, analysis, and effective application of individualized patient data. This field is constantly developing and has a broad scope, making use of digital technologies such as wearable devices, mobile health, telehealth, health information technology, telemedicine, apps, sensors, data analysis, and other digital solutions to improve the delivery of healthcare services, raise the quality of patient care, and optimize healthcare management [230,231]. For example, the use of digital devices such as smartphones not only facilitates communication but also provides a wide range of applications capable of monitoring blood pressure, recording blood glucose levels, ensuring adherence to drug treatment, and tracking levels of physical activity [231]. These capabilities demonstrate that the adoption of digital medicine enables patients to monitor their health and well-being more precisely, collecting real-time data and making it an essential pillar in contemporary medical practice [232,233]. Another goal of digital health is improving the experience of each patient, as well as the experience of the doctor and other non-medical providers. The final objective is to address health disparities and improve them with an individualized view of each patient [234,235].

Remote sensing and wearables, telemedicine and health information, data analytics and intelligence, predictive modeling, health and wellness behavior modification tools, bioinformatics tools (-omics), medical social media, digitized health record platforms, physician–patient portals, do-it-yourself (DIY) diagnostics, compliance and treatments, decision support systems, and imaging are included in the categories of products and services that digital health has to offer [229].

The continuous collection of individual biomedical data, such as genomics, proteomics, mobile health data, and EHRs, is fundamental. This data is essential for understanding a patient's unique characteristics and genetic predisposition to disease. This database may be then subjected to advanced analysis using techniques such as ML and AI to identify patterns, trends, and associations in large volumes of patient data, which can be used to personalize treatments [236,237]. A notable example of this process is genomic medicine. Digital health makes it possible to sequence a patient's genome more affordably and efficiently. This means that doctors can analyze a patient's DNA to identify genetic variations that can influence the response to specific drugs and treatments [236]. Based on the data collected and the genetic information, doctors can then tailor treatments according to each patient's specific needs, including the choice of drugs, dosages, and treatment strategies. In addition, digital health may be used to predict individual disease risks based on these data, allowing doctors to develop targeted prevention strategies. To keep a close eye on a patient's progress, such devices, including wearables and medical sensors, enable continuous health monitoring. This not only helps with current treatment but also with the early identification of health problems. Patients are involved in their own care through health apps and online platforms, allowing them to monitor their progress and make informed decisions [236].

Moreover, digital communication technologies facilitate the exchange of information between clinicians and patients, enabling more effective communication and the sharing of relevant data. This reduces the occurrence of unwanted side effects and leads to better prevention and a more comprehensive approach to patient well-being [234].

The EHR is a digital system that stores medical information and patient health information (e.g., medical history, test results, prescriptions, allergy information) in electronic format (Table 4).

Table 4. The uses and benefits of EHRs. Adapted from [168].

EHR Benefits	Integration of EHR in Healthcare
Information access and sharing	EHRs facilitate quick and secure access to patients' medical information, allowing healthcare professionals to make informed decisions and order care.
Better care management	EHRs help you better manage the care of chronic patients by enabling continuous monitoring and adjustment of treatment plans based on real-time data.
Integration and coordination	The integration of RSE (remote sensing and earth observation) into healthcare systems allows for more efficient coordination between different healthcare providers, improving continuity of care.
Clinical research	RSE data can be used in clinical research to identify health trends, evaluate the effectiveness of treatments, and improve evidence-based medicine. Furthermore, omics data, which encompasses genomic, transcriptomic, proteomic, and metabolomic information, plays a crucial role in precision medicine. This data enables the personalization of treatments based on the genetics and individual characteristics of each patient, improving the effectiveness of care. Omics data analysis also helps identify genetic markers of diseases, enabling early prevention and diagnosis.

Taken together, the incorporation of EHRs and omics data into digital health enables a more personalized, evidence-based approach to healthcare, improving the diagnosis, treatment, and prevention of disease. This convergence represents a significant advance in the ability to use digital information to improve people's health and well-being.

Further, wearable devices play a fundamental role in digital health, offering a variety of functions that help monitor the health and well-being of individuals (Table 5).

Table 5. Wearable devices used in digital health and their uses. Adapted from [168].

Wearable Devices	Properties, Capabilities, and Applications
Smartwatches	Monitor heart rate, measure blood pressure, track physical activity, count steps, monitor sleep quality, and send reminders to move, drink water or perform exercises
Fitness trackers	Monitor steps, distance traveled, calories burned, heart rate, and even track specific exercises like running and swimming
Glucose-monitoring devices	For people with diabetes, devices such as continuous glucose monitors (CGM) offer the ability to monitor blood glucose levels in real-time. They can send alerts when glucose levels are out of ideal range
Portable electrocardiogram (ECG) devices	Some smartwatches can perform ECGs. They can detect abnormal heart rhythms, such as atrial fibrillation
Sleep-monitoring devices	These devices record sleep patterns, duration, and quality. They provide insights into improving sleep habits
Breath-monitoring devices	Can monitor respiratory rate and blood oxygen saturation. This is useful for monitoring breathing problems such as sleep apnea
Virtual and augmented reality (VR/AR) Devices	In rehabilitation areas and therapy, VR and AR devices create virtual environments for therapeutic purposes, such as rehabilitation after injuries or strokes
Smart glasses	These are used in medical settings for access to clinical information, real-time documentation, and telehealth
Physiological activity-monitoring devices	In addition to the most well-known devices, some wearables monitor specific physiological activities, such as body temperature, exposure to UV light, hydration, and much more
Wearable sensors for clinical research	In clinical research, wearable sensors are used to collect objective and accurate data about the health of patients in clinical studies, enabling a deeper understanding of different medical conditions
Augmented reality glasses for surgery	In medicine, augmented reality glasses are used by surgeons to provide real-time information during surgical procedures, making them more accurate and safer

These examples illustrate the diversity of wearable devices in the area of digital health. Each of these devices is designed to meet specific health monitoring and care needs, and many of them are constantly evolving as technology advances. These devices play an important role in collecting real-time data, supporting medical diagnoses, promoting a healthy lifestyle, and improving healthcare [171]. In the context of wearable devices, the variability in sensors and inconsistency in data collection pose challenges in coordinating and assessing quality. User-related issues significantly impact the reliability of digital health data. These include digital health service accessibility, accuracy of the data, consistency of data input by users, and contextual validity of data to relevant aspects. Addressing these issues is crucial for improving the quality, usability, and acceptability of digital health interventions [56].

Furthermore, precision medicine, driven by the collection and analysis of this data, promotes innovation and collaboration in digital health technologies. The idea of multidisciplinarity continues to be essential. Facilitating the integration of personalized biomedical data collection and precision medicine into society requires public education, training for healthcare professionals, collaboration between experts in different areas, clear regulations, financial incentives, academic partnerships to drive innovation and develop patient-friendly technologies, and universal access and respect of ethical principles.

It is also important to ensure data security, privacy, and interoperability for effective integration into precision medicine workflows. This involves implementing robust security measures, appropriate regulation, and informed consent from patients for the use of their data. By doing so, we can harness the potential of digital health technologies and wearable devices to improve the quality of healthcare and promote a more personalized, evidence-based approach to medical treatment [238].

8. Clinical Trials and Study Design

The design of clinical trials has experienced a profound transformation in response to the medical paradigm shift, which recognizes that traditional one-size-fits-all treatments are often ineffective or produce negative effects in patients [239,240]. Hence, the next generation of trials must be a symbiosis between patient-centered strategies, where the therapeutic interventions are tailored to patient-specific biomarkers, and conventional drug-centered strategies, focused on evaluating the efficacy, safety, and pharmacological properties of the drug under study.

In fact, driven by fast advancements in omics, recent biomarker-based clinical trials have emerged as a very promising approach in this new era. In addition, advanced computational tools have revolutionized the way clinical trial data is analyzed. There is a wide variety of in silico methods that allow accurate data processing.

As patient-centered trial designs, master protocols have arisen, classified into basket trials, umbrella trials, and platform trials (Figure 4) [241–244]. They have been increasingly implemented, particularly in the field of oncology. According to Park et al. [241], at the time of publication (2019), there has been a rapid increase in the number of master protocols. Basket trials consist of evaluating a targeted therapy against multiple diseases sharing common molecular alterations. Umbrella trials, on the other hand, involve multiple interventions for a single disease stratified into subgroups according to molecular alteration. In turn, platform trials evaluate several treatments against a common control group [240,245–247]. Another innovative approach is adaptive design, which enables the dynamic evolution of studies [159]. This method allows for the early discontinuation of ineffective treatment arms while increasing randomization to more promising therapies. Nevertheless, some limitations associated with the early elimination of treatment may be listed, including the lack of consistent data on safety.

Although less common, home-based clinical trials are being conducted [248], especially in patients with cancer and limiting diseases. This site-less clinical trial design simplifies patient recruitment, enables the inclusion of more diverse populations, and increases participants' enrolment rates. However, these trials also pose some challenges and risks in terms of data reliability. The quality of data collected from home-based clinical trials depends on the validity and reliability of the instruments used for data collection, such as questionnaires, diaries, sensors, or devices. These instruments need to be designed carefully to ensure that they capture the relevant aspects of the patient's situation and outcomes and that they are easy to understand and complete by the patients. They also need to be tested for accuracy, completeness, consistency, and contextual validity before being used in clinical trials. The security of data collected from home-based clinical trials is crucial to protect the privacy and confidentiality of the patients. Researchers need to work with information technology professionals to ensure that data collection is safe and secure while maintaining patient privacy during decentralized trials. This may involve using encryption, authentication, authorization, backup, and recovery methods [249].

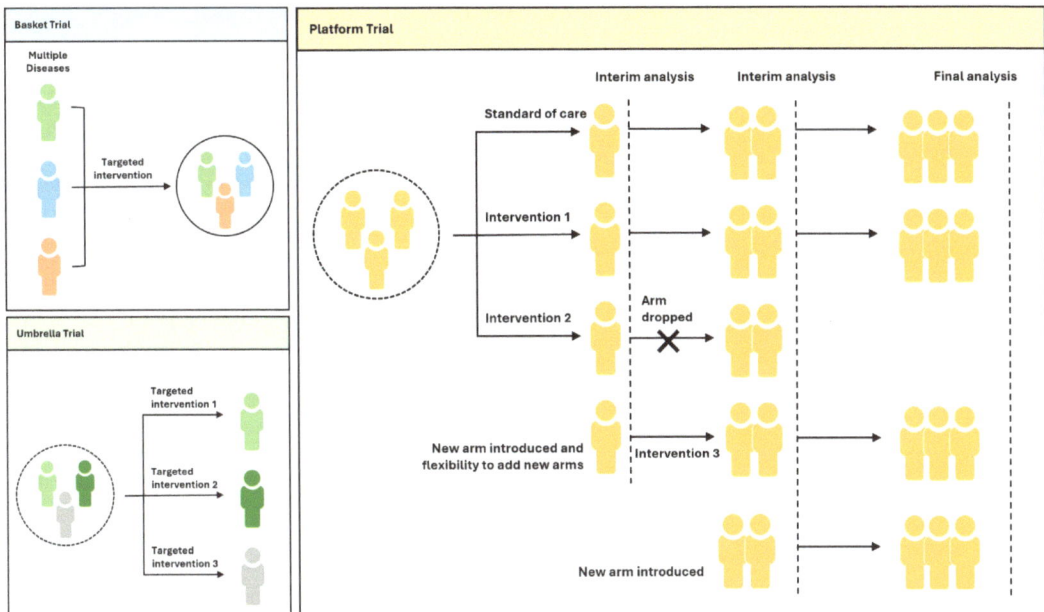

Figure 4. Representation of basket trials, umbrella trials, and platform trials. Created with SMART—Servier Medical ART. Available online: https://smart.servier.com (accessed on 22 September 2023).

Another emerging trend in the clinical trial landscape involves the integration of digital health technologies, such as mobile devices, mobile apps, and remote monitoring devices, directly into the study's framework. These innovative studies are often referred to as virtual clinical trials (VCTs), as they leverage digital tools to remotely gather data from participants instead of requiring in-person visits to research facilities. There are several digital tools currently available: eConsent, a digital method of obtaining informed consent from participants; electronic patient-reported outcomes (ePRO), which represent health-related outcomes (symptoms, adverse effects) directly reported by the patient and collected electronically; and sensors and wearable devices [250]. The most evident advantage of these studies is the increased participant adherence, as they participate from the convenience of their home. Moreover, data collected through digital devices may enable continuous real-time data acquisition rather than periodic data collection during in-person visits.

The ease of digital data collection has led to a huge amount of information, requiring complex and time-intensive analysis [240]. The analysis of real-world data using advanced computer methods provides real-world evidence. This is where AI and ML algorithms can be used to address this challenge and rapidly discover new therapies. Interestingly, real-world data has already practical uses, since the FDA has approved at least two cancer drugs developed using it [251,252]. Also, real-world data holds particular significance in assessing drug efficacy and safety in patient populations frequently excluded from randomized clinical trials, such as patients with limited performance status, older patients, patients with serious comorbidities, or underserved populations who may not be able to travel to an academic centre for a clinical trial [240].

In summary, these clinical trials offer great potential for improving treatment outcomes and reducing adverse effects, ultimately leading to a transformative era of personalized healthcare. There are still, however, opportunities for further evolution.

9. Future Perspectives: Integration of In Silico Tools in Hospital Settings

Expectation arising from the application of computational methods, such as ML, deep neural networks, and multi-modal biomedical AI, has been the reinvigoration of clinical research, including drug discovery, image interpretation, streamlining EHRs, improving workflow, and, over time, advancing public health [239]. Therapeutic monitoring and clinical decision-making constitute a multifaceted process in today's hospital settings. Healthcare professionals employ clinical assessments, interacting with patients to collect vital information about their medical history and current symptoms, guiding subsequent steps. We believe that we are moving towards a reality in which all these technologies will be applied in the context of clinical practice. However, before that, there are issues that must be overcome.

Collaborative care teams, comprising various healthcare professionals, including doctors, nurses, pharmacists, and specialists, collaborate on patient care plans to leverage collective expertise for more informed clinical decisions. Since patient engagement is a fundamental aspect of modern healthcare, hospitals need to actively involve patients in their care by providing information, discussing treatment options, and considering individual preferences during decision-making.

Despite exponential growth in acquiring healthcare data, the capacity to integrate such data to improve health outcomes presently fails to meet technological advances. These challenges can be overcome with the use of AI and other computing technologies in health services workflows. Genomic sequencing, providing detailed information about an individual's genetic makeup, has particularly benefited oncology and genetics, especially because of the several approvals for biomarker-based targeted therapies and immunotherapy [229,253,254]. Omics-based assays can be used to study the complex interactions in severe diseases, facilitating early-stage intervention and the selection of the most fit treatment.

EHRs streamline the management of health data by providing a centralized, comprehensive, and up-to-date repository of patient information [255,256]. This potentially eliminates the need for paper-based records, reducing errors associated with manual data entry and retrieval. Therefore, EHRs contribute to the creation of medical knowledge in two ways: (a) they enable the aggregation and analysis of large volumes of patient data for research, epidemiological studies, and the discovery of patterns and trends that inform medical practices; (b) CDS provides evidence-based guidelines and alerts to clinicians, contributing to better health outcomes. As such, EHRs are fundamental to the advancement of precision medicine. Key advantages in this context include genomic integration with clinical data and facilitation of personalized treatment plans by providing a comprehensive view of a patient's medical history, lab results, and other data. This enables healthcare providers to select treatments that are most likely to be effective for a specific patient.

Interoperability is critical for EHRs to fulfill their potential and ensure continuity of care. Patients can receive consistent care even if they change healthcare providers or facilities once their records can be accessed and updated from different systems. Unfortunately, non-interoperability is currently one of the biggest limitations on the exchange of data between different systems.

Alongside the uniformization of EHRs, the integration of CDS systems in hospitals' workflows is crucial in precision medicine. The healthcare providers need real-time, data-driven recommendations based on patients' specificities, including genomic data, risk assessment and predictive modelling, DDI alerts, clinical guideline adherence, continuous learning and improvement, and patient engagement. However, besides an infrastructural challenge, the use of CDS systems also demands training staff to accurately introduce and interpret information; keeping CDS systems up-to-date with evolving medical knowledge and technology can be resource-intensive, and evaluating the actual impact of CDS systems on patient outcomes can be challenging.

Therapeutic drug monitoring (TDM) is particularly important for medication management, involving regular assessments of drug levels in the bloodstream to optimize dosages and ensure safe and effective treatment. For example, in the case of a patient taking anticoagulant medication, regular TDM may be conducted to ensure the medication is within the therapeutic range and effectively prevent blood clots. In this context, pharmacometrics is a powerful tool. Besides this, the integration of pharmacogenomic data with pharmacometric models allows for even more precise dosing recommendations based on a patient's genetic profile.

All stakeholders must be involved in change. Healthcare providers need to develop trust in the information generated by AI applications (and other computational methods) and to face AI and advanced robotic systems as professional partners; legislators must speed up regulatory policies that clarify boundaries and guarantee patient safety and privacy; IT departments are critical to ensure robust IT infrastructure to support data transfer, integration, and analysis as well as to integrate CDS systems into EHR systems for seamless use in clinical workflows. Nowadays, clinical workflows do not consider big data-driven approaches. Consequently, the main priorities for the integration of in silico tools in hospital settings are the development of IT infrastructure capable of aligning big data with clinical practice, standardized protocols and boundary-setting, and the design of comprehensive training programs for healthcare professionals.

10. Conclusions

The integration of omics, biomarkers, pharmacometrics, ML, and digital wearables into healthcare presents a transformative potential for precision medicine and patient care. These methods offer numerous advantages, such as improved diagnostic accuracy, tailored treatment plans, and enhanced patient monitoring.

Among these methods, in silico approaches, which involve computer simulations and modeling, are gaining traction, reducing the need for costly and time-consuming physical examination, speeding up drug development, and enhancing disease understanding. They also hold promise for conducting virtual clinical trials, which can streamline the evaluation of medical interventions. User-friendly, seamless integration with existing healthcare systems and clear insights are crucial for broad adoption.

The education of clinicians and patients in the interpretation of genomic data and the use of wearable technologies is crucial for the successful implementation of these methods. Specialized training modules, integration with EHRs, and informative informatic systems can play a key role. These systems, accessible anytime and anywhere, can include interactive elements, making them cost-effective alternatives to traditional courses. Collaboration with healthcare professionals, educators, and technology experts will be essential to developing systems that meet the needs of both clinicians and patients.

Ethical considerations, funding, and legislative changes are indeed significant factors that could influence the adoption of these healthcare technologies. Ethical challenges include ensuring patient privacy, data protection, and equitable access to these technologies. Adequate funding is necessary to support the development and implementation of these methods, while legislative changes may be required to address regulatory and compliance issues. It is essential for stakeholders to work collaboratively to navigate these challenges and create an environment that supports innovation while safeguarding ethical principles and patient rights.

Author Contributions: Conceptualization, N.V. and B.C.; methodology L.M., B.C., M.P., A.S., J.S., L.S. and I.S.; formal analysis, L.M., B.C., M.P., A.S., J.S., L.S., I.S. and N.V.; investigation, L.M., B.C.; M.P., A.S., J.S., L.S., I.S., P.M., S.S. and N.V.; writing—original draft preparation, L.M., B.C., M.P., A.S., J.S., L.S. and I.S.; writing—review and editing, L.M., B.C., P.M., S.S. and N.V.; supervision, N.V.; project administration, N.V.; funding acquisition, N.V. All authors have read and agreed to the published version of the manuscript.

Funding: This work was financed by FEDER—Fundo Europeu de Desenvolimento Regional through the COMPETE 2020—*Operational Programme for Competitiveness and Internationalization* (POCI), Portugal 2020, and by Portuguese funds through FCT—*Fundação para a Ciência e a Tecnologia*, in a framework of the projects in CINTESIS, R&D Unit (reference UIDB/4255/2020) and within the scope of the project "RISE—LA/P/0053/2020". N.V. is also thankful for support from FCT and FEDER (European Union), award number IF/00092/2014/CP1255/CT0004 and CHAIR in Onco-Innovation at FMUP.

Institutional Review Board Statement: Not applicable.

Informed Consent Statement: Not applicable.

Data Availability Statement: Not applicable.

Acknowledgments: N.V. is thankful for support from FCT and FEDER (European Union), award number IF/00092/2014/CP1255/CT0004 and CHAIR in Onco-Innovation from FMUP.

Conflicts of Interest: The authors declare no conflict of interest.

References

1. Visvikis-Siest, S.; Theodoridou, D.; Kontoe, M.S.; Kumar, S.; Marschler, M. Milestones in Personalized Medicine: From the Ancient Time to Nowadays—The Provocation of COVID-19. *Front. Genet.* **2020**, *11*, 569175. [CrossRef]
2. The Changing Landscape of Precision Medicine. Available online: https://www.astrazeneca.com/what-science-can-do/topics/technologies/precision-medicine-history.html (accessed on 10 October 2023).
3. Akhoon, N. Precision Medicine: A New Paradigm in Therapeutics. *Int. J. Prev. Med.* **2021**, *12*, 12.
4. Gameiro, G.R.; Sinkunas, V.; Liguori, G.R.; Auler-Júnior, J.O.C. Precision Medicine: Changing the Way We Think about Healthcare. *Clinics* **2018**, *73*, e723. [CrossRef]
5. Denny, J.C.; Collins, F.S. Precision Medicine in 2030—Seven Ways to Transform Healthcare. *Cell* **2021**, *184*, 1415–1419. [CrossRef]
6. Grissinger, M. The Five Rights: A Destination Without a Map. *Pharm. Ther.* **2010**, *35*, 542.
7. National Research Council. *Toward Precision Medicine*; National Academies Press: Cambridge, MA, USA, 2011; ISBN 0309222222.
8. Delpierre, C.; Lefèvre, T. Precision and Personalized Medicine: What Their Current Definition Says and Silences about the Model of Health They Promote. Implication for the Development of Personalized Health. *Front. Sociol.* **2023**, *8*, 1112159. [CrossRef]
9. Baiardini, I.; Heffler, E. *The Patient-Centered Decision System as per the 4Ps of Precision Medicine*; Elsevier Inc.: Amsterdam, The Netherlands, 2018; ISBN 9780128134719.
10. Kim, H.J.; Kim, H.J.; Park, Y.; Lee, W.S.; Lim, Y.; Kim, J.H. Clinical Genome Data Model (CGDM) Provides Interactive Clinical Decision Support for Precision Medicine. *Sci. Rep.* **2020**, *10*, 1414. [CrossRef] [PubMed]
11. Yadav, S.P. The Wholeness in Suffix -Omics, -Omes, and the Word Om. *J. Biomol. Tech.* **2007**, *18*, 277.
12. Hasanzad, M.; Sarhangi, N.; Chimeh, S.E.; Ayati, N.; Afzali, M.; Khatami, F.; Nikfar, S.; Meybodi, H. Precision Medicine Journey through Omics Approach. *J. Diabetes Metab. Disord.* **2022**, *21*, 881–888. [CrossRef] [PubMed]
13. De Maria Marchiano, R.; Di Sante, G.; Piro, G.; Carbone, C.; Tortora, G.; Boldrini, L.; Pietragalla, A.; Daniele, G.; Tredicine, M.; Cesario, A.; et al. Translational Research in the Era of Precision Medicine: Where We Are and Where We Will Go. *J. Pers. Med.* **2021**, *11*, 216. [CrossRef] [PubMed]
14. Tebani, A.; Afonso, C.; Marret, S.; Bekri, S. Omics-Based Strategies in Precision Medicine: Toward a Paradigm Shift in Inborn Errors of Metabolism Investigations. *Int. J. Mol. Sci.* **2016**, *17*, 1555. [CrossRef]
15. Ahmed, Z. Precision Medicine with Multi-Omics Strategies, Deep Phenotyping, and Predictive Analysis. *Prog. Mol. Biol. Transl. Sci.* **2022**, *190*, 101–125. [CrossRef]
16. Kwon, Y.W.; Jo, H.S.; Bae, S.; Seo, Y.; Song, P.; Song, M.; Yoon, J.H. Application of Proteomics in Cancer: Recent Trends and Approaches for Biomarkers Discovery. *Front. Med.* **2021**, *8*, 747333. [CrossRef]
17. Giannitsis, E.; Katus, H.A. Biomarkers for Clinical Decision-Making in the Management of Pulmonary Embolism. *Clin. Chem.* **2017**, *63*, 91–100. [CrossRef]
18. Wafi, A.; Mirnezami, R. Translational –Omics: Future Potential and Current Challenges in Precision Medicine. *Methods* **2018**, *151*, 3–11. [CrossRef]
19. Hu, C.; Jia, W. Multi-Omics Profiling: The Way toward Precision Medicine in Metabolic. *J. Mol. Cell Biol.* **2021**, *13*, 576. [CrossRef]
20. Pirmohamed, M. Pharmacogenomics: Current Status and Future Perspectives. *Nat. Rev. Genet.* **2023**, *24*, 350–362. [CrossRef] [PubMed]
21. Badary, O.A. Pharmacogenomics and COVID-19: Clinical Implications of Human Genome Interactions with Repurposed Drugs. *Pharmacogenom. J.* **2021**, *21*, 275–284. [CrossRef] [PubMed]
22. Miteva-Marcheva, N.N.; Ivanov, H.Y.; Dimitrov, D.K.; Stoyanova, V.K. Application of Pharmacogenetics in Oncology. *Biomark. Res.* **2020**, *8*, 32. [CrossRef] [PubMed]
23. Licinio, J.; Wong, M.-L. Pharmacogenomics of Antidepressant Treatment Effects. *Dialogues Clin. Neurosci.* **2011**, *13*, 63–71. [CrossRef] [PubMed]
24. McDonough, C.W. Pharmacogenomics in Cardiovascular Diseases. *Curr. Protoc.* **2021**, *1*, e189. [CrossRef]
25. Mallal, S.; Phillips, E.; Carosi, G.; Molina, J.-M.; Workman, C.; Tomažič, J.; Jägel-Guedes, E.; Rugina, S.; Kozyrev, O.; Cid, J.F.; et al. HLA-B*5701 Screening for Hypersensitivity to Abacavir. *N. Engl. J. Med.* **2008**, *358*, 568–579. [CrossRef] [PubMed]

26. Lecomte, T.; Ferraz, J.-M.; Zinzindohoué, F.; Loriot, M.-A.; Tregouet, D.-A.; Landi, B.; Berger, A.; Cugnenc, P.-H.; Jian, R.; Beaune, P.; et al. Thymidylate Synthase Gene Polymorphism Predicts Toxicity in Colorectal Cancer Patients Receiving 5-Fluorouracil-Based Chemotherapy. *Clin. Cancer Res.* **2004**, *10*, 5880–5888. [CrossRef]
27. Flockhart, D.A.; O'Kane, D.; Williams, M.S.; Watson, M.S.; Flockhart, D.A.; Gage, B.; Gandolfi, R.; King, R.; Lyon, E.; Nussbaum, R.; et al. Pharmacogenetic Testing of CYP2C9 and VKORC1 Alleles for Warfarin. *Genet. Med.* **2008**, *10*, 139–150. [CrossRef]
28. Ferrell, P.B.; McLeod, H.L. Carbamazepine, *HLA-B*1502* and Risk of Stevens–Johnson Syndrome and Toxic Epidermal Necrolysis: US FDA Recommendations. *Pharmacogenomics* **2008**, *9*, 1543–1546. [CrossRef] [PubMed]
29. de Souza, J.A.; Olopade, O.I. CYP2D6 Genotyping and Tamoxifen: An Unfinished Story in the Quest for Personalized Medicine. *Semin. Oncol.* **2011**, *38*, 263–273. [CrossRef] [PubMed]
30. D'Adamo, G.L.; Widdop, J.T.; Giles, E.M. The Future Is Now? Clinical and Translational Aspects of "Omics" Technologies. *Immunol. Cell Biol.* **2021**, *99*, 168–176. [CrossRef]
31. Vogeser, M.; Bendt, A.K. From Research Cohorts to the Patient—A Role for "Omics" in Diagnostics and Laboratory Medicine? *Clin. Chem. Lab. Med.* **2023**, *61*, 974–980. [CrossRef]
32. Castaneda, C.; Nalley, K.; Mannion, C.; Bhattacharyya, P.; Blake, P.; Pecora, A.; Goy, A.; Suh, K.S. Clinical Decision Support Systems for Improving Diagnostic Accuracy and Achieving Precision Medicine. *J. Clin. Bioinform.* **2015**, *5*, 4. [CrossRef]
33. Sperber, N.R.; Dong, O.M.; Roberts, M.C.; Dexter, P.; Elsey, A.R.; Ginsburg, G.S.; Horowitz, C.R.; Johnson, J.A.; Levy, K.D.; Ong, H.; et al. Strategies to Integrate Genomic Medicine into Clinical Care: Evidence from the IGNITE Network. *J. Pers. Med.* **2021**, *11*, 647. [CrossRef]
34. FDA Label Search. Available online: https://labels.fda.gov/ (accessed on 16 October 2023).
35. The Personalized Medicine Coalition. Available online: https://www.personalizedmedicinecoalition.org/ (accessed on 16 October 2023).
36. Precision Medicine | FDA. Available online: https://www.fda.gov/medical-devices/in-vitro-diagnostics/precision-medicine (accessed on 10 October 2023).
37. Nimmesgern, E.; Benediktsson, I.; Norstedt, I. Personalized Medicine in Europe. *Clin. Transl. Sci.* **2017**, *10*, 61–63. [CrossRef]
38. Aronson, J.K.; Ferner, R.E. Biomarkers—A General Review. *Curr. Protoc. Pharmacol.* **2017**, *2017*, 9.23.1–9.23.17. [CrossRef] [PubMed]
39. Ho, D.; Quake, S.R.; McCabe, E.R.B.; Chng, W.J.; Chow, E.K.; Ding, X.; Gelb, B.D.; Ginsburg, G.S.; Hassenstab, J.; Ho, C.M.; et al. Enabling Technologies for Personalized and Precision Medicine. *Trends Biotechnol.* **2020**, *38*, 497–518. [CrossRef]
40. Mokondjimobe, E.; Longo-Mbenza, B.; Akiana, J.; Ndalla, U.O.; Dossou-Yovo, R.; Mboussa, J.; Parra, H.J. Biomarkers of Oxidative Stress and Personalized Treatment of Pulmonary Tuberculosis: Emerging Role of Gamma-Glutamyltransferase. *Adv. Pharmacol. Sci.* **2012**, *2012*, 465634. [CrossRef]
41. Kirkwood, S.C.; Hockett, R.D. Pharmacogenomic Biomarkers. *Dis. Markers* **2002**, *18*, 63–71. [CrossRef] [PubMed]
42. Mendrick, D.L. Genomic and Genetic Biomarkers of Toxicity. *Toxicology* **2008**, *245*, 175–181. [CrossRef]
43. Karaulov, A.V.; Garib, V.; Garib, F.; Valenta, R. Protein Biomarkers in Asthma. *Int. Arch. Allergy Immunol.* **2018**, *175*, 189–208. [CrossRef]
44. Sigdel, T.K.; Gao, X.; Sarwal, M.M. Protein and Peptide Biomarkers in Organ Transplantation. *Biomark. Med.* **2012**, *6*, 259–271. [CrossRef] [PubMed]
45. Gao, J.; Garulacan, L.A.; Storm, S.M.; Hefta, S.A.; Opiteck, G.J.; Lin, J.H.; Moulin, F.; Dambach, D.M. Identification of in Vitro Protein Biomarkers of Idiosyncratic Liver Toxicity. *Toxicol. Vitr.* **2004**, *18*, 533–541. [CrossRef]
46. Grondman, I.; Pirvu, A.; Riza, A.; Ioana, M.; Netea, M.G. Biomarkers of Inflammation and the Etiology of Sepsis. *Biochem. Soc. Trans.* **2020**, *48*, 1–14. [CrossRef]
47. Johnson, C.H.; Ivanisevic, J.; Siuzdak, G. Metabolomics: Beyond Biomarkers and towards Mechanisms. *Nat. Rev. Mol. Cell Biol.* **2016**, *17*, 451–459. [CrossRef] [PubMed]
48. Costa-pinheiro, P.; Montezuma, D. Diagnostic and Prognostic Epigenetic Biomarkers in Cancer. *Epigenomics* **2015**, *7*, 1003–1015. [CrossRef] [PubMed]
49. Hoque, M.O.; Begum, S.; Topaloglu, O.; Jeronimo, C.; Mambo, E.; Westra, W.H.; Califano, J.A.; Sidransky, D. Quantitative Detection of Promoter Hypermethylation of Multiple Genes in the Tumor, Urine, and Serum DNA of Patients with Renal Cancer. *Cancer Res.* **2004**, *64*, 5511–5517. [CrossRef]
50. Javitt, G.H.; Vollebregt, E.R. Regulation of Molecular Diagnostics. *Annu. Rev. Genom. Hum. Genet.* **2022**, *23*, 653–673. [CrossRef]
51. Sun, L.; Pfeifer, J.D. Pitfalls in Molecular Diagnostics. *Semin. Diagn. Pathol.* **2019**, *36*, 342–354. [CrossRef] [PubMed]
52. Chien, J.Y.; Friedrich, S.; Heathman, M.A.; de Alwis, D.P.; Sinha, V. Pharmacokinetics/Pharmacodynamics and the Stages of Drug Development: Role of Modeling and Simulation. *AAPS J.* **2005**, *7*, E544–E559. [CrossRef]
53. McComb, M.; Ramanathan, M. Generalized Pharmacometric Modeling, a Novel Paradigm for Integrating Machine Learning Algorithms: A Case Study of Metabolomic Biomarkers. *Clin. Pharmacol. Ther.* **2020**, *107*, 1343–1351. [CrossRef]
54. Goetz, L.H.; Schork, N.J. Personalized Medicine: Motivation, Challenges, and Progress. *Fertil. Steril.* **2018**, *109*, 952–963. [CrossRef]
55. Rigatti, S.J. Random Forest. *J. Insur. Med.* **2017**, *47*, 31–39. [CrossRef]
56. Al-kaabawi, Z.; Wei, Y.; Moyeed, R. Bayesian Hierarchical Models for Linear Networks. *J. Appl. Stat.* **2022**, *49*, 1421–1448. [CrossRef]

57. Leil, T.A.; Kasichayanula, S.; Boulton, D.W.; LaCreta, F. Evaluation of 4β-Hydroxycholesterol as a Clinical Biomarker of CYP3A4 Drug Interactions Using a Bayesian Mechanism-Based Pharmacometric Model. *CPT Pharmacomet. Syst. Pharmacol.* **2014**, *3*, 1–10. [CrossRef]
58. Diczfalusy, U.; Nylén, H.; Elander, P.; Bertilsson, L. 4β-Hydroxycholesterol, an Endogenous Marker of CYP3A4/5 Activity in Humans. *Br. J. Clin. Pharmacol.* **2011**, *71*, 183–189. [CrossRef]
59. Kathman, S.J.; Williams, D.H.; Hodge, J.P.; Dar, M. A Bayesian Population PK-PD Model of Ispinesib-Induced Myelosuppression. *Clin. Pharmacol. Ther.* **2007**, *81*, 88–94. [CrossRef]
60. Bauer, R.J.; Guzy, S.; Ng, C. A Survey of Population Analysis Methods and Software for Complex Pharmacokinetic and Pharmacodynamic Models with Examples. *AAPS J.* **2007**, *9*, E60–E83. [CrossRef]
61. Terranova, N.; Venkatakrishnan, K.; Benincosa, L.J. Application of Machine Learning in Translational Medicine: Current Status and Future Opportunities. *AAPS J.* **2021**, *23*, 1–10. [CrossRef]
62. Wang, R.; Shao, X.; Zheng, J.; Saci, A.; Qian, X.; Pak, I.; Roy, A.; Bello, A.; Rizzo, J.I.; Hosein, F.; et al. A Machine-Learning Approach to Identify a Prognostic Cytokine Signature That Is Associated With Nivolumab Clearance in Patients With Advanced Melanoma. *Clin. Pharmacol. Ther.* **2019**, *107*, 978–987. [CrossRef]
63. Feng, Y.; Wang, X.; Bajaj, G.; Agrawal, S.; Bello, A.; Lestini, B.; Finckenstein, F.G.; Park, J.; Roy, A. Nivolumab Exposure—Response Analyses of Ef Fi Cacy and Safety in Previously Treated Squamous or Nonsquamous Non—Small Cell Lung Cancer. *Clin. Cancer Res.* **2017**, *23*, 5394–5406. [CrossRef] [PubMed]
64. Data, T.A.; Gillies, R.J.; Kinahan, P.E.; Hricak, H. Radiomics: Images Are More Than. *Radiology* **2016**, *278*, 563–577.
65. Terranova, N.; Girard, P.; Ioannou, K.; Klinkhardt, U.; Munafo, A. Assessing Similarity among Individual Tumor Size Lesion Dynamics: The CICIL Methodology. *CPT Pharmacomet. Syst. Pharmacol.* **2018**, *7*, 228–236. [CrossRef] [PubMed]
66. Terranova, N.; Girard, P.; Klinkhardt, U.; Munafo, A. Resistance Development: A Major Piece in the Jigsaw Puzzle of Tumor Size Modeling. *CPT Pharmacomet. Syst. Pharmacol.* **2015**, *4*, 320–323. [CrossRef] [PubMed]
67. Sands, B.E.; Chen, J.; Feagan, B.G.; Penney, M.; Rees, W.A.; Ph, D.; Danese, S.; Higgins, P.D.R. *Efficacy and Safety of MEDI2070, an Antibody Against Interleukin 23, Patients with Moderate to Severe Crohn's Disease: A Phase 2a Study*; Elsevier Inc.: Amsterdam, The Netherlands, 2017; ISBN 6465378647.
68. Zhang, N.; Liang, M.; Jing, C.; Philip, L.; Bo, Z.B.; Vainshtein, I.; Roskos, L.K.; Faggioni, R.; Savic, R.M. Combining Pharmacometric Models with Predictive and Prognostic Biomarkers for Precision Therapy in Crohn's Disease: A Case Study of Brazikumab. *CPT Pharmacomet. Syst. Pharmacol.* **2023**, *12*, 1945–1959. [CrossRef] [PubMed]
69. Best, W.R.; Becktel, J.M.; Signleton, J.W.; Kern, F. Development of a Crohn's Disease Activity Index. National Cooperative Crohn's Disease Study. *Gastroenterology* **1976**, *70*, 439–444. [CrossRef] [PubMed]
70. Miyazaki, T.; Watanabe, K.; Kojima, K.; Koshiba, R.; Fujimoto, K.; Sato, T.; Kawai, M.; Kamikozuru, K.; Yokoyama, Y.; Hida, N.; et al. Efficacies and Related Issues of Ustekinumab in Japanese Patients with Crohn's Disease: A Preliminary Study. *Digestion* **2019**, *101*, 53–59. [CrossRef] [PubMed]
71. Hendrikse, N.M.; Llinares Garcia, J.; Vetter, T.; Humphreys, A.J.; Ehmann, F. Biomarkers in Medicines Development—From Discovery to Regulatory Qualification and Beyond. *Front. Med.* **2022**, *9*, 878942. [CrossRef] [PubMed]
72. Cheng, F.; Ma, Y.; Uzzi, B.; Loscalzo, J. Importance of Scientific Collaboration in Contemporary Drug Discovery and Development: A Detailed Network Analysis. *BMC Biol.* **2020**, *18*, 138. [CrossRef]
73. Initiative, I.M. IMI Mission and Objectives. Available online: https://www.imi.europa.eu/about-imi/mission-objectives (accessed on 22 September 2023).
74. Zheng, Q.S.; Li, L.J. Pharmacometrics: A Quantitative Tool of Pharmacological Research. *Acta Pharmacol. Sin.* **2012**, *33*, 1337–1338. [CrossRef]
75. Bandeira, L.C.; Pinto, L.; Carneiro, C.M. Pharmacometrics: The Already-Present Future of Precision Pharmacology. *Ther. Innov. Regul. Sci.* **2022**, *57*, 57–69. [CrossRef]
76. Himstedt, A.; Bäckman, P.; Borghardt, J.M. Physiologically-Based Pharmacokinetic Modeling after Drug Inhalation. In *Inhaled Medicines: Optimizing Development through Integration of In Silico, In Vitro and In Vivo Approaches*; Academic Press: Cambridge, MA, USA, 2021; pp. 319–358. [CrossRef]
77. Usman, M.; Rasheed, H.; Pharmacokinetics, P.B.; Creation, D. Pharmacometrics and Its Application in Clinical Practice. *Encycl. Pharm. Pract. Clin. Pharm.* **2019**, *3B*, 227–238.
78. Division of Pharmacometrics | FDA. Available online: https://www.fda.gov/about-fda/center-drug-evaluation-and-research-cder/division-pharmacometrics (accessed on 10 October 2023).
79. Sheiner, L.B.; Rosenberg, B.; Marathe, V.V. Estimation of Population Characteristics of Pharmacokinetic Parameters from Routine Clinical Data. *J. Pharmacokinet. Biopharm.* **1977**, *5*, 445–479. [CrossRef]
80. Dollery, C.T. Clinical Pharmacology—The First 75 Years and a View of the Future. *Br. J. Clin. Pharmacol.* **2006**, *61*, 650–665. [CrossRef]
81. Usman, M.; Khadka, S.; Saleem, M.; Rasheed, H.; Kunwar, B.; Ali, M. Pharmacometrics: A New Era of Pharmacotherapy and Drug Development in Low- and Middle-Income Countries. *Adv. Pharmacol. Pharm. Sci.* **2023**, *2023*, 3081422. [CrossRef] [PubMed]
82. Lewis, B. Sheiner Lecturer Award. Available online: https://go-isop.org/awards/lewis-b-sheiner-award/ (accessed on 10 October 2023).

83. Dagenais, S.; Russo, L.; Madsen, A.; Webster, J.; Becnel, L. Use of Real-World Evidence to Drive Drug Development Strategy and Inform Clinical Trial Design. *Clin. Pharmacol. Ther.* **2022**, *111*, 77–89. [CrossRef] [PubMed]
84. Ette, E.I.; Williams, P.J. Population Pharmacokinetics I: Background, Concepts, and Models. *Ann. Pharmacother.* **2004**, *38*, 1702–1706. [CrossRef] [PubMed]
85. Abouir, K.; Samer, C.F.; Gloor, Y.; Desmeules, J.A.; Daali, Y. Reviewing Data Integrated for PBPK Model Development to Predict Metabolic Drug-Drug Interactions: Shifting Perspectives and Emerging Trends. *Front. Pharmacol.* **2021**, *12*, 708299. [CrossRef]
86. Siebinga, H.; de Wit-Van der Veen, B.J.; Stokkel, M.D.M.; Huitema, A.D.R.; Hendrikx, J.J.M.A. Current Use and Future Potential of (Physiologically Based) Pharmacokinetic Modelling of Radiopharmaceuticals: A Review. *Theranostics* **2022**, *12*, 7804–7820. [CrossRef]
87. Pfister, M.; D'Argenio, D.Z. The Emerging Scientific Discipline of Pharmacometrics. *J. Clin. Pharmacol.* **2010**, *50*, 6S. [CrossRef] [PubMed]
88. Stone, J.A.; Banfield, C.; Pfister, M.; Tannenbaum, S.; Allerheiligen, S.; Wetherington, J.D.; Krishna, R.; Grasela, D.M. Model-Based Drug Development Survey Finds Pharmacometrics Impacting Decision Making in the Pharmaceutical Industry. *J. Clin. Pharmacol.* **2010**, *50*, 20S–30S. [CrossRef]
89. Zou, H.; Banerjee, P.; Leung, S.S.Y.; Yan, X. Application of Pharmacokinetic-Pharmacodynamic Modeling in Drug Delivery: Development and Challenges. *Front. Pharmacol.* **2020**, *11*, 997. [CrossRef]
90. Meibohm, B.; Derendorf, H. Basic Concepts of Pharmacokinetic/Pharmacodynamic (PK/PD) Modelling. *Int. J. Clin. Pharmacol. Ther.* **1997**, *35*, 401–413.
91. Upton, R.N.; Mould, D.R. Basic Concepts in Population Modeling, Simulation, and Model-Based Drug Development: Part 3-Introduction to Pharmacodynamic Modeling Methods. *CPT Pharmacomet. Syst. Pharmacol.* **2014**, *3*, 1–16. [CrossRef]
92. Salahudeen, M.S.; Nishtala, P.S. An Overview of Pharmacodynamic Modelling, Ligand-Binding Approach and Its Application in Clinical Practice. *Saudi Pharm. J.* **2017**, *25*, 165–175. [CrossRef]
93. Felmlee, M.A.; Morris, M.E.; Mager, D.E. Mechanism-Based Pharmacodynamic Modeling. *Comput. Toxicol.* **2012**, *1*, 583–600. [CrossRef]
94. Lin, L.H.; Ghasemi, M.; Burke, S.M.; Mavis, C.K.; Nichols, J.R.; Torka, P.; Mager, D.E.; Hernandez-Ilizaliturri, F.J.; Goey, A.K.L. Population Pharmacokinetics and Pharmacodynamics of Carfilzomib in Combination with Rituximab, Ifosfamide, Carboplatin, and Etoposide in Adult Patients with Relapsed/Refractory Diffuse Large B Cell Lymphoma. *Target Oncol.* **2023**, *18*, 685–695. [CrossRef] [PubMed]
95. Palmer, M.E.; Andrews, L.J.; Abbey, T.C.; Dahlquist, A.E.; Wenzler, E. The Importance of Pharmacokinetics and Pharmacodynamics in Antimicrobial Drug Development and Their Influence on the Success of Agents Developed to Combat Resistant Gram Negative Pathogens: A Review. *Front. Pharmacol.* **2022**, *13*, 888079. [CrossRef] [PubMed]
96. Derendorf, H.; Möllmann, H.; Hochhaus, G.; Meibohm, B.; Barth, J. Clinical PK/PD Modelling as a Tool in Drug Development of Corticosteroids. *Int. J. Clin. Pharmacol. Ther.* **1997**, *35*, 481–488. [PubMed]
97. Tuntland, T.; Ethell, B.; Kosaka, T.; Blasco, F.; Zang, R.; Jain, M.; Gould, T.; Hoffmaster, K. Implementation of Pharmacokinetic and Pharmacodynamic Strategies in Early Research Phases of Drug Discovery and Development at Novartis Institute of Biomedical Research. *Front. Pharmacol.* **2014**, *5*, 174. [CrossRef] [PubMed]
98. Qusai, U.; Hameed, A.; Rasheed, K.H. Compartmental and Non-Compartmental Pharmacokinetic Analysis of Extended Release Diclofenac Sodium Tablet. *Coll. Eng. J.* **2016**, *19*, 161–165.
99. Gabrielsson, J.; Weiner, D. Non-Compartmental Analysis. *Comput. Toxicol.* **2012**, *929*, 377–389. [CrossRef]
100. Foster, D.M. *Noncompartmental versus Compartmental Approaches to Pharmacokinetic Analysis*, 2nd ed.; Elsevier Inc.: Amsterdam, The Netherlands, 2006; ISBN 9780123694171.
101. Noncompartmental vs. Compartmental PK Analysis. Available online: https://www.allucent.com/resources/blog/what-noncompartmental-pharmacokinetic-analysis (accessed on 10 October 2023).
102. Osipova, N.; Budko, A.; Maksimenko, O.; Shipulo, E.; Vanchugova, L.; Chen, W.; Gelperina, S.; Wacker, M.G. Comparison of Compartmental and Non-Compartmental Analysis to Detect Biopharmaceutical Similarity of Intravenous Nanomaterial-Based Rifabutin Formulations. *Pharmaceutics* **2023**, *15*, 1258. [CrossRef]
103. Hosseini, I.; Gajjala, A.; Bumbaca Yadav, D.; Sukumaran, S.; Ramanujan, S.; Paxson, R.; Gadkar, K. GPKPDSim: A SimBiology®-Based GUI Application for PKPD Modeling in Drug Development. *J. Pharmacokinet. Pharmacodyn.* **2018**, *45*, 259–275. [CrossRef]
104. World Health Organization. Characterization and Application of Physiologically Based Pharmacokinetic Models. *Int. Programme Chem. Saf.* **2010**, *9*, 16–37.
105. Tan, Y.M.; Worley, R.R.; Leonard, J.A.; Fisher, J.W. Challenges Associated with Applying Physiologically Based Pharmacokinetic Modeling for Public Health Decision-Making. *Toxicol. Sci.* **2018**, *162*, 341–348. [CrossRef] [PubMed]
106. Teorell, T. Kinetics of Distribution of Substances Administered to the Body, I: The Extravascular Modes of Administration. *Arch. Int. Pharmacodyn. Ther.* **1937**, *57*, 205–225.
107. Zhuang, X.; Lu, C. PBPK Modeling and Simulation in Drug Research and Development. *Acta Pharm. Sin. B* **2016**, *6*, 430–440. [CrossRef] [PubMed]
108. Jones, H.M.; Rowland-Yeo, K. Basic Concepts in Physiologically Based Pharmacokinetic Modeling in Drug Discovery and Development. *CPT Pharmacomet. Syst. Pharmacol.* **2013**, *2*, 1–12. [CrossRef]

109. Umehara, K.; Huth, F.; Jin, Y.; Schiller, H.; Aslanis, V.; Heimbach, T.; He, H. Drug-Drug Interaction (DDI) Assessments of Ruxolitinib, a Dual Substrate of CYP3A4 and CYP2C9, Using a Verified Physiologically Based Pharmacokinetic (PBPK) Model to Support Regulatory Submissions. *Drug Metab. Pers. Ther.* **2019**, *34*, 20180042. [CrossRef] [PubMed]
110. Marques, L.; Vale, N. Prediction of CYP-Mediated Drug Interaction Using Physiologically Based Pharmacokinetic Modeling: A Case Study of Salbutamol and Fluvoxamine. *Pharmaceutics* **2023**, *15*, 1586. [CrossRef]
111. Zamir, A.; Rasool, M.F.; Imran, I.; Saeed, H.; Khalid, S.; Majeed, A.; Rehman, A.U.; Ahmad, T.; Alasmari, F.; Alqahtani, F. Physiologically Based Pharmacokinetic Model To Predict Metoprolol Disposition in Healthy and Disease Populations. *ACS Omega* **2023**, *8*, 29302–29313. [CrossRef]
112. Amaeze, O.U.; Isoherranen, N. Application of a Physiologically Based Pharmacokinetic Model to Predict Isoniazid Disposition during Pregnancy. *Clin. Transl. Sci.* **2023**, *16*, 2163–2176. [CrossRef]
113. Mould, D.R.; Upton, R.N. Basic Concepts in Population Modeling, Simulation, and Model-Based Drug Development—Part 2: Introduction to Pharmacokinetic Modeling Methods. *CPT Pharmacomet. Syst. Pharmacol.* **2013**, *2*, 1–14. [CrossRef]
114. Li, A.; Mak, W.Y.; Ruan, T.; Dong, F.; Zheng, N.; Gu, M.; Guo, W.; Zhang, J.; Cheng, H.; Ruan, C.; et al. Population Pharmacokinetics of Amisulpride in Chinese Patients with Schizophrenia with External Validation: The Impact of Renal Function. *Front. Pharmacol.* **2023**, *14*, 1215065. [CrossRef]
115. He, S.; Zhao, J.; Bian, J.; Zhao, Y.; Li, Y.; Guo, N.; Hu, L.; Liu, B.; Shao, Q.; He, H.; et al. Population Pharmacokinetics and Pharmacogenetics Analyses of Dasatinib in Chinese Patients with Chronic Myeloid Leukemia. *Pharm. Res.* **2023**, *40*, 2413–2422. [CrossRef]
116. Verma, M.; Gall, L.; Biasetti, J.; Di Veroli, G.Y.; Pichardo-Almarza, C.; Gibbs, M.A.; Kimko, H. Quantitative Systems Modeling Approaches towards Model-Informed Drug Development: Perspective through Case Studies. *Front. Syst. Biol.* **2023**, *2*, 1063308. [CrossRef]
117. Chen, Y.; Li, J.; Li, D.; Hu, C. Pharmacokinetic Modeling and Predictive Performance: Practical Considerations for Therapeutic Monoclonal Antibodies. *Eur. J. Drug Metab. Pharmacokinet.* **2021**, *46*, 595–600. [CrossRef]
118. Krivelevich, I.; Lin, S. Visualization of Sparse PK Concentration Sampling Data, Step by Step (Improvement by Improvement) STEP 1: STARTING BOXPLOT First, Let's Draw a Simple Boxplot as a Starting Point. *Appl. Below Simple SAS Code PROC* **2021**, *1*, 1–14.
119. Choi, L.; Crainiceanu, C.M.; Caffo, B.S. Practical Recommendations for Population PK Studies with Sampling Time Errors. *Eur. J. Clin. Pharmacol.* **2013**, *69*, 2055. [CrossRef]
120. Alizadeh, E.A.; Rast, G.; Cantow, C.; Schiwon, J.; Krause, F.; De Meyer, G.R.Y.; Guns, P.J.; Guth, B.D.; Markert, M. Optimization of Bioanalysis of Dried Blood Samples. *J. Pharmacol. Toxicol. Methods* **2023**, *123*, 107296. [CrossRef] [PubMed]
121. Sheiner, L.B.; Beal, S.L. Evaluation of Methods for Estimating Population Pharmacokinetic Parameters. III. Monoexponential Model: Routine Clinical Pharmacokinetic Data. *J. Pharmacokinet. Biopharm.* **1983**, *11*, 303–319. [CrossRef] [PubMed]
122. Sheiner, L.B.; Beal, S.L. Evaluation of Methods for Estimating Population Pharmacokinetic Parameters II. Biexponential Model and Experimental Pharmacokinetic Data. *J. Pharmacokinet. Biopharm.* **1981**, *9*, 635–651. [CrossRef] [PubMed]
123. Brocks, D.; Hamdy, D. Bayesian Estimation of Pharmacokinetic Parameters: An Important Component to Include in the Teaching of Clinical Pharmacokinetics and Therapeutic Drug Monitoring. *Res. Pharm. Sci.* **2020**, *15*, 503–514. [CrossRef] [PubMed]
124. Gennemark, P.; Danis, A.; Nyberg, J.; Hooker, A.C.; Tucker, W. Optimal Design in Population Kinetic Experiments by Set-Valued Methods. *AAPS J.* **2011**, *13*, 495–507. [CrossRef] [PubMed]
125. Sherwin, C.M.T.; Kiang, T.K.L.; Spigarelli, M.G.; Ensom, M.H.H. Fundamentals of Population Pharmacokinetic Modelling. *Clin. Pharmacokinet.* **2012**, *51*, 573–590. [CrossRef] [PubMed]
126. Su, J.; Kang, J.J. *Challenges and Strategies in PKPD Programming PKNCA Data Other Deliverables CHALLENGES IN PKPD PROGRAMMING Challenges Due to Source Data Multiple Data Sources*; Merck & Co., Inc.: Rahway, NJ, USA, 2018; pp. 1–6.
127. Schmidt, H.; Radivojevic, A. Enhancing Population Pharmacokinetic Modeling Efficiency and Quality Using an Integrated Workflow. *J. Pharmacokinet. Pharmacodyn.* **2014**, *41*, 319–334. [CrossRef]
128. Lin, W.; Chen, Y.; Unadkat, J.D.; Zhang, X.; Wu, D.; Heimbach, T. Applications, Challenges, and Outlook for PBPK Modeling and Simulation: A Regulatory, Industrial and Academic Perspective. *Pharm. Res.* **2022**, *39*, 1701–1731. [CrossRef]
129. Peters, S.A.; Dolgos, H. Requirements to Establishing Confidence in Physiologically Based Pharmacokinetic (PBPK) Models and Overcoming Some of the Challenges to Meeting Them. *Clin. Pharmacokinet.* **2019**, *58*, 1355–1371. [CrossRef]
130. Binuya, M.A.E.; Engelhardt, E.G.; Schats, W.; Schmidt, M.K.; Steyerberg, E.W. Methodological Guidance for the Evaluation and Updating of Clinical Prediction Models: A Systematic Review. *BMC Med. Res. Methodol.* **2022**, *22*, 316. [CrossRef] [PubMed]
131. Cook, S.F.; Bies, R.R. Disease Progression Modeling: Key Concepts and Recent Developments. *Curr. Pharmacol. Rep.* **2016**, *2*, 221–230. [CrossRef]
132. Tyson, R.J.; Park, C.C.; Powell, J.R.; Patterson, J.H.; Weiner, D.; Watkins, P.B.; Gonzalez, D. Precision Dosing Priority Criteria: Drug, Disease, and Patient Population Variables. *Front. Pharmacol.* **2020**, *11*, 420. [CrossRef]
133. Arida-Moody, L.; Moody, J.B.; Renaud, J.M.; Poitrasson-Rivière, A.; Hagio, T.; Smith, A.M.; Ficaro, E.P.; Murthy, V.L. Effects of Two Patient-Specific Dosing Protocols on Measurement of Myocardial Blood Flow with 3D 82Rb Cardiac PET. *Eur. J. Nucl. Med. Mol. Imaging* **2021**, *48*, 3835–3846. [CrossRef]
134. Reyner, E.; Lum, B.; Jing, J.; Kagedal, M.; Ware, J.A.; Dickmann, L.J. Intrinsic and Extrinsic Pharmacokinetic Variability of Small Molecule Targeted Cancer Therapy. *Clin. Transl. Sci.* **2020**, *13*, 410–418. [CrossRef]

135. Fabbiani, M.; Di Giambenedetto, S.; Bracciale, L.; Bacarelli, A.; Ragazzoni, E.; Cauda, R.; Navarra, P.; De Luca, A. Pharmacokinetic Variability of Antiretroviral Drugs and Correlation with Virological Outcome: 2 Years of Experience in Routine Clinical Practice. *J. Antimicrob. Chemother.* **2009**, *64*, 109–117. [CrossRef]
136. Rao, P.S.; Modi, N.; Nguyen, N.T.T.; Vu, D.H.; Xie, Y.L.; Gandhi, M.; Gerona, R.; Metcalfe, J.; Heysell, S.K.; Alffenaar, J.W.C. Alternative Methods for Therapeutic Drug Monitoring and Dose Adjustment of Tuberculosis Treatment in Clinical Settings: A Systematic Review. *Clin. Pharmacokinet.* **2023**, *62*, 375–398. [CrossRef]
137. Kriegova, E.; Kudelka, M.; Radvansky, M.; Gallo, J. A Theoretical Model of Health Management Using Data-Driven Decision-Making: The Future of Precision Medicine and Health. *J. Transl. Med.* **2021**, *19*, 68. [CrossRef] [PubMed]
138. Martínez-García, M.; Hernández-Lemus, E. Data Integration Challenges for Machine Learning in Precision Medicine. *Front. Med.* **2022**, *8*, 784455. [CrossRef] [PubMed]
139. Naithani, N.; Sinha, S.; Misra, P.; Vasudevan, B.; Sahu, R. Precision Medicine: Concept and Tools. *Med. J. Armed Forces India* **2021**, *77*, 249–257. [CrossRef]
140. Giordano, C.; Brennan, M.; Mohamed, B.; Rashidi, P.; Modave, F.; Tighe, P. Accessing Artificial Intelligence for Clinical Decision-Making. *Front. Digit. Health* **2021**, *3*, 645232. [CrossRef] [PubMed]
141. Ghaffar Nia, N.; Kaplanoglu, E.; Nasab, A. Evaluation of Artificial Intelligence Techniques in Disease Diagnosis and Prediction. *Discov. Artif. Intell.* **2023**, *3*, 5. [CrossRef]
142. Xie, Y.; Meng, W.Y.; Li, R.Z.; Wang, Y.W.; Qian, X.; Chan, C.; Yu, Z.F.; Fan, X.X.; Pan, H.D.; Xie, C. Early Lung Cancer Diagnostic Biomarker Discovery by Machine Learning Methods. *Transl. Oncol.* **2021**, *14*, 100907. [CrossRef] [PubMed]
143. Goenka, N.; Tiwari, S. *Deep Learning for Alzheimer Prediction Using Brain Biomarkers*; Springer: Dordrecht, The Netherlands, 2021; Volume 54, ISBN 1046202110016.
144. Jarada, T.N.; Rokne, J.G.; Alhajj, R. A Review of Computational Drug Repositioning: Strategies, Approaches, Opportunities, Challenges, and Directions. *J. Cheminform.* **2020**, *12*, 46. [CrossRef]
145. Lauschke, V.M.; Zhou, Y.; Ingelman-Sundberg, M. Novel Genetic and Epigenetic Factors of Importance for Inter-Individual Differences in Drug Disposition, Response and Toxicity. *Pharmacol. Ther.* **2019**, *197*, 122–152. [CrossRef]
146. Dagliati, A.; Tibollo, V.; Sacchi, L.; Malovini, A.; Limongelli, I.; Gabetta, M.; Napolitano, C.; Mazzanti, A.; De Cata, P.; Chiovato, L.; et al. Big Data as a Driver for Clinical Decision Support Systems: A Learning Health Systems Perspective. *Front. Digit. Humanit.* **2018**, *5*, 8. [CrossRef]
147. Sarker, I.H. Machine Learning: Algorithms, Real-World Applications and Research Directions. *SN Comput. Sci.* **2021**, *2*, 160. [CrossRef]
148. Vermeulen, E.; van den Anker, J.N.; Della Pasqua, O.; Hoppu, K.; van der Lee, J.H. How to Optimise Drug Study Design: Pharmacokinetics and Pharmacodynamics Studies Introduced to Paediatricians. *J. Pharm. Pharmacol.* **2017**, *69*, 439–447. [CrossRef]
149. Wedagedera, J.R.; Afuape, A.; Chirumamilla, S.K.; Momiji, H.; Leary, R.; Dunlavey, M.; Matthews, R.; Abduljalil, K.; Jamei, M.; Bois, F.Y. Population PBPK Modeling Using Parametric and Nonparametric Methods of the Simcyp Simulator, and Bayesian Samplers. *CPT Pharmacomet. Syst. Pharmacol.* **2022**, *11*, 755–765. [CrossRef]
150. Ménard, T.; Barmaz, Y.; Koneswarakantha, B.; Bowling, R.; Popko, L. Enabling Data-Driven Clinical Quality Assurance: Predicting Adverse Event Reporting in Clinical Trials Using Machine Learning. *Drug Saf.* **2019**, *42*, 1045–1053. [CrossRef] [PubMed]
151. Phillips, R.; Sauzet, O.; Cornelius, V. Statistical Methods for the Analysis of Adverse Event Data in Randomised Controlled Trials: A Scoping Review and Taxonomy. *BMC Med. Res. Methodol.* **2020**, *20*, 288. [CrossRef] [PubMed]
152. Ferrer, F.; Chauvin, J.; Deville, J.L.; Ciccolini, J. Adaptive Dosing of Sunitinib in a Metastatic Renal Cell Carcinoma Patient: When in Silico Modeling Helps to Go Quicker to the Point. *Cancer Chemother. Pharmacol.* **2022**, *89*, 565–569. [CrossRef] [PubMed]
153. Ferrer, F.; Chauvin, J.; De Victor, B.; Lacarelle, B.; Deville, J.L.; Ciccolini, J. Clinical-Based vs. Model-Based Adaptive Dosing Strategy: Retrospective Comparison in Real-World MRCC Patients Treated with Sunitinib. *Pharmaceuticals* **2021**, *14*, 494. [CrossRef] [PubMed]
154. Sun, D.; Gao, W.; Hu, H.; Zhou, S. Why 90% of Clinical Drug Development Fails and How to Improve It? *Acta Pharm. Sin. B* **2022**, *12*, 3049–3062. [CrossRef] [PubMed]
155. Polasek, T.M.; Kirkpatrick, C.M.J.; Rostami-Hodjegan, A. Precision Dosing to Avoid Adverse Drug Reactions. *Ther. Adv. Drug Saf.* **2019**, *10*, 2042098619894147. [CrossRef] [PubMed]
156. Miller, N.A.; Reddy, M.B.; Heikkinen, A.T.; Lukacova, V.; Parrott, N. Physiologically Based Pharmacokinetic Modelling for First-In-Human Predictions: An Updated Model Building Strategy Illustrated with Challenging Industry Case Studies. *Clin. Pharmacokinet.* **2019**, *58*, 727–746. [CrossRef]
157. Mao, J.; Chen, Y.; Xu, L.; Chen, W.; Chen, B.; Fang, Z.; Qin, W.; Zhong, M. Applying Machine Learning to the Pharmacokinetic Modeling of Cyclosporine in Adult Renal Transplant Recipients: A Multi-Method Comparison. *Front. Pharmacol.* **2022**, *13*, 1016399. [CrossRef] [PubMed]
158. Phe, K.; Heil, E.L.; Tam, V.H. Optimizing Pharmacokinetics-Pharmacodynamics of Antimicrobial Management in Patients with Sepsis: A Review. *J. Infect. Dis.* **2021**, *222*, S132–S141. [CrossRef] [PubMed]
159. Pallmann, P.; Bedding, A.W.; Choodari-Oskooei, B.; Dimairo, M.; Flight, L.; Hampson, L.V.; Holmes, J.; Mander, A.P.; Odondi, L.; Sydes, M.R.; et al. Adaptive Designs in Clinical Trials: Why Use Them, and How to Run and Report Them. *BMC Med.* **2018**, *16*, 29. [CrossRef] [PubMed]
160. Shortliffe, E.H.; Buchanan, B.G. A Model of Inexact Reasoning in Medicine. *Math. Biosci.* **1975**, *23*, 351–379. [CrossRef]

161. Miller, R.A.; Pople, H.E.; Myers, J.D. Internist, an Experimental Computer-Based Diagnostic Consultant for General Internal Medicine. *N. Engl. J. Med.* **1982**, *307*, 468–476. [CrossRef] [PubMed]
162. Poweleit, E.A.; Vinks, A.A.; Mizuno, T. Artificial Intelligence and Machine Learning Approaches to Facilitate Therapeutic Drug Management and Model-Informed Precision Dosing. *Ther. Drug Monit.* **2023**, *45*, 143–150. [CrossRef] [PubMed]
163. Keutzer, L.; You, H.; Farnoud, A.; Nyberg, J.; Wicha, S.G.; Maher-Edwards, G.; Vlasakakis, G.; Moghaddam, G.K.; Svensson, E.M.; Menden, M.P.; et al. Machine Learning and Pharmacometrics for Prediction of Pharmacokinetic Data: Differences, Similarities and Challenges Illustrated with Rifampicin. *Pharmaceutics* **2022**, *14*, 1530. [CrossRef]
164. Mould, D.R.; Upton, R.N. Basic Concepts in Population Modeling, Simulation, and Model-Based Drug Development. *CPT Pharmacomet. Syst. Pharmacol.* **2012**, *1*, e6. [CrossRef]
165. Gobburu, J.V.S.; Chen, E.P. Artificial Neural Networks as a Novel Approach to Integrated Pharmacokinetic-Pharmacodynamic Analysis. *J. Pharm. Sci.* **1996**, *85*, 505–510. [CrossRef]
166. Veng-Pedersen, P.; Modi, N.B. Neural Networks in Pharmacodynamic Modeling. Is Current Modeling Practice of Complex Kinetic Systems at a Dead End? *J. Pharmacokinet. Biopharm.* **1992**, *20*, 397–412. [CrossRef] [PubMed]
167. Cucurull-Sanchez, L.; Chappell, M.J.; Chelliah, V.; Amy Cheung, S.Y.; Derks, G.; Penney, M.; Phipps, A.; Malik-Sheriff, R.S.; Timmis, J.; Tindall, M.J.; et al. Best Practices to Maximize the Use and Reuse of Quantitative and Systems Pharmacology Models: Recommendations From the United Kingdom Quantitative and Systems Pharmacology Network. *CPT Pharmacomet. Syst. Pharmacol.* **2019**, *8*, 259–272. [CrossRef] [PubMed]
168. McComb, M.; Bies, R.; Ramanathan, M. Machine Learning in Pharmacometrics: Opportunities and Challenges. *Br. J. Clin. Pharmacol.* **2022**, *88*, 1482–1499. [CrossRef] [PubMed]
169. Collin, C.B.; Gebhardt, T.; Golebiewski, M.; Karaderi, T.; Hillemanns, M.; Khan, F.M.; Salehzadeh-Yazdi, A.; Kirschner, M.; Krobitsch, S.; Kuepfer, L. Computational Models for Clinical Applications in Personalized Medicine—Guidelines and Recommendations for Data Integration and Model Validation. *J. Pers. Med.* **2022**, *12*, 166. [CrossRef] [PubMed]
170. Niazi, S.K. The Coming of Age of AI/ML in Drug Discovery, Development, Clinical Testing, and Manufacturing: The FDA Perspectives. *Drug Des. Dev. Ther.* **2023**, *17*, 2691–2725. [CrossRef]
171. El-Alti, L.; Sandman, L.; Munthe, C. Person Centered Care and Personalized Medicine: Irreconcilable Opposites or Potential Companions? *Health Care Anal.* **2019**, *27*, 45–59. [CrossRef]
172. Vicente, A.M.; Ballensiefen, W.; Jönsson, J.I. How Personalised Medicine Will Transform Healthcare by 2030: The ICPerMed Vision. *J. Transl. Med.* **2020**, *18*, 180. [CrossRef]
173. Brnabic, A.; Hess, L.M. Systematic Literature Review of Machine Learning Methods Used in the Analysis of Real-World Data for Patient-Provider Decision Making. *BMC Med. Inform. Decis. Mak.* **2021**, *21*, 54. [CrossRef] [PubMed]
174. Freriksen, J.J.M.; van der Heijden, J.E.M.; de Hoop-Sommen, M.A.; Greupink, R.; de Wildt, S.N. Physiologically Based Pharmacokinetic (PBPK) Model-Informed Dosing Guidelines for Pediatric Clinical Care: A Pragmatic Approach for a Special Population. *Paediatr. Drugs* **2023**, *25*, 5–11. [CrossRef]
175. Weissler, E.H.; Naumann, T.; Andersson, T.; Ranganath, R.; Elemento, O.; Luo, Y.; Freitag, D.F.; Benoit, J.; Hughes, M.C.; Khan, F.; et al. The Role of Machine Learning in Clinical Research: Transforming the Future of Evidence Generation. *Trials* **2021**, *22*, 537. [CrossRef]
176. Gallo, J.M. Pharmacokinetic/Pharmacodynamic-Driven Drug Development. *Mount Sinai J. Med.* **2010**, *77*, 381–388. [CrossRef]
177. Gao, H.; Wang, W.; Dong, J.; Ye, Z.; Ouyang, D. An Integrated Computational Methodology with Data-Driven Machine Learning, Molecular Modeling and PBPK Modeling to Accelerate Solid Dispersion Formulation Design. *Eur. J. Pharm. Biopharm.* **2021**, *158*, 336–346. [CrossRef]
178. Joerger, M. Covariate Pharmacokinetic Model Building in Oncology and Its Potential Clinical Relevance. *AAPS J.* **2012**, *14*, 119–132. [CrossRef]
179. Zhu, X.; Zhang, M.; Wen, Y.; Shang, D. Machine Learning Advances the Integration of Covariates in Population Pharmacokinetic Models: Valproic Acid as an Example. *Front. Pharmacol.* **2022**, *13*, 994665. [CrossRef]
180. Fendt, R.; Hofmann, U.; Schneider, A.R.P.; Schaeffeler, E.; Burghaus, R.; Yilmaz, A.; Blank, L.M.; Kerb, R.; Lippert, J.; Schlender, J.F.; et al. Data-Driven Personalization of a Physiologically Based Pharmacokinetic Model for Caffeine: A Systematic Assessment. *CPT Pharmacomet. Syst. Pharmacol.* **2021**, *10*, 782–793. [CrossRef] [PubMed]
181. Schaefer, J.; Lehne, M.; Schepers, J.; Prasser, F.; Thun, S. The Use of Machine Learning in Rare Diseases: A Scoping Review. *Orphanet J. Rare Dis.* **2020**, *15*, 145. [CrossRef]
182. Weaver, R.J.; Valentin, J.P. Today's Challenges to De-Risk and Predict Drug Safety in Human "Mind-The-Gap". *Toxicol. Sci.* **2019**, *167*, 307–321. [CrossRef] [PubMed]
183. Trifirò, G.; Crisafulli, S. A New Era of Pharmacovigilance: Future Challenges and Opportunities. *Front. Drug Saf. Regul.* **2022**, *2*, 2020–2023. [CrossRef]
184. Kolluri, S.; Lin, J.; Liu, R.; Zhang, Y.; Zhang, W. Machine Learning and Artificial Intelligence in Pharmaceutical Research and Development: A Review. *AAPS J.* **2022**, *24*, 19. [CrossRef] [PubMed]
185. Seyhan, A.A. Lost in Translation: The Valley of Death across Preclinical and Clinical Divide—Identification of Problems and Overcoming Obstacles. *Transl. Med. Commun.* **2019**, *4*, 18. [CrossRef]
186. Cole, S.; Hay, J.L.; Luzon, E.; Nordmark, A.; Rusten, I.S. European Regulatory Perspective on Pediatric Physiologically Based Pharmacokinetic Models. *Int. J. Pharmacokinet.* **2017**, *2*, 113–124. [CrossRef]

187. Wu, F.; Shah, H.; Li, M.; Duan, P.; Zhao, P.; Suarez, S.; Raines, K.; Zhao, Y.; Wang, M.; Lin, H.P.; et al. Biopharmaceutics Applications of Physiologically Based Pharmacokinetic Absorption Modeling and Simulation in Regulatory Submissions to the U.S. Food and Drug Administration for New Drugs. *AAPS J.* **2021**, *23*, 31. [CrossRef] [PubMed]
188. Woillard, J.B.; Labriffe, M.; Prémaud, A.; Marquet, P. Estimation of Drug Exposure by Machine Learning Based on Simulations from Published Pharmacokinetic Models: The Example of Tacrolimus. *Pharmacol. Res.* **2021**, *167*, 105578. [CrossRef] [PubMed]
189. Woillard, J.B.; Labriffe, M.; Debord, J.; Marquet, P. Tacrolimus Exposure Prediction Using Machine Learning. *Clin. Pharmacol. Ther.* **2021**, *110*, 361–369. [CrossRef] [PubMed]
190. Woillard, J.B.; Labriffe, M.; Debord, J.; Marquet, P. Mycophenolic Acid Exposure Prediction Using Machine Learning. *Clin. Pharmacol. Ther.* **2021**, *110*, 370–379. [CrossRef] [PubMed]
191. Uster, D.W.; Stocker, S.L.; Carland, J.E.; Brett, J.; Marriott, D.J.E.; Day, R.O.; Wicha, S.G. A Model Averaging/Selection Approach Improves the Predictive Performance of Model-Informed Precision Dosing: Vancomycin as a Case Study. *Clin. Pharmacol. Ther.* **2021**, *109*, 175–183. [CrossRef] [PubMed]
192. Bououda, M.; Uster, D.W.; Sidorov, E.; Labriffe, M.; Marquet, P.; Wicha, S.G.; Woillard, J.B. A Machine Learning Approach to Predict Interdose Vancomycin Exposure. *Pharm. Res.* **2022**, *39*, 721–731. [CrossRef] [PubMed]
193. Zhu, X.; Huang, W.; Lu, H.; Wang, Z.; Ni, X.; Hu, J.; Deng, S.; Tan, Y.; Li, L.; Zhang, M.; et al. A Machine Learning Approach to Personalized Dose Adjustment of Lamotrigine Using Noninvasive Clinical Parameters. *Sci. Rep.* **2021**, *11*, 5568. [CrossRef]
194. Roche-Lima, A.; Roman-Santiago, A.; Feliu-Maldonado, R.; Rodriguez-Maldonado, J.; Nieves-Rodriguez, B.G.; Carrasquillo-Carrion, K.; Ramos, C.M.; Da Luz Sant'Ana, I.; Massey, S.E.; Duconge, J. Machine Learning Algorithm for Predicting Warfarin Dose in Caribbean Hispanics Using Pharmacogenetic Data. *Front. Pharmacol.* **2020**, *10*, 1550. [CrossRef]
195. Gill, J.; Moullet, M.; Martinsson, A.; Miljković, F.; Williamson, B.; Arends, R.H.; Pilla Reddy, V. Evaluating the Performance of Machine-Learning Regression Models for Pharmacokinetic Drug-Drug Interactions. *CPT Pharmacomet. Syst. Pharmacol.* **2023**, *12*, 122–134. [CrossRef]
196. Harun, R.; Yang, E.; Kassir, N.; Zhang, W.; Lu, J. Machine Learning for Exposure-Response Analysis: Methodological Considerations and Confirmation of Their Importance via Computational Experimentations. *Pharmaceutics* **2023**, *15*, 1381. [CrossRef] [PubMed]
197. Song, D.; Chen, Y.; Min, Q.; Sun, Q.; Ye, K.; Zhou, C.; Yuan, S.; Sun, Z.; Liao, J. Similarity-Based Machine Learning Support Vector Machine Predictor of Drug-Drug Interactions with Improved Accuracies. *J. Clin. Pharm. Ther.* **2019**, *44*, 268–275. [CrossRef]
198. Liu, C.; Xu, Y.; Liu, Q.; Zhu, H.; Wang, Y. Application of Machine Learning Based Methods in Exposure–Response Analysis. *J. Pharmacokinet. Pharmacodyn.* **2022**, *49*, 401–410. [CrossRef] [PubMed]
199. Bonate, P.L.; Barrett, J.S.; Ait-Oudhia, S.; Brundage, R.; Corrigan, B.; Duffull, S.; Gastonguay, M.; Karlsson, M.O.; Kijima, S.; Krause, A.; et al. Training the next Generation of Pharmacometric Modelers: A Multisector Perspective. *J. Pharmacokinet. Pharmacodyn.* **2023**, *51*, 5–31. [CrossRef]
200. Karatza, E.; Yakovleva, T.; Adams, K.; Rao, G.G.; Ait-Oudhia, S. Knowledge Dissemination and Central Indexing of Resources in Pharmacometrics: An ISOP Education Working Group Initiative. *J. Pharmacokinet. Pharmacodyn.* **2022**, *49*, 397–400. [CrossRef] [PubMed]
201. Ismail, M.; Sale, M.; Yu, Y.; Pillai, N.; Liu, S.; Pflug, B.; Bies, R. Development of a Genetic Algorithm and NONMEM Workbench for Automating and Improving Population Pharmacokinetic/Pharmacodynamic Model Selection. *J. Pharmacokinet. Pharmacodyn.* **2022**, *49*, 243–256. [CrossRef]
202. Sibieude, E.; Khandelwal, A.; Girard, P.; Hesthaven, J.S.; Terranova, N. Population Pharmacokinetic Model Selection Assisted by Machine Learning. *J. Pharmacokinet. Pharmacodyn.* **2022**, *49*, 257–270. [CrossRef]
203. Liu, Q.; Huang, R.; Hsieh, J.; Zhu, H.; Tiwari, M.; Liu, G.; Jean, D.; ElZarrad, M.K.; Fakhouri, T.; Berman, S.; et al. Landscape Analysis of the Application of Artificial Intelligence and Machine Learning in Regulatory Submissions for Drug Development From 2016 to 2021. *Clin. Pharmacol. Ther.* **2023**, *113*, 771–774. [CrossRef]
204. Mallon, A.M.; Häring, D.A.; Dahlke, F.; Aarden, P.; Afyouni, S.; Delbarre, D.; El Emam, K.; Ganjgahi, H.; Gardiner, S.; Kwok, C.H.; et al. Advancing Data Science in Drug Development through an Innovative Computational Framework for Data Sharing and Statistical Analysis. *BMC Med. Res. Methodol.* **2021**, *21*, 250. [CrossRef]
205. Danese, M.D.; Halperin, M.; Duryea, J.; Duryea, R. The Generalized Data Model for Clinical Research. *BMC Med. Inform. Decis. Mak.* **2019**, *19*, 117. [CrossRef]
206. Danilov, G.; Kotik, K.; Shifrin, M.; Strunina, Y.; Pronkina, T.; Tsukanova, T.; Nepomnyashiy, V.; Konovalov, N.; Danilov, V.; Potapov, A. Data Quality Estimation Via Model Performance: Machine Learning as a Validation Tool. *Stud. Health Technol. Inform.* **2023**, *305*, 369–372. [CrossRef]
207. Castro-Alamancos, M.A. A System to Easily Manage Metadata in Biomedical Research Labs Based on Open-Source Software. *Bio Protoc.* **2022**, *12*, e4404. [CrossRef]
208. Xiang, D.; Cai, W. Privacy Protection and Secondary Use of Health Data: Strategies and Methods. *Biomed. Res. Int.* **2021**, *2021*, 6967166. [CrossRef]
209. Schmidt, B.M.; Colvin, C.J.; Hohlfeld, A.; Leon, N. Definitions, Components and Processes of Data Harmonisation in Healthcare: A Scoping Review. *BMC Med. Inform. Decis. Mak.* **2020**, *20*, 222. [CrossRef]
210. Aldoseri, A.; Al-Khalifa, K.N.; Magid Hamouda, A. Re-Thinking Data Strategy and Integration for Artificial Intelligence: Concepts, Opportunities, and Challenges. *Appl. Sci.* **2023**, *13*, 7082. [CrossRef]

211. Chiruvella, V.; Guddati, A.K. Ethical Issues in Patient Data Ownership. *Interact. J. Med. Res.* **2021**, *10*, e22269. [CrossRef]
212. Siala, H.; Wang, Y. SHIFTing Artificial Intelligence to Be Responsible in Healthcare: A Systematic Review. *Soc. Sci. Med.* **2022**, *296*, 114782. [CrossRef] [PubMed]
213. Lee, J.; Jeong, J.; Jung, S.; Moon, J.; Rho, S. Verification of De-Identification Techniques for Personal Information Using Tree-Based Methods with Shapley Values. *J. Pers. Med.* **2022**, *12*, 190. [CrossRef] [PubMed]
214. Hassija, V.; Chamola, V.; Mahapatra, A.; Singal, A.; Goel, D.; Huang, K.; Scardapane, S.; Spinelli, I.; Mahmud, M.; Hussain, A. Interpreting Black-Box Models: A Review on Explainable Artificial Intelligence. *Cognit Comput.* **2023**, *1*, 45–74. [CrossRef]
215. Rasheed, K.; Qayyum, A.; Ghaly, M.; Al-Fuqaha, A.; Razi, A.; Qadir, J. Explainable, Trustworthy, and Ethical Machine Learning for Healthcare: A Survey. *Comput. Biol. Med.* **2022**, *149*, 106043. [CrossRef]
216. McCarron, T.L.; Moffat, K.; Wilkinson, G.; Zelinsky, S.; Boyd, J.M.; White, D.; Hassay, D.; Lorenzetti, D.L.; Marlett, N.J.; Noseworthy, T. Understanding Patient Engagement in Health System Decision-Making: A Co-Designed Scoping Review. *Syst. Rev.* **2019**, *8*, 97. [CrossRef] [PubMed]
217. Becker, C.; Gross, S.; Gamp, M.; Beck, K.; Amacher, S.A.; Mueller, J.; Bohren, C.; Blatter, R.; Schaefert, R.; Schuetz, P.; et al. Patients' Preference for Participation in Medical Decision-Making: Secondary Analysis of the BEDSIDE-OUTSIDE Trial. *J. Gen. Intern. Med.* **2023**, *38*, 1180–1189. [CrossRef] [PubMed]
218. Lu, S.C.; Swisher, C.L.; Chung, C.; Jaffray, D.; Sidey-Gibbons, C. On the Importance of Interpretable Machine Learning Predictions to Inform Clinical Decision Making in Oncology. *Front. Oncol.* **2023**, *13*, 1129380. [CrossRef] [PubMed]
219. Rodríguez-Pérez, R.; Bajorath, J. Interpretation of Machine Learning Models Using Shapley Values: Application to Compound Potency and Multi-Target Activity Predictions. *J. Comput. Aided Mol. Des.* **2020**, *34*, 1013–1026. [CrossRef] [PubMed]
220. Tajgardoon, M.; Samayamuthu, M.J.; Calzoni, L.; Visweswaran, S. Patient-Specific Explanations for Predictions of Clinical Outcomes. *ACI Open* **2019**, *3*, e88–e97. [CrossRef] [PubMed]
221. Sun, H.; Depraetere, K.; Meesseman, L.; Silva, P.C.; Szymanowsky, R.; Fliegenschmidt, J.; Hulde, N.; Von Dossow, V.; Vanbiervliet, M.; De Baerdemaeker, J.; et al. Machine Learning-Based Prediction Models for Different Clinical Risks in Different Hospitals: Evaluation of Live Performance. *J. Med. Internet Res.* **2022**, *24*, e34295. [CrossRef]
222. Petersson, L.; Larsson, I.; Nygren, J.M.; Nilsen, P.; Neher, M.; Reed, J.E.; Tyskbo, D.; Svedberg, P. Challenges to Implementing Artificial Intelligence in Healthcare: A Qualitative Interview Study with Healthcare Leaders in Sweden. *BMC Health Serv. Res.* **2022**, *22*, 850. [CrossRef]
223. Nugent, B.M.; Madabushi, R.; Buch, B.; Peiris, V.; Crentsil, V.; Miller, V.M.; Bull, J.R.; Jenkins, M. Heterogeneity in Treatment Effects across Diverse Populations. *Pharm. Stat.* **2021**, *20*, 929–938. [CrossRef]
224. He, Z.; Tang, X.; Yang, X.; Guo, Y.; George, T.J.; Charness, N.; Quan Hem, K.B.; Hogan, W.; Bian, J. Clinical Trial Generalizability Assessment in the Big Data Era: A Review. *Clin. Transl. Sci.* **2020**, *13*, 675–684. [CrossRef] [PubMed]
225. Norori, N.; Hu, Q.; Aellen, F.M.; Faraci, F.D.; Tzovara, A. Addressing Bias in Big Data and AI for Health Care: A Call for Open Science. *Patterns* **2021**, *2*, 100347. [CrossRef]
226. Drabiak, K. Leveraging Law and Ethics to Promote Safe and Reliable AI/ML in Healthcare. *Front. Nucl. Med.* **2022**, *2*, 983340. [CrossRef]
227. Koppad, S.; Gkoutos, G.V.; Acharjee, A. Cloud Computing Enabled Big Multi-Omics Data Analytics. *Bioinform. Biol. Insights* **2021**, *15*, 11779322211035921. [CrossRef]
228. Hofer, I.S.; Burns, M.; Kendale, S.; Wanderer, J.P. Realistically Integrating Machine Learning Into Clinical Practice: A Road Map of Opportunities, Challenges, and a Potential Future. *Anesth. Analg.* **2020**, *130*, 1115–1118. [CrossRef]
229. Digital Health—StatPearls—NCBI Bookshelf. Available online: https://www.ncbi.nlm.nih.gov/books/NBK470260/ (accessed on 11 October 2023).
230. Dunn, P.; Hazzard, E. Technology Approaches to Digital Health Literacy. *Int. J. Cardiol.* **2019**, *293*, 294–296. [CrossRef]
231. Jandoo, T. WHO Guidance for Digital Health: What It Means for Researchers. *Digit. Health* **2020**, *6*, 2055207619898984. [CrossRef] [PubMed]
232. Johnson, K.B.; Wei, W.Q.; Weeraratne, D.; Frisse, M.E.; Misulis, K.; Rhee, K.; Zhao, J.; Snowdon, J.L. Precision Medicine, AI, and the Future of Personalized Health Care. *Clin. Transl. Sci.* **2021**, *14*, 86–93. [CrossRef] [PubMed]
233. Fernandez-Luque, L.; Al Herbish, A.; Al Shammari, R.; Argente, J.; Bin-Abbas, B.; Deeb, A.; Dixon, D.; Zary, N.; Koledova, E.; Savage, M.O. Digital Health for Supporting Precision Medicine in Pediatric Endocrine Disorders: Opportunities for Improved Patient Care. *Front. Pediatr.* **2021**, *9*, 715705. [CrossRef] [PubMed]
234. What Is Digital Health (Digital Healthcare) and Why Is It Important? Available online: https://www.techtarget.com/searchhealthit/definition/digital-health-digital-healthcare (accessed on 11 October 2023).
235. Woods, L.; Dendere, R.; Eden, R.; Grantham, B.; Krivit, J.; Pearce, A.; McNeil, K.; Green, D.; Sullivan, C. Perceived Impact of Digital Health Maturity on Patient Experience, Population Health, Health Care Costs, and Provider Experience: Mixed Methods Case Study. *J. Med. Internet Res.* **2023**, *25*, e4584. [CrossRef] [PubMed]
236. Kulynych, J.; Greely, H.T. Clinical Genomics, Big Data, and Electronic Medical Records: Reconciling Patient Rights with Research When Privacy and Science Collide. *J. Law. Biosci.* **2017**, *4*, 94–132. [CrossRef] [PubMed]
237. Syed, R.; Eden, R.; Makasi, T.; Chukwudi, I.; Mamudu, A.; Kamalpour, M.; Kapugama Geeganage, D.; Sadeghianasl, S.; Leemans, S.J.J.; Goel, K.; et al. Digital Health Data Quality Issues: Systematic Review. *J. Med. Internet Res.* **2023**, *25*, e42615. [CrossRef] [PubMed]

238. Paul, M.; Maglaras, L.; Ferrag, M.A.; Almomani, I. Digitization of Healthcare Sector: A Study on Privacy and Security Concerns. *ICT Express* **2023**, *9*, 571–588. [CrossRef]
239. Subbiah, V. The next Generation of Evidence-Based Medicine. *Nat. Med.* **2023**, *29*, 49–58. [CrossRef]
240. Fountzilas, E.; Tsimberidou, A.M.; Vo, H.H.; Kurzrock, R. Clinical Trial Design in the Era of Precision Medicine. *Genome Med.* **2022**, *14*, 101. [CrossRef]
241. Hirakawa, A.; Asano, J.; Sato, H.; Teramukai, S. Master Protocol Trials in Oncology: Review and New Trial Designs. *Contemp. Clin. Trials Commun.* **2018**, *12*, 1–8. [CrossRef] [PubMed]
242. Redman, M.W.; Allegra, C.J. The Master Protocol Concept. *Semin. Oncol.* **2015**, *42*, 724–730. [CrossRef] [PubMed]
243. Woodcock, J.; LaVange, L.M. Master Protocols to Study Multiple Therapies, Multiple Diseases, or Both. *N. Engl. J. Med.* **2017**, *377*, 62–70. [CrossRef]
244. Renfro, L.A.; Sargent, D.J. Statistical Controversies in Clinical Research: Basket Trials, Umbrella Trials, and Other Master Protocols: A Review and Examples. *Ann. Oncol.* **2017**, *28*, 34–43. [CrossRef]
245. Food and Drug Administration. *FDA Modernizes Clinical Trials with Master Protocols*; CDER SBIA Chronicles: Silver Spring, MD, USA, 2019; pp. 1–2.
246. Basket Clinical Trial Designs: The Key to Testing Innovative Therapies Is Innovation in Study Design and Conduct—ACRP. Available online: https://www.acrpnet.org/2020/02/basket-clinical-trial-designs-the-key-to-testing-innovative-therapies-is-innovation-in-study-design-and-conduct/ (accessed on 11 October 2023).
247. Park, J.J.H.; Siden, E.; Zoratti, M.J.; Dron, L.; Harari, O.; Singer, J.; Lester, R.T.; Thorlund, K.; Mills, E.J. Systematic Review of Basket Trials, Umbrella Trials, and Platform Trials: A Landscape Analysis of Master Protocols. *Trials* **2019**, *20*, 572. [CrossRef] [PubMed]
248. Home-Based Clinical Studies—A Paradigm Shift?—Clinical Trials Arena. Available online: https://www.clinicaltrialsarena.com/comment/home-based-clinical-studies-a-paradigm-shift-6094192-2/ (accessed on 11 October 2023).
249. Franklin, M.; Thorn, J. Self-Reported and Routinely Collected Electronic Healthcare Resource-Use Data for Trial-Based Economic Evaluations: The Current State of Play in England and Considerations for the Future. *BMC Med. Res. Methodol.* **2019**, *19*, 8. [CrossRef]
250. Virtual Clinical Trials | ObvioHealth. Available online: https://www.obviohealth.com/resources/how-virtual-clinical-trials-are-revolutionizing-health-research (accessed on 11 October 2023).
251. FDA Grants Accelerated Approval to Pembrolizumab for First Tissue/Site Agnostic Indication | FDA. Available online: https://www.fda.gov/drugs/resources-information-approved-drugs/fda-grants-accelerated-approval-pembrolizumab-first-tissuesite-agnostic-indication (accessed on 11 October 2023).
252. Wedam, S.; Fashoyin-Aje, L.; Bloomquist, E.; Tang, S.; Sridhara, R.; Goldberg, K.B.; Theoret, M.R.; Amiri-Kordestani, L.; Pazdur, R.; Beaver, J.A. FDA Approval Summary: Palbociclib for Male Patients with Metastatic Breast Cancer. *Clin. Cancer Res.* **2020**, *26*, 1208–1212. [CrossRef]
253. Nice, E.C. The Omics Revolution: Beyond Genomics. A Meeting Report. *Clin. Proteomics* **2020**, *17*, 1. [CrossRef] [PubMed]
254. Ochoa, D.; Karim, M.; Ghoussaini, M.; Hulcoop, D.G.; McDonagh, E.M.; Dunham, I. Human Genetics Evidence Supports Two-Thirds of the 2021 FDA-Approved Drugs. *Nat. Rev. Drug Discov.* **2022**, *21*, 551. [CrossRef] [PubMed]
255. Abul-Husn, N.S.; Kenny, E.E. Personalized Medicine and the Power of Electronic Health Records. *Cell* **2019**, *177*, 58–69. [CrossRef] [PubMed]
256. Sitapati, A.; Kim, H.; Berkovich, B.; Marmor, R.; Singh, S.; El-Kareh, R.; Clay, B.; Ohno-Machado, L. Integrated Precision Medicine: The Role of Electronic Health Records in Delivering Personalized Treatment. *Wiley Interdiscip. Rev. Syst. Biol. Med.* **2017**, *9*, e1378. [CrossRef]

Disclaimer/Publisher's Note: The statements, opinions and data contained in all publications are solely those of the individual author(s) and contributor(s) and not of MDPI and/or the editor(s). MDPI and/or the editor(s) disclaim responsibility for any injury to people or property resulting from any ideas, methods, instructions or products referred to in the content.

Article

Exploring the Impact of Model-Informed Precision Dosing on Procalcitonin Concentrations in Critically Ill Patients: A Secondary Analysis of the DOLPHIN Trial

Sarah Dräger [1,2,3,*], Tim M. J. Ewoldt [1,2,4], Alan Abdulla [1,2], Wim J. R. Rietdijk [1,5], Nelianne Verkaik [6], Christian Ramakers [7], Evelien de Jong [8], Michael Osthoff [3], Birgit C. P. Koch [1,2] and Henrik Endeman [4] on behalf of the DOLPHIN Investigators

1. Department of Hospital Pharmacy, Erasmus University Medical Center, 3015 GD Rotterdam, The Netherlands
2. Rotterdam Clinical Pharmacometrics Group, 3015 GD Rotterdam, The Netherlands
3. Department of Internal Medicine, University Hospital Basel, 4031 Basel, Switzerland
4. Department of Intensive Care Medicine, Erasmus University Medical Center, 3015 GD Rotterdam, The Netherlands; h.endeman@erasmusmc.nl
5. Department of Institutional Affairs, Vrije Universiteit Amsterdam, 1081 HV Amsterdam, The Netherlands
6. Department of Medical Microbiology and Infectious Diseases, Erasmus Medical Center, 3015 GD Rotterdam, The Netherlands
7. Department of Clinical Chemistry, Erasmus Medical Center, 3015 GD Rotterdam, The Netherlands
8. Department of Intensive Care, Rode Kruis Ziekenhuis, 1942 LE Beverwijk, The Netherlands
* Correspondence: s.drager@erasmusmc.nl; Tel.: +31-650032142

Abstract: Model-informed precision dosing (MIPD) might be used to optimize antibiotic treatment. Procalcitonin (PCT) is a biomarker for severity of infection and response to antibiotic treatment. The aim of this study was to assess the impact of MIPD on the course of PCT and to investigate the association of PCT with pharmacodynamic target (PDT) attainment in critically ill patients. This is a secondary analysis of the DOLPHIN trial, a multicentre, open-label, randomised controlled trial. Patients with a PCT value available at day 1 (T1), day 3 (T3), or day 5 (T5) after randomisation were included. The primary outcome was the absolute difference in PCT concentration at T1, T3, and T5 between the MIPD and the standard dosing group. In total, 662 PCT concentrations from 351 critically ill patients were analysed. There was no statistically significant difference in PCT concentration between the trial arms at T1, T3, or T5. The median PCT concentration was highest in patients who exceeded 10× PDT at T1 [13.15 ng/mL (IQR 5.43–22.75)]. In 28-day non-survivors and in patients that exceeded PDT at T1, PCT decreased significantly between T1 and T3, but plateaued between T3 and T5. PCT concentrations were not significantly different between patients receiving antibiotic treatment with or without MIPD guidance. The potential of PCT to guide antibiotic dosing merits further investigation.

Keywords: model-informed precision dosing; procalcitonin; inflammation; biomarker; antibiotics; critically ill; pharmacodynamic target attainment

1. Introduction

Sepsis and septic shock are potentially life-threatening conditions in critically ill patients in whom timely initiation of antibiotic treatment is important to improve survival [1]. In the intensive care unit (ICU), 40–60% of the patients fail to achieve the currently recommended pharmacodynamic target (PDT) of antibiotics [2–5]. Due to extensive pathophysiological alterations, they are at risk of both over- and underdosing, increasing the chance of significant adverse events and therapeutic failure [6,7].

Therapeutic drug monitoring (TDM) is optimizing antibiotic dosing using measurements of plasma concentrations and could provide individualized dosing recommendations, especially when combined with model-informed precision dosing (MIPD) [8,9].

MIPD is an approach that uses population pharmacokinetic (PK) models to optimize initial dosing and integrates TDM results using pharmacokinetic software to guide subsequent patient-individualized dosing. Different MIPD software has been developed to facilitate its use in clinical practice [10]. However, individualization of antibiotic dosing might not be limited to TDM or MIPD. Biomarkers might provide additional information about treatment response and toxicity. Procalcitonin (PCT) is a biomarker that indicates the presence of bacterial infection and is a marker for severity of disease and resolution of infection [11–15]. Additionally, some studies have demonstrated its potential utility in guiding antibiotic treatment duration, with subsequent decrease in antibiotic consumption [16–22].

Pharmacokinetic/pharmacodynamic (PK/PD) relationships of beta-lactam antibiotics and fluoroquinolones are based on the relation between the minimum inhibitory concentration (MIC) of the underlying pathogen and a measure of antibiotic exposure as time above the MIC ($T_{>MIC}$) for beta-lactam antibiotics or area under the concentration–time curve (AUC) for fluoroquinolones [9,23]. Current studies mainly focus on the relationship between PK/PD and the MIC of the pathogen, but rarely take into account the host and its immune response to antibiotic treatment as influencing factor. Consequently, the relationship between PK/PDs of antibiotics, plasma drug exposure and the host's immune response as reflected by biomarkers such as PCT has rarely been described [9]. However, biomarker-guided antibiotic dosing could be a promising next step towards a patient-individual dosing strategy [9,24].

This study aims to explore the association of MIPD with the course of PCT, and the association of PCT with PDT attainment of antibiotics in critically ill patients. For this purpose, we performed a secondary analysis of a multicentre, randomised controlled trial, the DOLPHIN trial, that investigated the impact of TDM and MIPD on clinical outcome of ICU patients [25,26].

2. Material and Methods

2.1. Study Design

We performed a secondary analysis on data collected from 388 ICU patients of the DOLPHIN trial, a multicentre, open-label randomised controlled trial [25]. The trial aimed to assess whether early MIPD of beta-lactam antibiotics and ciprofloxacin decreases ICU length of stay (LOS) compared to standard dosing. The trial was conducted between October 2018 and September 2021 in eight ICUs in the Netherlands. The study was conducted in accordance with the Declaration of Helsinki and approved by the Medical Ethics Committee of the Erasmus University Medical Center (Erasmus MC) Rotterdam (registration number MEC-2017-568, 9 March 2018, title: "Dose Individualization on Antibiotics in ICU patients: to TDM or not to TDM and the effects on outcome (DOLPHIN trial)"; EudraCT 2017-004677-14). Informed consent was obtained from all subjects or their legal representatives involved in the study before randomisation. The measurement of PCT was included into the study protocol [26]. Patients were included and randomised within 36 h of the initial administration of the antibiotic (T0). For patients randomised to the MIPD group, the first TDM (T1) was performed within 36 h after randomisation followed by a dosing recommendation within the subsequent 12 h. Subsequently, TDM was performed at day 3 (T3), day 5 (T5), and day 7 (T7) combined with dosage recommendations after T3 and T5. PCT measurements were performed retrospectively, in batches, at the Erasmus MC Rotterdam in patient samples available according to the TDM schedule at T1, T3, T5, and T7. In both trial arms, antibiotic treatment was initiated using standard dosages [25].

2.2. Study Populations

Study population I (n = 351): Inclusion criteria for this study population were all patients who participated in the DOLPHIN trial and who had at least one PCT measurement performed at T1, T3, or T5.

Study population II (n = 306): Inclusion criteria for this study population were all patients who participated in the DOLPHIN trial and who had a PCT measurement performed at T1.

Neither T0 nor T7 were included in the study, given the limited significance related to the study setting that investigated the impact of early MIPD and the limited number of measurements available.

2.3. Data Collection and Definitions

The demographic data were prospectively collected in the electronic Case Report Form of the original DOLPHIN trial and have been used for this secondary analysis. Clinical characteristics were collected at the time of initiation of antibiotic treatment. The definition of sepsis and septic shock was based on the sepsis III criteria [27]. Sequential Organ Failure Assessment (SOFA) score and laboratory results were assessed at each sample collection. The percentage of PCT decrease (delta PCT) between T1 and T3 and T1 and T5 was calculated as $\frac{T3-T1}{T3} \times 100$ and $\frac{T5-T1}{T5} \times 100$. Target attainment was defined as achieving PDT of the respective antibiotic after reaching a steady state. The following formula was used to assess PDT for beta-lactam antibiotics:

$$\frac{\frac{C_{free}}{C_{total}} \times C_{min} \text{ steady state}}{\text{Epidemiologic cutoff value (ECOFF)}}$$

C_{free}: unbound antibiotic concentration; C_{total}: total antibiotic concentration; C_{min}: minimal concentration, ECOFF: epidemiological cut-off value.

Values < 1 were defined as "below target", values 1–10 were considered "attained target", and values > 10 were defined as "above target" corresponding to 100% $fT_{>1 \times ECOFF}$, 100% $fT_{>1 to 10 \times ECOFF}$, and 100% $fT_{>10 \times ECOFF}$. The ECOFFs were used according to the original study [25]. For the analysis of the association between PDT attainment and PCT, patients were allocated to the "above target"/"attained target"/"below target" group at T1 and remained allocated to the corresponding group at T3 and T5. This approach aimed to analyse PCT concentration over time according to the initial PDT. For ciprofloxacin, an AUC over 24 h to the ECOFF (AUC 0–24 h/ECOFF) was used to define PDT. A ratio < 125 h was defined as "below target", 125–500 h as "attained target", and >500 h as "above target".

2.4. Laboratory Methods

EDTA samples were stored at -80 °C in a biobank at the Erasmus MC. After the study termination, PCT was measured in batches in all EDTA samples available at T1, T3, T5, and T7. The measurements were performed using an electrochemiluminescence Brahms PCT immunoassay on a Cobas E801 analyser (Roche Diagnostics, Rotkreuz, Switzerland).

2.5. Outcomes

The primary outcome was the absolute difference in PCT concentration at T1, T3, and T5 between the MIPD and the standard dosing group Secondary outcomes included (i) the relative difference of PCT decrease (delta PCT) between T1 and T3 and between T1 and T5 between the study groups, (ii) the percentage of patients who experienced an $\geq$80% decrease of PCT concentrations between T1 and T3, and between T1 and T5 or who reached an absolute PCT value < 0.5 ng/mL at T1, T3, or T5 in the MIPD and standard dosing group, respectively, indicating resolution of infection according to the literature [28], (iii) the absolute difference in PCT concentrations at T1, T3, and T5, when only patients with PCT > 0.5 ng/mL were included, (iv) the association between PCT concentrations at T1, T3, and T5 and 28 d mortality presented as 28-day survivors and non-survivors, and (v) the association of PCT concentrations with PDT.

2.6. Statistical Analyses

Continuous data were summarized or as medians with interquartile ranges (IQR). Normality of distribution of PCT at T1, T3, and T5 was tested using the Kolmogorov–Smirnov test due to an appropriately large sample size. As the *p*-value of the Kolmogorov–Smirnov test was <0.001 for T1, T3, and T5, PCT values were log-transformed for further analyses and for the figures. Categorical variables were described using frequencies and percentages. To assess differences between the MIPD and the standard dosing arm, χ^2 tests were used for categorical data, independent *t*-tests for continuous normally distributed variables, and Mann–Whitney U tests for continuous non-normally distributed variables. To assess differences between two dependent variables (e.g., PCT values at two points in time in one study arm), Wilcoxon signed rank test was used. The primary outcome and the secondary outcome were presented as median with IQR. A two-sided *p*-value < 0.05 was considered statistically significant. All analyses were performed in the R statistical software (version 4.2.1) and Prism Version 9 (GraphPad Software, San Diego, CA, USA). During the analysis phase, we found a downward slope trend in PCT over the study period, though there was no statistically significant difference between the standard dosing and the MIPD study arm. For the analyses between PCT and PDT attainment at T1, and the course of PCT in 28-day survivors and non-survivors, we therefore decided to pool the data from both treatment groups.

3. Results

3.1. Patient Characteristics

In total, 662 PCT measurements in 351 patients (study population I) were analysed: 336/662 (50.8%) PCT concentrations in 177 patients were allocated to the standard dosing, and 326/662 (49.2%) PCT concentrations in 174 patients were allocated to the MIPD group, respectively. In this study population, patient characteristics were balanced between both groups (Table 1).

Table 1. Baseline characteristics of the study population I.

	Standard Dosing (*n* = 177)	MIPD (*n* = 174)	Total (*n* = 351)	*p*-Value
Age, median (IQR)	64 (54–70)	65 (56–72)	64 (55–71)	0.301
Female sex, *n* (%)	66 (37.3)	66 (37.9)	132 (37.6)	0.913
BMI, median (IQR), kg/m^2	25.9 (23.0–29.4)	26.3 (23.4–31.1)	26.1 (23.1–30.6)	0.292
CCI, median (IQR)	3 (2–5)	3 (2–4)	3 (2–5)	0.222
APACHE IV Score, median (IQR)	70 (51–90)	70 (51–89)	70 (51–89)	0.703
SOFA Score T1, median (IQR)	7 (4–9)	7 (4–10)	7 (4–10)	0.363
SOFA Score T3, median (IQR)	4 (2–8)	5 (2–8)	5 (2–8)	0.425
SOFA Score T5, median (IQR)	1.5 (0–6)	3 (0–6)	2 (0–6)	0.057
Sepsis, *n* (%)				0.333
No	77 (44)	84 (48)	161 (46)	
Sepsis	56 (32)	58 (33)	114 (33)	
Septic shock	44 (25)	32 (18)	76 (22)	
Antibiotic class, *n* (%)				0.901
Beta-lactam	135 (76)	131 (75)	266 (76)	
Fluoroquinolone	42 (24)	43 (25)	85 (24)	
Main focus of infection, *n* (%)				0.921
Pulmonary	117 (66)	117 (67)	234 (67)	
Intra-abdominal	27 (15)	29 (17)	56 (16)	
Skin and soft tissue	6 (3)	3 (2)	9 (3)	
Central nervous system	5 (3)	4 (2)	9 (3)	
Urinary tract	3 (2)	6 (3)	9 (3)	
Bacteraemia	6 (3)	2 (1)	8 (2)	
Catheter-related infection	2 (1)	2 (1)	4 (1)	
Ear, nose, throat	1 (1)	2 (1)	3 (1)	
Endocarditis	1 (1)	1 (1)	2 (1)	
Unknown focus	6 (3)	5 (3)	11 (3)	
Other	3 (2)	3 (2)	6 (2)	

Table 1. *Cont.*

	Standard Dosing (n = 177)	MIPD (n = 174)	Total (n = 351)	p-Value
Laboratory values, median (IQR)				
PCT T1, ng/mL	3.22 (0.71–14.0) *	1.92 (0.41–16.2) **	2.35 (0.54–14.25)	0.153
PCT T3, ng/mL	1.83 (0.39–5.30) *	0.7 (0.26–4.43) **	1.15 (0.34–4.96)	0.057
PCT T5, ng/mL	0.91 (0.29–4.44) *	0.72 (0.24–2.42) **	0.89 (0.25–3.35)	0.333
WBC T1, $\times 10^9$/L	13.0 (9.2–18.0)	13.6 (8.8–17.4)	13.2 (8.9–17.7)	0.978
WBC T3, $\times 10^9$/L	12.6 (8.7–16.0)	11.7 (8.7–18.0)	12.2 (8.7–17.1)	0.918
WBC T5, $\times 10^9$/L	12.8 (9.8–16.6)	13.5 (9.8–18.7)	13.1 (9.7–18.3)	0.439
CRP T1, mg/L	216 (123–329)	197 (104–304)	213 (110–321)	0.176
CRP T3, mg/L	128 (71–223)	122.5 (67–191)	123 (68–200)	0.536
CRP T5, mg/L	84 (42–180)	80 (43–160)	82 (42–169)	0.801
Creatinine T1, μmol/L	94 (63–146)	89 (58–163)	91 (60–153)	0.602
Creatinine T3, μmol/L	85 (59–128)	75 (54–140)	80 (55–135)	0.742
Creatinine T5, μmol/L	84 (55–119)	70 (50–122)	77 (53–120)	0.424
Outcome				
ICU LOS, median (IQR)	8 (3–19)	11 (5–20.75)	10 (4–20)	0.052
Hospital LOS, median (IQR)	21 (10–36.25)	26 (14–43.75)	23 (12.00, 40.75)	0.035
Mortality 28 days, n (%)	44 (24.9)	45 (25.9)	89 (25.4)	0.902
Mortality 6 months, n (%)	57 (32.2)	62 (35.6)	119 (33.9)	0.501

Patients had a least one PCT measurement available at T1, T3, or T5. MIPD: Model-informed precision dosing; IQR: interquartile range; BMI: body mass index; CCI: Charlson Comorbidity Score; APACHE IV: Acute Physiology and Chronic Health Evaluation version 4; SOFA: sequential organ failure assessment; PCT: procalcitonin, CRP: C-reactive protein; WBC: white blood cell count; ICU LOS: intensive care unit length of stay. * Number of PCT values available: T1 = 161, T3 = 114, T5 = 61. ** Number of PCT values available: T1 = 146, T3 = 108, T5 = 7.

The median age was 64 years (IQR 55–71) and 132/351 patients (37.6%) were female. There was no significant difference in severity of disease between the patients at admission in regard to APACHE IV score [70 (IQR 51–90) vs. 70 (IQR 51–89), $p = 0.703$] or SOFA score [8 (IQR 5–10) vs. 8 (IQR 5–11), $p = 0.909$]. In total, 200/351 (57.0%) patients presented with sepsis or septic shock. The main focus of infection was the respiratory tract in 234/351 (66.7%) patients and the majority received a beta-lactam antibiotic as empirical treatment (Table 1). There was a slightly, but not statistically significant, shorter median ICU LOS in the standard dosing group compared to the MIPD group (8 days (IQR 3–19) vs. 11 days (IQR 5–20.75), $p = 0.052$), but no significant difference in 28-day mortality (24.9% vs. 25.9%, $p = 0.902$) or 6-month mortality (32.2% vs. 35.6%, $p = 0.501$) (Table 1).

3.2. The Course of PCT

The median PCT concentration at T1 was 3.2 ng/mL (IQR 0.7–14.1) in the standard dosing group and 1.9 ng/mL (IQR 0.4–16.6) in the MIPD group. Although the difference in PCT concentrations was not statistically significant between the groups ($p = 0.153$), a tendency towards a higher median PCT concentration in the standard dosing group could be observed (Figure 1).

In both study arms, PCT decreased significantly over time. Between the study allocations, no significant difference in PCT concentrations could be observed at T3 and T5. There was a slightly greater, but statistically not significant, difference in PCT concentrations between the MIPD and standard dosing group at T3 [PCT standard dosing group 1.83 ng/mL (IQR 0.39–5.30) vs. PCT MIPD group 0.7 ng/mL (IQR 0.26–4.43), $p = 0.057$], which was no longer observed at T5 [PCT standard dosing group 0.91 ng/mL (IQR 0.29–4.44) vs. PCT MIPD group 0.72 ng/mL (IQR 0.24–2.42), $p = 0.333$]. Furthermore, there was no significant difference in the median CRP and white blood cell counts between T1, T3, and T5 in both study arms (Table 1). A PCT value < 0.5 ng/mL at T1 was observed in 75/306 patients (24.5%) at T1. When excluding them from the primary analysis, still no differences in the absolute PCT concentrations between the standard dosing and the MIPD group could be observed, either at T1, T3, or T5. (e.g., PCT T1 standard dosing arm: 6.20 ng/mL (IQR

2.0–18.2) vs. MIPD group 4.44 ng/mL (IQR 1.44–22.93), *p*-value: 0.50) (Supplementary Figure S1).

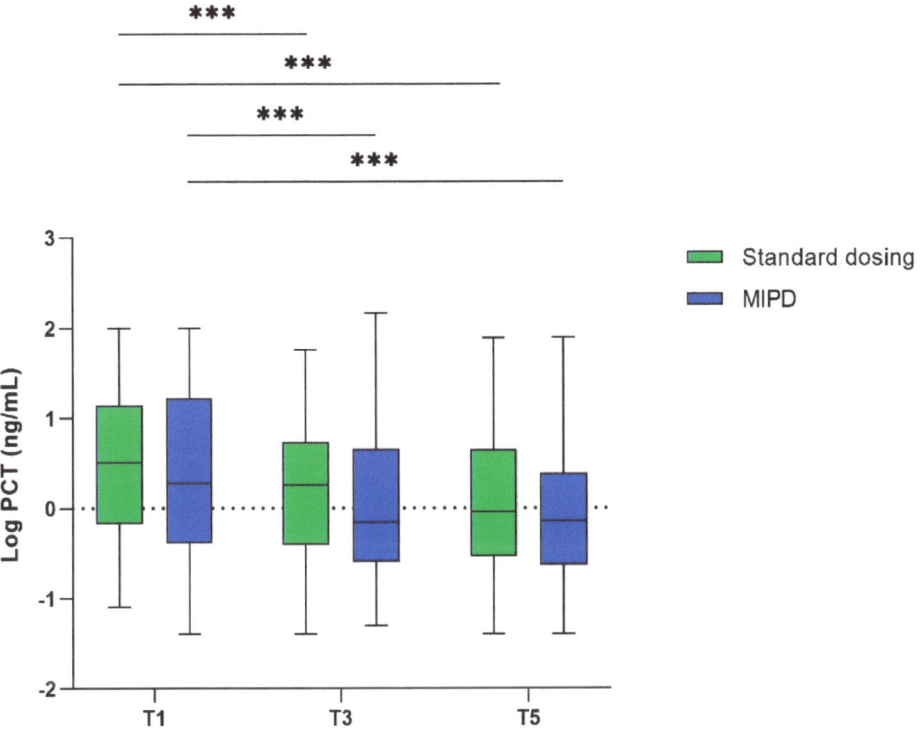

Figure 1. Median procalcitonin concentration at T1, T3, and T5 according to the trial arm. Due to non-normal distributed data, logPCT values are provided. Asterisks indicating statistical significance (<0.0001). PCT: procalcitonin, MIPD: model-informed precision dosing.

In total, there were 184 and 108 PCT pairs available to assess delta PCT between T1 and T3, and between T1 and T5, respectively. The median PCT decrease was 46% (IQR 13–55) between T1 and T3, and 58% (IQR 31–81) between T1 and T5. There was no difference in PCT decrease (delta PCT in %) between the standard dosing and MIPD group during these periods (Figure 2). Overall, a PCT decrease of ≥80%, which indicates resolution of infection, was observed in 9/184 (4.9%) patients (6 patients in the standard dosing, and 3 patients in the MIPD group) between T1 and T3 and in 29/108 (26.9%) patients (18 patients in the standard dosing and 11 patients in the MIPD group) between T1 and T5.

3.3. Course of PCT in 28-Day Survivors and Non-Survivors (Study Population I)

In study population I, there was a statistically significant difference in the median PCT concentration between patients who survived until day 28 and those who died before day 28, at every point in time (Figure 3). In 28-day survivors, the PCT concentration decreased significantly over time between T1 and T3, T1 and T5, and T3 and T5. In contrast, PCT decreased significantly between T1 and T3 ($p = 0.0001$) in 28-day non-survivors, but not between T3 and T5 ($p = 0.39$) (Figure 3). This observation was consistent when analysing the MIPD and standard dosing group separately (Supplementary Figure S2).

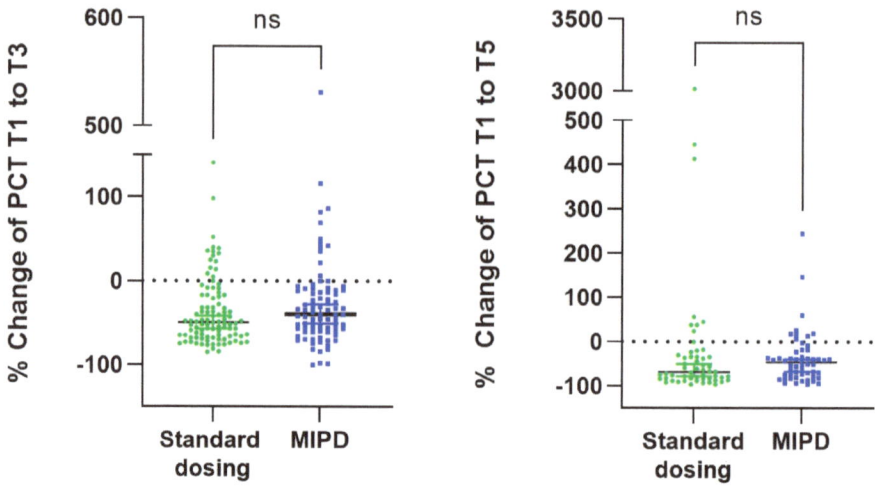

Figure 2. Change of PCT in % in the standard dosing and the MIPD group. ns: not statistically significant. PCT: procalcitonin, MIPD: model-informed precision dosing.

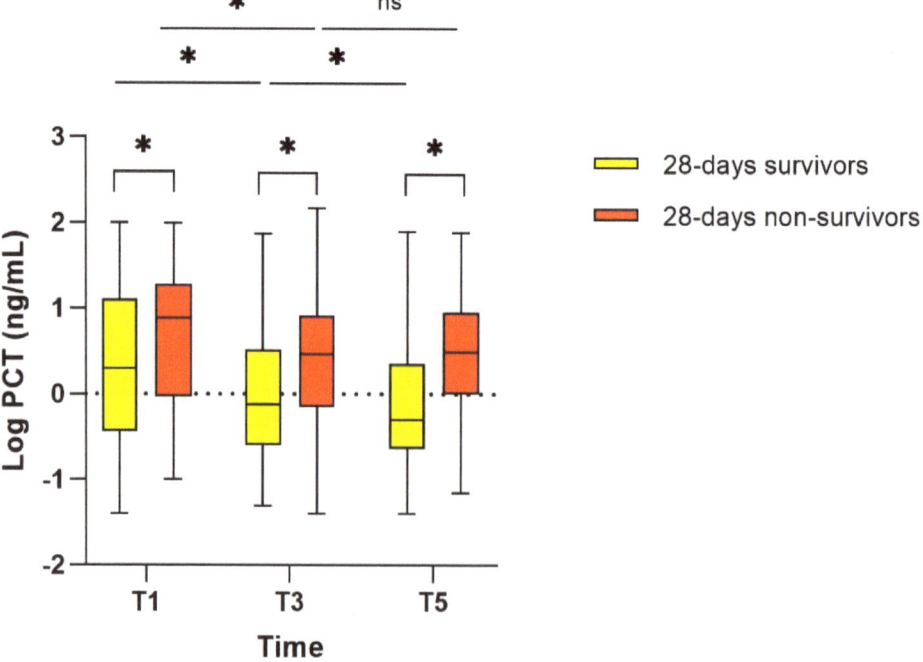

Figure 3. Course of PCT in 28-day survivors and non-survivors. Due to non-normal distributed data, log PCT values are provided. Asterisks indicating statistically significant change. Number of observations (PCT pairs available) 28-day survivors: T1/T3: 140, T1/T5: 81, T3/T5: 89. 28-day non-survivors: T1/T3: 44, T1/T5: 27, T3/T5: 28. ns: not statistically significant. PCT: procalcitonin.

3.4. Association of PCT with Pharmacodynamic Target Attainment (Study Population II)

We included 306 patients (study population II) who had a PCT measurement available at T1 into this analysis. One patient out of the initial 307 patients had a PCT measurement available at T1, but did not have any TDM and MIPD performed and was subsequently excluded from this analysis. Baseline characteristics are summarized in Table 2. Of the 306 patients, 178/306 (58.2%) attained PDT, 100/306 (32.7%) were below, and 28/306 (9.2%) exceeded PDT. The median PCT concentration differed significantly between the three PDT groups at T1: the median PCT was 3.35 ng/mL (IQR 0.80–17.52) in patients who attained PDT, 0.76 ng/mL (IQR 0.29–2.41) in patients below, and 13.15 ng/mL (IQR 5.43–22.75) in patients above PDT ($p < 0.001$) (Figure 4 and Table 2). In patients who either achieved or fell below PDT, a significant decrease in PCT over time was observed. However, patients who exceeded PDT at T1 showed a significant difference in PCT between T1 and T3 ($p = 0.001$), but not between T3 and T5 ($p = 0.578$). Similar results were observed when analysing each trial arm separately, although this analysis was limited by the smaller number of observations (Supplementary Figure S3).

Table 2. Baseline characteristics of the study population II (n = 306 patients) with a PCT available at T1 allocated to the according target attainment group.

	Below Target (n = 100)	Attained Target (n = 178)	Above Target (n = 28)	Total (n = 306)	p Value
Age, median (IQR)	61 (49–68)	65 (57–70)	68 (61–73)	64 (55–71)	0.003
Female sex, n (%)	33 (33.0)	69 (38.8)	15 (53.6)	117 (38.2)	0.141
BMI, median (IQR), kg/m^2	25.7 (23.0–29.5)	26.5 (23.2–30.9)	24.0 (20.2–26.2)	26.2 (22.9–30.6)	0.063
CCI, median (IQR)	2 (1–4)	3 (2–4)	4 (3–5)	3 (2–4)	<0.001
APACHE IV Score, median (IQR)	64 (48–85)	73 (56–89)	78 (60–95)	70 (51–89)	0.046
SOFA Score T0, median (IQR)	6 (4–8)	8 (5–11)	9 (8–11)	8 (5–10)	<0.001
SOFA Score T1, median (IQR)	5 (4–8)	8 (4–11)	7 (5–9)	7 (4–10)	<0.001
SOFA Score T3, median (IQR)	4 (2–6)	6 (3–11)	6 (4–10)	5 (3–9)	<0.001
SOFA Score T5, median (IQR)	3 (2–5)	6 (3–10)	6 (3–9)	5 (3–8)	<0.001
Sepsis, n (%)					<0.001
No	64 (64)	69 (39)	12 (43)	145 (47)	
Sepsis	29 (29)	63 (35)	9 (32)	101 (33)	
Septic shock	7 (7)	46 (26)	7 (25)	60 (20)	
Antibiotic class, n (%)					<0.001
Beta-lactam	53 (53)	147 (83)	28 (100)	228 (75)	
Fluoroquinolone	47 (47)	31 (17)	0 (0)	78 (26)	
Main focus of infection, n (%)					<0.001
Pulmonary	82 (82)	113 (64)	11 (39)	206 (67)	
Intra-abdominal	4 (4)	33 (19)	10 (36)	47 (15)	
Skin and soft tissue	3 (3)	5 (3)	1 (4)	9 (3)	
Central nervous system	2 (2)	6 (3)	0 (0)	8 (3)	
Urinary tract	1 (1)	6 (3)	1 (4)	8 (3)	
Bacteraemia	0 (0)	4 (2)	2 (7)	6 (2)	
Catheter-related infection	0 (0)	4 (2)	0 (0)	4 (1)	
Ear, nose, throat	1 (1)	1 (1)	1 (4)	3 (1)	
Endocarditis	1 (1)	1 (1)	0 (0)	2 (1)	
Other	3 (3)	1 (1)	2 (7)	6 (2)	
Unknown focus	3 (3)	4 (2)	0 (0)	7 (2)	
Laboratory values, median (IQR)					
PCT T1, ng/mL	0.76 (0.29–2.41) *	3.35 (0.80–17.52) **	13.15 (5.43–22.75) ***	2.34 (0.53–14.28)	<0.001
PCT T3, ng/mL	0.42 (0.22–1.80) *	1.46 (0.46–5.92) **	3.96 (2.82–10.82) ***	1.07 (0.33–4.18)	<0.001
PCT T5, ng/mL	0.27 (0.17–0.84) *	1.04 (0.28–3.61) **	1.07 (0.89–1.70) ***	0.78 (0.23–2.36)	<0.001
WBC T1, ×10^9/L	13.6 (9.3–17.8)	12.85 (8.8–17.3)	16.1 (13.6–22.0)	13.6 (9.2–17.9)	0.02
WBC T3, ×10^9/L	12.0 (8.8–15.4)	12.1 (8.5–17.6)	16.6 (12.3–20.3)	12.4 (8.7–17.2)	0.039
WBC T5, ×10^9/L	13 (10.3–16.3)	13.7 (9.9–18.9)	16.7 (12.5–24.7)	13.4 (10.0–18.7)	0.169
CRP T1, mg/L	188 (94–288)	214 (107–332)	245 (195–307)	213 (110–322)	0.117
CRP T3, mg/L	112 (58–204)	129 (72–198)	114 (89–177)	121 (67–193)	0.658
CRP T5, mg/L	70 (39–162)	82 (42–175)	78 (68–119)	76 (42–165)	0.875
Creatinine T1, µmol/L	64 (52–91)	105 (68–155)	173 (97–233)	90 (60–149)	<0.001
Creatinine T3, µmol/L	60 (48–82)	89 (59–135)	144 (87–236)	78 (54–128)	<0.001
Creatinine T5, µmol/L	59 (44–81)	82 (56–120)	191 (142–253)	76 (52–118)	<0.001
Outcome					
ICU LOS, median (IQR)	10 (4–19)	10 (4–21)	4 (2.75–9)	9.5 (3.25–19)	0.006
ICU LOS, median (IQR) 28 d survivors	11 (4–21.5)	10 (3–21.5)	4 (2–6.25) $	10 (3–20.5)	0.028

Table 2. Cont.

	Below Target (n = 100)	Attained Target (n = 178)	Above Target (n = 28)	Total (n = 306)	p Value
Hospital LOS, median (IQR)	25 (12.5–41.0)	24 (12.25–43.0)	14.5 (8.5–22.25) $	23 (12.0–41.0)	0.027
Hospital LOS, median (IQR) 28 d survivors	28 (14.25–44.5)	29 (15–49)	18 (11.5–38)	28.5 (14.25–47.75)	0.336
Mortality 28 d, n (%)	17 (17)	50 (28.1)	12 (42.9)	79 (25.8)	0.010
Mortality 6 months, n (%)	21 (21)	71 (39.9)	14 (50.0)	106 (34.6)	<0.001

BMI: body mass index, APACHE IV: Acute Physiology and Chronic Health Evaluation version 4; SOFA: sequential organ failure assessment; ICU LOS: intensive care unit length of stay; CNS: central nervous system; CRP C-reactive protein; WBC white blood cell count. * Number of PCT values available: T1 = 100, T3 = 61, T5 = 36. ** Number of PCT values available: T1 = 178, T3 = 110, T5 = 66. *** Number of PCT values available: T1 = 28, T3 = 12, T5 = 5. $ Number of observations = 16.

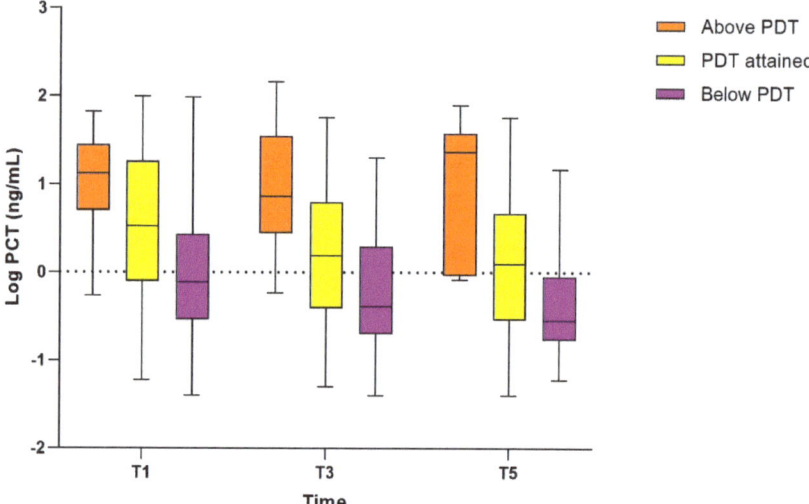

Figure 4. Median procalcitonin concentration at T1, T3, and T5 according to pharmacodynamic target attainment at T1. n = 306 patients. Patients were allocated to the PDT group at T1 and were not re-classified at T3 or T5. Due to non-normal distributed data, logPCT values are provided. PCT: procalcitonin; PDT: pharmacodynamic target.

Patients who either achieved or exceeded PDT at T1 exhibited higher disease severity, as indicated by higher median APACHE IV and SOFA scores upon admission (Table 2). There was a significant difference in the mortality rate between the PDT groups. Patients that were below PDT had a 28-day mortality rate of 17% (17/100), whereas patients that were on or above PDT demonstrated a 28-day mortality rate of 28.1% (50/178) and 42.9% (12/28), respectively ($p = 0.01$).

4. Discussion

We performed a secondary analysis on data from the DOLPHIN trial, in which we observed a significant decrease in PCT over the study period in the MIPD and the standard dosing study arm. In addition, patients exceeding the predefined PDT at T1 were found to have higher PCT concentrations in the blood, had poorer clinical outcome, and showed persistant elevated PCT values after an initial response to antibiotic treatment.

We did not find a difference in absolute PCT concentrations or the decrease of PCT over time in critically ill patients who received antibiotic treatment with or without MIPD and TDM guidance. Although not statistically significant, we observed a lower PCT concentration two to three days after the initiation of the antibiotic treatment in the MIPD group, pointing towards a potential impact of MIPD on a faster resolution of infection. However, the lack of any significant impact of MIPD on the course of PCT is in line with the results of the main study, in which no difference between the study arms was observed with regard to ICU LOS as the primary outcome parameter and mortality [25]. The limitation of the DOLPHIN trial, i.e., the heterogeneity of patients included and the trial design, are still relevant in this secondary analysis and potentially masking a greater effect of MIPD on the PCT decrease, i.e., the resolution of infection [29–31].

Although the association between the PK/PD of antibiotics and the host response has been discussed in the literature [9,13,23,24,32], clinical studies investigating this relationship are scarce, with no large prospective observational or randomised controlled trial data available to date. Aldaz et al. conducted a retrospective, observational, controlled cohort study with 96 patients in total, in which the decrease of PCT $\geq$ 80% until the end of treatment was assessed to describe the effectiveness of TDM-guided meropenem treatment [33]. A significantly higher proportion of patients in the TDM-guided group (71%) showed a PCT decrease of $\geq$80% by the end of the treatment compared to those who received meropenem treatment without TDM guidance (53%; $p = 0.02$). In contrast, our study did not reveal any difference in PCT decrease between the study arms. Moreover, a decrease of PCT $\geq$ 80% until T3 could only be observed in 9%, and in 25% of the patients until T5, being substantially lower compared to the results of Aldaz et al. [33]. However, comparability of the two studies is limited due to the different time points used to assess the PCT decline, the different antibiotics investigated, and the different study designs. In our study, we observed that approximately a quarter of the patients had a PCT < 0.5 ng/mL at T1. Although the use of PCT to guide initiation of antibiotic treatment is still debated [28], and its use in guiding the moment to stop antibiotic treatment is more accepted [15,34], PCT values < 0.5 ng/mL may be associated with a lower probability of bacterial infection in sepsis patients [28]. Overall, this group of patients with PCT values < 0.5 ng/mL might have had less benefit from antibiotic treatment and subsequently from TDM and MIPD.

We found that patients who had a high initial PCT value were at risk of exceeding the 10× PDT and of experiencing potential drug toxicity. Additionally, these patients represented the sickest subgroup of patients, reflected in a high APACHE Score, low eGFR, and high PCT values. Subsequently, they showed a significantly higher 28-day and 6-month mortality rate. This may underline the role of PCT as marker of severity of disease and to predict mortality [35]. Severity of disease is characterized by multi-organ failure due to a hyper-inflammatory status reflected in, e.g., high PCT concentrations, and at the same time decreased hepatic and renal function leading to a decrease of antibiotic clearance [36]. Therefore, it is a risk factor for excessive plasma concentrations of beta-lactam antibiotics, which, in turn, has been shown to be present with higher mortality rates [5,37,38]. However, previous findings were mainly based on clinical scores and altered renal function, but not on biomarker concentrations. Our results underscore the value of PCT as marker of severity of disease and show that higher PCT values are more frequently present in patients exceeding PDT. Additionally, although beta-lactams are known to have a wide therapeutic window, it is unclear if they may cause more toxic side effects than actually presumed [39,40].

It is noteworthy that PCT values plateaued between T3 and T5 in two distinct patient groups, the 28-day non-survivors and those exceeding PDT at T1. Antibiotic treatment seemed to have less impact on the course of PCT in the latter patients in the later state of the infection compared to patients who attained PDT or remained below PDT. The elevated PCT concentrations in these patients may not be, or only partially be, associated with a bacterial infection and be responsive to antibiotic treatment. Hence, it remains unclear if the optimization of antibiotic treatment may result in an improvement of clinical outcome or if it represents a hyper-inflammatory status that requires another treatment approach, e.g., the use of anti-inflammatory drugs which might have a greater impact on a favourable course of the disease. Conversely, patients with lower PCT values might benefit more from TDM and MIPD guided treatment, especially as they frequently did not achieve PDT. Proteomic and metabolomic studies to detect sepsis phenotypes might improve the understanding of the origin of inflammation and the classification of sepsis patients to different subclasses to identify those who may benefit the most from MIPD [41,42]. Furthermore, studies investigating the longitudinal trends of PCT during the course of infection and treatment are required to better understand the dynamics and the role of persisting high PCT plasma concentrations beyond the first phase of treatment.

To better understand the impact of MIPD on infection resolution and the PCT trajectory, prospective studies incorporating PCT measurements in their design are required. Given its more widespread availability compared to TDM and MIPD and its availability as point-of-care test, PCT could play an important role for future TDM trials and dosing strategies, e.g., helping to identify patients being at risk to exceed PDT combined with its role as marker for bacterial infections and severity of inflammation and disease. Furthermore, more research is needed to describe the relationship between inflammation biomarkers, i.e., the host's immune response, PK/PD parameters and TDM, more precisely. Gatti et al. has shown that inflammation reflected in high plasma CRP and PCT concentrations may down-regulate the metabolism of voriconazole in patients with COVID-19-associated aspergillosis, resulting in potentially toxic voriconazole concentrations [43]. In antibiotics, exposure–response relationships using modelling approaches have been described in pharmacodynamics of vancomycin and CRP in adults [44], of teicoplanin and CRP in neonates [45] or in animal studies [23]. Aulin et al. described the pharmacodynamics of PCT in patients with sepsis who had a daily PCT measurement performed and showed a significant variation of its dynamics as response to antibiotic treatment [24]. We present first data from a large clinical trial providing more insights of the association between PCT and antibiotic PDT attainment underlining the need for future prospective studies.

This study has several limitations. First, approximately 10% of the patients of the DOLPHIN trial could not be included in this secondary analysis due to the lack of samples available to determine PCT. This may have introduced some selection bias. PCT was not available in all patients at all points in time. Therefore, longitudinal, paired analyses were limited to the patients in whom at least two PCT measurements were available. Due to the study design, PCT was rarely available at T0, the initiation of antibiotic treatment, and therefore was not included into the analysis. We did not include microbiological data to support the role of PCT as a marker of bacterial infection due to its inconsistent collection and limited availability. Furthermore, data regarding concurrent treatments with drugs that could potentially influence the course of PCT were not available. Finally, we used a similar PCT threshold throughout the study population, although it may vary in patients with chronic renal dysfunction or congestive heart failure [18].

5. Conclusions

MIPD was not shown to have a significant impact on the course of PCT over time in critically ill patients. Patients with higher PCT values were more likely to exceed PDT and had a higher mortality rate. More severely ill patients demonstrated persistant elevated PCT concentrations after initial response to antibiotic treatment. The potential of PCT as biomarker for the identification of patients who are at risk to exceed PDT, and the use of PCT to guide antibiotic dosing, should be focus of future prospective trials.

Supplementary Materials: The following supporting information can be downloaded at: https://www.mdpi.com/article/10.3390/pharmaceutics16020270/s1: Figure S1. Median procalcitonin concentration at T1, T3, and T5 in patients with a PCT > 0.5 ng/mL at T1 according to the trial arm. Due to non-normal distributed data, logPCT values are provided. Asterisks indicating statistical significance (<0.0001). ns: not statistically significant. PCT: procalcitonin, MIPD: model-informed precision dosing. Figure S2. Course of procalcitonin in 28-day survivors and non-survivors according to the trial arm. Due to non-normal distributed data, log PCT values are provided. PCT: procalcitonin, MIPD: model-informed precision dosing. Figure S3. Course of procalcitonin according to the pharmacodynamic target attained at T1 and according to the trial arm. Due to the limited number of observations, we refrained from further statistical tests. PCT: procalcitonin, MIPD: model-informed precision dosing, PDT: pharmacodynamic target.

Author Contributions: Conceptualization, S.D., T.M.J.E., A.A., W.J.R.R., B.C.P.K. and H.E. Formal analysis, S.D. and W.J.R.R. Funding acquisition, S.D., B.C.P.K. and H.E. Investigation, S.D., T.M.J.E. and A.A. Methodology, S.D. and W.J.R.R. Project administration, B.C.P.K. and H.E. Resources, C.R., B.C.P.K. and H.E. Supervision, N.V., E.d.J., M.O., B.C.P.K. and H.E. Validation, T.M.J.E. Visualization, S.D. and W.J.R.R. Writing—original draft, S.D. Writing—review and editing, T.M.J.E., A.A., W.J.R.R., N.V., C.R., E.d.J., M.O., B.C.P.K. and H.E. All authors have read and agreed to the published version of the manuscript.

Funding: This project has received funding from the Dutch Organization for Health Research and Development ZonMw (grant 848017008), Stichting de Merel, and Erasmus MC MRace Grant. S.D. was supported by the "Research Fund of the University of Basel for Excellent Junior Researchers" (Number 3MS1093) and reports Travel Grant of the "ESCMID PK/PD of Anti-Infectives Study Group" (EPASG). The funders of the study had no role in study design, data collection, data analysis, data interpretation or writing of the report.

Institutional Review Board Statement: The study was conducted in accordance with the Declaration of Helsinki and approved by the Medical Ethics Committee of the Erasmus University Medical Center (Erasmus MC) in Rotterdam (registration number MEC-2017-568, 9 March 2018, Title: "Dose individualization on Antibiotics in ICU patients: to TDM or not to TDM and the effects on outcome (DOLPHIN trial); EudraCT 2017-004677-14).

Informed Consent Statement: Informed consent was obtained from all subjects or their legal representatives involved in the study before randomisation.

Data Availability Statement: The data that support the findings of this study are available from the corresponding author upon reasonable request.

Acknowledgments: We would like to thank the laboratory staff of the Division of Laboratory Medicine of the Erasmus University Medical Centre for determining the PCT concentrations. Results from the current study were presented at the 33rd European Congress of Clinical Microbiology & Infectious Diseases, Copenhagen, Denmark (Poster LB056).

Conflicts of Interest: B.C.P.K. reports grants or contracts unrelated to this work from IMI, European Union and Prinses Beatrix Foundation; Foundation Coolsingel; a role as unpaid Board member for IATDMCT, ESCMID EPASG, SWAB. The funders had no role in the design of the study; in the collection, analyses, or interpretation of data; in the writing of the manuscript; or in the decision to publish the results. All other authors declare no conflict of interest.

Abbreviations

APACHE IV	Acute physiology and chronic health evaluation version 4
BMI	Body mass index
CRP	C-reactive protein
GFR	Glomerular filtration rate
ICU	Intensive Care Unit
LOS	Length of stay
MIC	Minimal inhibitory concentration
MIPD	Model informed precision dosing
PCT	Procalcitonin
PK/PD	pharmacokinetic/pharmacodynamic
PDT	pharmacodynamic target
RCT	Randomised controlled trial
SOFA	Sequential organ failure assessment
TDM	Therapeutic drug monitoring

References

1. Rhodes, A.; Evans, L.E.; Alhazzani, W.; Levy, M.M.; Antonelli, M.; Ferrer, R.; Kumar, A.; Sevransky, J.E.; Sprung, C.L.; Nunnally, M.E.; et al. Surviving Sepsis Campaign: International Guidelines for Management of Sepsis and Septic Shock: 2016. *Intensive Care Med.* **2017**, *43*, 304–377. [CrossRef] [PubMed]

2. Roberts, J.A.; Paul, S.K.; Akova, M.; Bassetti, M.; De Waele, J.J.; Dimopoulos, G.; Kaukonen, K.M.; Koulenti, D.; Martin, C.; Montravers, P.; et al. DALI: Defining antibiotic levels in intensive care unit patients: Are current beta-lactam antibiotic doses sufficient for critically ill patients? *Clin. Infect. Dis.* **2014**, *58*, 1072–1083. [CrossRef] [PubMed]
3. Smekal, A.K.; Furebring, M.; Eliasson, E.; Lipcsey, M. Low attainment to PK/PD-targets for beta-lactams in a multi-center study on the first 72 h of treatment in ICU patients. *Sci. Rep.* **2022**, *12*, 21891. [CrossRef] [PubMed]
4. Haeseker, M.; Stolk, L.; Nieman, F.; Hoebe, C.; Neef, C.; Bruggeman, C.; Verbon, A. The ciprofloxacin target AUC: MIC ratio is not reached in hospitalized patients with the recommended dosing regimens. *Br. J. Clin. Pharmacol.* **2013**, *75*, 180–185. [CrossRef] [PubMed]
5. Hagel, S.; Bach, F.; Brenner, T.; Bracht, H.; Brinkmann, A.; Annecke, T.; Hohn, A.; Weigand, M.; Michels, G.; Kluge, S.; et al. Effect of therapeutic drug monitoring-based dose optimization of piperacillin/tazobactam on sepsis-related organ dysfunction in patients with sepsis: A randomized controlled trial. *Intensive Care Med.* **2022**, *48*, 311–321. [CrossRef] [PubMed]
6. Abdul-Aziz, M.H.; Lipman, J.; Mouton, J.W.; Hope, W.W.; Roberts, J.A. Applying pharmacokinetic/pharmacodynamic principles in critically ill patients: Optimizing efficacy and reducing resistance development. *Semin. Respir. Crit. Care Med.* **2015**, *36*, 136–153. [CrossRef] [PubMed]
7. Huttner, A.; Von Dach, E.; Renzoni, A.; Huttner, B.D.; Affaticati, M.; Pagani, L.; Daali, Y.; Pugin, J.; Karmime, A.; Fathi, M.; et al. Augmented renal clearance, low beta-lactam concentrations and clinical outcomes in the critically ill: An observational prospective cohort study. *Int. J. Antimicrob. Agents* **2015**, *45*, 385–392. [CrossRef] [PubMed]
8. Tangden, T.; Ramos Martin, V.; Felton, T.W.; Nielsen, E.I.; Marchand, S.; Bruggemann, R.J.; Bulitta, J.B.; Bassetti, M.; Theuretzbacher, U.; Tsuji, B.T.; et al. The role of infection models and PK/PD modelling for optimising care of critically ill patients with severe infections. *Intensive Care Med.* **2017**, *43*, 1021–1032. [CrossRef]
9. Wicha, S.G.; Martson, A.G.; Nielsen, E.I.; Koch, B.C.P.; Friberg, L.E.; Alffenaar, J.W.; Minichmayr, I.K.; International Society of Anti-Infective Pharmacology (ISAP), the PK/PD Study Group of the European Society of Clinical Microbiology, Infectious Diseases (EPASG). From Therapeutic Drug Monitoring to Model-Informed Precision Dosing for Antibiotics. *Clin. Pharmacol. Ther.* **2021**, *109*, 928–941. [CrossRef]
10. Del Valle-Moreno, P.; Suarez-Casillas, P.; Mejias-Trueba, M.; Ciudad-Gutierrez, P.; Guisado-Gil, A.B.; Gil-Navarro, M.V.; Herrera-Hidalgo, L. Model-Informed Precision Dosing Software Tools for Dosage Regimen Individualization: A Scoping Review. *Pharmaceutics* **2023**, *15*, 1859. [CrossRef]
11. Scott, J.; Deresinski, S. Use of biomarkers to individualize antimicrobial therapy duration: A narrative review. *Clin. Microbiol. Infect.* **2023**, *29*, 160–164. [CrossRef] [PubMed]
12. Azzini, A.M.; Dorizzi, R.M.; Sette, P.; Vecchi, M.; Coledan, I.; Righi, E.; Tacconelli, E. A 2020 review on the role of procalcitonin in different clinical settings: An update conducted with the tools of the Evidence Based Laboratory Medicine. *Ann. Transl. Med.* **2020**, *8*, 610. [CrossRef] [PubMed]
13. Heffernan, A.J.; Sime, F.B.; Lipman, J.; Roberts, J.A. Individualising Therapy to Minimize Bacterial Multidrug Resistance. *Drugs* **2018**, *78*, 621–641. [CrossRef] [PubMed]
14. van Nieuwkoop, C.; Bonten, T.N.; van't Wout, J.W.; Kuijper, E.J.; Groeneveld, G.H.; Becker, M.J.; Koster, T.; Wattel-Louis, G.H.; Delfos, N.M.; Ablij, H.C.; et al. Procalcitonin reflects bacteremia and bacterial load in urosepsis syndrome: A prospective observational study. *Crit. Care* **2010**, *14*, R206. [CrossRef] [PubMed]
15. de Jong, E.; van Oers, J.A.; Beishuizen, A.; Vos, P.; Vermeijden, W.J.; Haas, L.E.; Loef, B.G.; Dormans, T.; van Melsen, G.C.; Kluiters, Y.C.; et al. Efficacy and safety of procalcitonin guidance in reducing the duration of antibiotic treatment in critically ill patients: A randomised, controlled, open-label trial. *Lancet Infect. Dis.* **2016**, *16*, 819–827. [CrossRef] [PubMed]
16. Gregoriano, C.; Heilmann, E.; Molitor, A.; Schuetz, P. Role of procalcitonin use in the management of sepsis. *J. Thorac. Dis.* **2020**, *12*, S5–S15. [CrossRef] [PubMed]
17. Rhee, C. Using Procalcitonin to Guide Antibiotic Therapy. *Open Forum Infect. Dis.* **2017**, *4*, ofw249. [CrossRef]
18. Covington, E.W.; Roberts, M.Z.; Dong, J. Procalcitonin Monitoring as a Guide for Antimicrobial Therapy: A Review of Current Literature. *Pharmacotherapy* **2018**, *38*, 569–581. [CrossRef]
19. Velicer, C.M.; Heckbert, S.R.; Lampe, J.W.; Potter, J.D.; Robertson, C.A.; Taplin, S.H. Antibiotic use in relation to the risk of breast cancer. *JAMA* **2004**, *291*, 827–835. [CrossRef]
20. Garnacho-Montero, J.; Gutierrez-Pizarraya, A.; Escoresca-Ortega, A.; Corcia-Palomo, Y.; Fernandez-Delgado, E.; Herrera-Melero, I.; Ortiz-Leyba, C.; Marquez-Vacaro, J.A. De-escalation of empirical therapy is associated with lower mortality in patients with severe sepsis and septic shock. *Intensive Care Med.* **2014**, *40*, 32–40. [CrossRef]
21. Meier, M.A.; Branche, A.; Neeser, O.L.; Wirz, Y.; Haubitz, S.; Bouadma, L.; Wolff, M.; Luyt, C.E.; Chastre, J.; Tubach, F.; et al. Procalcitonin-guided Antibiotic Treatment in Patients With Positive Blood Cultures: A Patient-level Meta-analysis of Randomized Trials. *Clin. Infect. Dis.* **2019**, *69*, 388–396. [CrossRef] [PubMed]
22. Nobre, V.; Harbarth, S.; Graf, J.D.; Rohner, P.; Pugin, J. Use of procalcitonin to shorten antibiotic treatment duration in septic patients: A randomized trial. *Am. J. Respir. Crit. Care Med.* **2008**, *177*, 498–505. [CrossRef] [PubMed]
23. Thorsted, A.; Nielsen, E.I.; Friberg, L.E. Pharmacodynamics of immune response biomarkers of interest for evaluation of treatment effects in bacterial infections. *Int. J. Antimicrob. Agents* **2020**, *56*, 106059. [CrossRef] [PubMed]
24. Aulin, L.B.S.; de Lange, D.W.; Saleh, M.A.A.; van der Graaf, P.H.; Voller, S.; van Hasselt, J.G.C. Biomarker-Guided Individualization of Antibiotic Therapy. *Clin. Pharmacol. Ther.* **2021**, *110*, 346–360. [CrossRef] [PubMed]

25. Ewoldt, T.M.J.; Abdulla, A.; Rietdijk, W.J.R.; Muller, A.E.; de Winter, B.C.M.; Hunfeld, N.G.M.; Purmer, I.M.; van Vliet, P.; Wils, E.J.; Haringman, J.; et al. Model-informed precision dosing of beta-lactam antibiotics and ciprofloxacin in critically ill patients: A multicentre randomised clinical trial. *Intensive Care Med.* **2022**, *48*, 1760–1771. [CrossRef] [PubMed]
26. Abdulla, A.; Ewoldt, T.M.J.; Hunfeld, N.G.M.; Muller, A.E.; Rietdijk, W.J.R.; Polinder, S.; van Gelder, T.; Endeman, H.; Koch, B.C.P. The effect of therapeutic drug monitoring of beta-lactams and fluoroquinolones on clinical outcome in critically ill patients: The DOLPHIN trial protocol of a multi-centre randomised controlled trial. *BMC Infect. Dis.* **2020**, *20*, 57. [CrossRef] [PubMed]
27. Shankar-Hari, M.; Phillips, G.S.; Levy, M.L.; Seymour, C.W.; Liu, V.X.; Deutschman, C.S.; Angus, D.C.; Rubenfeld, G.D.; Singer, M.; Sepsis Definitions Task, F. Developing a New Definition and Assessing New Clinical Criteria for Septic Shock: For the Third International Consensus Definitions for Sepsis and Septic Shock (Sepsis-3). *JAMA* **2016**, *315*, 775–787. [CrossRef] [PubMed]
28. Schuetz, P.; Beishuizen, A.; Broyles, M.; Ferrer, R.; Gavazzi, G.; Gluck, E.H.; Gonzalez Del Castillo, J.; Jensen, J.U.; Kanizsai, P.L.; Kwa, A.L.H.; et al. Procalcitonin (PCT)-guided antibiotic stewardship: An international experts consensus on optimized clinical use. *Clin. Chem. Lab. Med.* **2019**, *57*, 1308–1318. [CrossRef]
29. Rietdijk, W.J.R.; Drager, S.; Endeman, H.; Koch, B.C.P. Beta-lactam therapeutic drug monitoring in critically ill patients: Learnings for future research. *Clin. Infect. Dis.* **2023**, *77*, 663–664. [CrossRef]
30. Liebchen, U.; Briegel, J.; Brinkmann, A.; Frey, O.; Wicha, S.G. Individualised dosing of antibiotics in ICU patients: Timing, target and model selection matter. *Intensive Care Med.* **2023**, *49*, 475–476. [CrossRef]
31. Cotta, M.O.; Lipman, J.; De Waele, J. Advancing precision-based antimicrobial dosing in critically ill patients. *Intensive Care Med.* **2023**, *49*, 324–326. [CrossRef]
32. Sanz-Codina, M.; Bozkir, H.O.; Jorda, A.; Zeitlinger, M. Individualized antimicrobial dose optimization: A systematic review and meta-analysis of randomized controlled trials. *Clin. Microbiol. Infect.* **2023**, *29*, 845–857. [CrossRef]
33. Aldaz, A.; Idoate Grijalba, A.I.; Ortega, A.; Aquerreta, I.; Monedero, P. Effectiveness of Pharmacokinetic/Pharmacodynamic-Guided Meropenem Treatment in Critically Ill Patients: A Comparative Cohort Study. *Ther. Drug Monit.* **2021**, *43*, 256–263. [CrossRef] [PubMed]
34. Hochreiter, M.; Kohler, T.; Schweiger, A.M.; Keck, F.S.; Bein, B.; von Spiegel, T.; Schroeder, S. Procalcitonin to guide duration of antibiotic therapy in intensive care patients: A randomized prospective controlled trial. *Crit. Care* **2009**, *13*, R83. [CrossRef] [PubMed]
35. Schuetz, P.; Birkhahn, R.; Sherwin, R.; Jones, A.E.; Singer, A.; Kline, J.A.; Runyon, M.S.; Self, W.H.; Courtney, D.M.; Nowak, R.M.; et al. Serial Procalcitonin Predicts Mortality in Severe Sepsis Patients: Results From the Multicenter Procalcitonin MOnitoring SEpsis (MOSES) Study. *Crit. Care Med.* **2017**, *45*, 781–789. [CrossRef] [PubMed]
36. Wanner, G.A.; Keel, M.; Steckholzer, U.; Beier, W.; Stocker, R.; Ertel, W. Relationship between procalcitonin plasma levels and severity of injury, sepsis, organ failure, and mortality in injured patients. *Crit. Care Med.* **2000**, *28*, 950–957. [CrossRef] [PubMed]
37. Moser, S.; Rehm, S.; Guertler, N.; Hinic, V.; Drager, S.; Bassetti, S.; Rentsch, K.M.; Sendi, P.; Osthoff, M. Probability of pharmacological target attainment with flucloxacillin in *Staphylococcus aureus* bloodstream infection: A prospective cohort study of unbound plasma and individual MICs. *J. Antimicrob. Chemother.* **2021**, *76*, 1845–1854. [CrossRef] [PubMed]
38. Richter, D.C.; Frey, O.; Rohr, A.; Roberts, J.A.; Koberer, A.; Fuchs, T.; Papadimas, N.; Heinzel-Gutenbrunner, M.; Brenner, T.; Lichtenstern, C.; et al. Therapeutic drug monitoring-guided continuous infusion of piperacillin/tazobactam significantly improves pharmacokinetic target attainment in critically ill patients: A retrospective analysis of four years of clinical experience. *Infection* **2019**, *47*, 1001–1011. [CrossRef] [PubMed]
39. Roger, C.; Louart, B. Beta-Lactams Toxicity in the Intensive Care Unit: An Underestimated Collateral Damage? *Microorganisms* **2021**, *9*, 1505. [CrossRef] [PubMed]
40. Imani, S.; Buscher, H.; Marriott, D.; Gentili, S.; Sandaradura, I. Too much of a good thing: A retrospective study of beta-lactam concentration-toxicity relationships. *J. Antimicrob. Chemother.* **2017**, *72*, 2891–2897. [CrossRef]
41. DeMerle, K.M.; Angus, D.C.; Baillie, J.K.; Brant, E.; Calfee, C.S.; Carcillo, J.; Chang, C.H.; Dickson, R.; Evans, I.; Gordon, A.C.; et al. Sepsis Subclasses: A Framework for Development and Interpretation. *Crit. Care Med.* **2021**, *49*, 748–759. [CrossRef] [PubMed]
42. Hussain, H.; Vutipongsatorn, K.; Jimenez, B.; Antcliffe, D.B. Patient Stratification in Sepsis: Using Metabolomics to Detect Clinical Phenotypes, Sub-Phenotypes and Therapeutic Response. *Metabolites* **2022**, *12*, 376. [CrossRef] [PubMed]
43. Gatti, M.; Fornaro, G.; Pasquini, Z.; Zanoni, A.; Bartoletti, M.; Viale, P.; Pea, F. Impact of Inflammation on Voriconazole Exposure in Critically ill Patients Affected by Probable COVID-19-Associated Pulmonary Aspergillosis. *Antibiotics* **2023**, *12*, 764. [CrossRef]
44. Rawson, T.M.; Charani, E.; Moore, L.S.P.; Gilchrist, M.; Georgiou, P.; Hope, W.; Holmes, A.H. Exploring the Use of C-Reactive Protein to Estimate the Pharmacodynamics of Vancomycin. *Ther. Drug Monit.* **2018**, *40*, 315–321. [CrossRef]
45. Ramos-Martin, V.; Neely, M.N.; McGowan, P.; Siner, S.; Padmore, K.; Peak, M.; Beresford, M.W.; Turner, M.A.; Paulus, S.; Hope, W.W. Population pharmacokinetics and pharmacodynamics of teicoplanin in neonates: Making better use of C-reactive protein to deliver individualized therapy. *J. Antimicrob. Chemother.* **2016**, *71*, 3168–3178. [CrossRef]

Disclaimer/Publisher's Note: The statements, opinions and data contained in all publications are solely those of the individual author(s) and contributor(s) and not of MDPI and/or the editor(s). MDPI and/or the editor(s) disclaim responsibility for any injury to people or property resulting from any ideas, methods, instructions or products referred to in the content.

Review

Treatment of Chronic Lymphocytic Leukemia in the Personalized Medicine Era

María Del Mar Sánchez Suárez [1], Alicia Martín Roldán [1], Carolina Alarcón-Payer [1,*], Miguel Ángel Rodríguez-Gil [2], Jaime Eduardo Poquet-Jornet [3], José Manuel Puerta Puerta [2] and Alberto Jiménez Morales [1]

[1] Servicio de Farmacia, Hospital Universitario Virgen de las Nieves, 18014 Granada, Granada, Spain; mariadmar157@gmail.com (M.D.M.S.S.); aliciamartinroldan@gmail.com (A.M.R.); alberto.jimenez.morales.sspa@juntadeandalucia.es (A.J.M.)

[2] Unidad de Gestión Clínica Hematología y Hemoterapia, Hospital Universitario Virgen de las Nieves, 18014 Granada, Granada, Spain; miguel.rodriguez.gil.sspa@juntadeandalucia.es (M.Á.R.-G.); josem.puerta.sspa@juntadeandalucia.es (J.M.P.P.)

[3] Servicio de Farmacia, Hospital de Dénia Marina Salud, 03700 Dénia, Alicante, Spain; jaime.poquet@marinasalud.es

* Correspondence: carolina.alarcon.sspa@juntadeandalucia.es

Abstract: Chronic lymphocytic leukemia is a lymphoproliferative disorder marked by the expansion of monoclonal, mature CD5+CD23+ B cells in peripheral blood, secondary lymphoid tissues, and bone marrow. The disease exhibits significant heterogeneity, with numerous somatic genetic alterations identified in the neoplastic clone, notably mutated TP53 and immunoglobulin heavy chain mutational statuses. Recent studies emphasize the pivotal roles of genetics and patient fragility in treatment decisions. This complexity underscores the need for a personalized approach, tailoring interventions to individual genetic profiles for heightened efficacy. The era of personalized treatment in CLL signifies a transformative shift, holding the potential for improved outcomes in the conquest of this intricate hematologic disorder. This review plays a role in elucidating the evolving CLL treatment landscape, encompassing all reported genetic factors. Through a comprehensive historical analysis, it provides insights into the evolution of CLL management. Beyond its retrospective nature, this review could be a valuable resource for clinicians, researchers, and stakeholders, offering a window into the latest advancements. In essence, it serves as a dynamic exploration of our current position and the promising prospects on the horizon.

Keywords: chronic lymphocytic leukemia; genetic alterations; inhibitors of Bruton tyrosine kinase; TP53 mutation; immunoglobulin heavy chain variable region mutated

1. Introduction

Chronic lymphocytic leukemia (CLL) or small lymphocytic lymphoma (SLL), the most common leukemia in adults, is characterized by the expansion of monoclonal CD5+CD23+ B cells in peripheral blood (PB), lymphoid tissues, and bone marrow. CLL and SLL share pathology but have different manifestations based on the location of abnormal cells, with CLL in the blood and SLL in lymph nodes. The age-adjusted incidence is 4.9 per 100,000 inhabitants yearly, peaking at a median age of 70, affecting more males than females [1–4].

Recent trends reveal an increased detection of early stages, allowing close monitoring for asymptomatic cases. CLL is often diagnosed during routine medical visits when a complete blood count shows an elevated lymphocyte count. If the expansion of lymphocytes continues, a flow cytometric analysis is conducted to check the number of CD5+CD19+ B cells, looking for an increased count of cells expressing specific markers [5].

During this asymptomatic phase, clinical history might not reveal much, but some patients may report weight loss, lethargy, night sweats, and complaints of "swollen glands".

Physical examination mainly focuses on identifying swollen lymph nodes, enlarged spleen or liver, and signs of low red blood cells or platelets [5].

As shown in Figure 1, the evolution of CLL treatment has witnessed significant advancements over the years. Traditionally, CLL management relied on conventional chemotherapy, often utilizing alkylating agents and purine analogs. In 2014, initial treatment was determined by age and comorbidities. Younger patients (<65 years) received chemoimmunotherapy (CIT) like fludarabine, cyclophosphamide, and rituximab (FCR), while those aged 65–75 were given bendamustine and rituximab (BR). Patients over 75 or with significant comorbidities received single-agent chlorambucil, with or without anti-CD20 monoclonal antibody treatment. Therapies targeting B-cell receptor (BCR) signaling have revolutionized CLL treatment, expanding options for high-risk patients with limited previous choices [6,7].

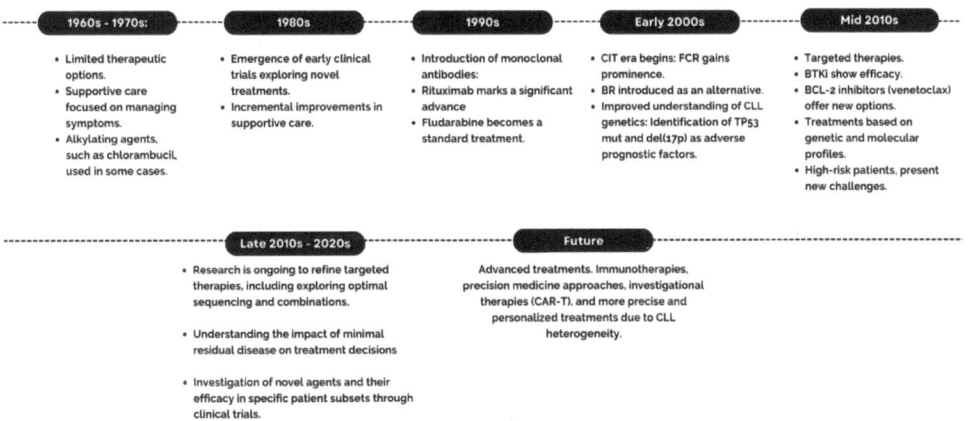

Figure 1. Timeline of the evolution of CLL treatments.

Patients with CLL fall into categories ranging from those minimally affected and not requiring therapy to those with aggressive diseases necessitating immediate treatment. Therapy is now reserved for those with active or symptomatic disease or advanced Binet or Rai stages. Options include venetoclax with obinutuzumab (VO), monotherapy with Bruton tyrosine kinase inhibitors (BTKi) (ibrutinib, acalabrutinib, and zanubrutinib), or CIT. On the other hand, patients with 17p deletion (del17p) or TP53 mutation (TP53mut) resistance to chemotherapy are treated with targeted agents [8,9]. This review aims to approach the therapeutic management of CLL patients from the point of view of personalized medicine. For this purpose, key recommendations from the main expert guidelines for the management of this patient group will be explored, with the treatment of refractory patients strongly influenced by prior treatment and TP53, del17, and immunoglobulin heavy chain variable region mutations (IGHVm) [8,9]. Finally, investigations into new therapeutic strategies for future improvements in CLL treatment outcomes will be highlighted.

2. Materials and Methods

For the following literature review, a comprehensive search was conducted in the PubMed and Web of Science databases for articles published within the last decade. Keywords related to CLL, treatment, genetics, mutations, prognosis, and therapy were used in various combinations. In addition, the citations of selected articles were included as supplementary sources. Articles published in English and Spanish were considered, with no restrictions on article type (clinical trials, original articles, reviews, etc.) or population size.

3. Pathogenesis

Advancements in our comprehension of the genetics and biology of CLL reveal its considerable heterogeneity. This enhanced understanding allows for a more profound insight into the diverse cell types that could serve as the origins of this malignancy, as well as the genetic elements associated with its pathogenesis. Over time, various cell types have been proposed as potential sources of CLL, building on an evolving comprehension of B-cell biology and differentiation.

CLL may initiate in the stem cell phase, resulting in an increased proportion of polyclonal pro-B cells. This progression may lead, over time, to the development of monoclonal or oligoclonal CD5+ B-cell populations bearing resemblance to monoclonal B-cell lymphocytosis (MBL). Through the acquisition of genetic and epigenetic alterations, hematopoietic stem cells might exhibit a fate bias towards the B-cell lineage. Subsequent antigenic stimulation could then drive the selection and expansion of mature B cells, culminating in the formation of oligoclonal populations. The causes of genetic and epigenetic variations are still unknown [10].

The identification of clonal rearrangements in immunoglobulin genes, coupled with the expression of distinct cell surface markers, has confirmed that CLL originates from a mature B cell. This B cell is notably characterized by low expression levels of B cell markers, including surface membrane immunoglobulins, CD19, and CD20. Additionally, it exhibits positivity for the expression of CD23 (also recognized as FcεRII, a marker present in B cells and dendritic cells) and the antigens CD200 and CD5 [11].

IGHVm CLLs originate from CD5+CD27+ B cells of the post-germinal center, which are transcriptionally like memory B cells and are most likely derived from CD5+CD27− B cells that have undergone the post-germinal center reaction. On the other hand, immunoglobulin heavy chain variable region unmutated (IGHVum) CLLs appear to arise from pre-CG CD5+CD27− B cells, which may be derived from naïve B cells or a separate lineage of precursor B cells. B-cell receptor stimulation, additional genetic and epigenetic abnormalities, and microenvironmental factors will contribute to the precursors of CLL, MBL, and frank monoclonal CLL [10,12].

3.1. Genetic Alterations

Several genetic features underlying the clinic-biological heterogeneity of CLL have been described, including immunogenetic features and somatic genetic alterations of the neoplastic clone. The genomic changes in CLL have been extensively investigated using traditional molecular cytogenetics as well as comprehensive approaches such as whole-exome sequencing and whole-genome next-generation sequencing (NGS) [13,14].

Approximately 80% of patients have genetic mutations for del(13q), del(11q), del(17p), or trisomy 12. In contrast, a smaller percentage of patients, around 10–20%, have a more heterogeneous low-frequency mutation profile [15]. Massive sequencing techniques have identified several mutations in different genes, with an average of 20 specific mutations detected per case of CLL, which is considered relatively low in relation to other tumors.

TP53mut is identified in 5–10% of CLL cases at the time of diagnosis, but this frequency escalates to 40–50% among refractory patients [16]. Being among the prevalent genetic alterations in various human cancers, TP53 serves both as a prognostic indicator and a target for treatment. TP53 is a tumor suppressor gene responsible for encoding the p53 protein, which plays a proapoptotic role in response to DNA damage. Positioned on the short arm of chromosome 17 (17p) [17], disruption of TP53 leads to heightened resistance to apoptosis induced by DNA-damaging agents, encompassing chemotherapy, thereby affecting the response to such treatments [18]. The most common genetic lesions of TP53 are somatic mutations and del(17p) [19]. More than 5211 different mutations have been observed in 40416 unique samples across 46 different tissue types, indicative of the genetic variability of TP53 [20].

A rare occurrence is the coexistence of del(17p) with MYC aberrations (translocations or gains) in a very limited number of patients, and this combination may be linked to an exceptionally unfavorable prognosis. However, it is crucial to note that existing studies are primarily retrospective cohorts, with most patients already undergoing treatment. Therefore, it is imperative to conduct further assessments of the TP53 mutational status to ascertain whether the poor prognosis is indeed a consequence of the combination of a TP53mut and not only del(17p) with a MYC aberration [21].

Due to the significant clinical impact, guidelines for the International Workshop on Chronic Lymphocytic Leukemia (iwCLL) recommend testing for del(17p) via fluorescence in situ hybridization (FISH) and TP53 mutation status via DNA sequencing prior to initiating treatment. The European Research Initiative on Chronic CLL (ERIC) advocates considering the application of NGS for the analysis of TP53mut. This approach is distinguished by its higher sensitivity compared to the conventional Sanger sequencing method [22].

As mentioned above, CLL can be divided into two molecular subgroups: (i) non-mutated IGHV CLL (approximately 40% of all CLL), reflecting mature B cells that have not undergone the GC reaction and have undergone T-cell independent maturation, and (ii) IGHVm CLL (60% of all CLL), where mature B cells have undergone the germinal centers (GC) reaction and have undergone the somatic hypermutation process [23]. These IGHVm gene CLLs are genetically developed by activation-induced cytidine deaminase (AID). AID also plays a crucial role in IGH rearrangements, specifically in processes such as class switch recombination (CSR) and recombination between switch Mu (Sµ) and the 3′ regulatory region (3′RR) (Sµ-3′RRrec). Given the predominant presence of unswitched CLL B-cells, an investigation into the blockade of IGH rearrangement in CLL was prompted [24]. Patients with somatic IGHVm with <98% germline homology are considered to have a better prognosis. In addition, it is important to emphasize that, as the mutational status of IGHV is stable throughout the course of the disease, it is not necessary to perform this study again [25].

The presence of TP53mut and the mutational status of IGHV guide treatment decisions by influencing the choice of therapeutic agents and the intensity of treatment. Targeted therapies and alternative approaches are often considered for patients with TP53mut due to chemotherapy resistance, while patients with mutated immunoglobulins may have a more favorable response to less aggressive treatment strategies. The individualized approach to treatment based on these molecular characteristics helps optimize outcomes for patients with CLL. Numerous mutations have been documented, and Table 1 delineates the features of the most significant ones. Currently, none of these mutations are factored into treatment decision making.

Table 1. Mutations implicated in CLL.

Mutation	Prevalence	Location	Signaling Pathway	Prognosis	References
TP53	5–10% at the beginning of treatment 40–50% in refractory patients	Chromosome 17	Resistance to apoptosis induced via DNA-damaging agents	Very poor prognosis	[17,18]
BIRC3	2–6%	Chromosome 11	NF-κB signaling	Poor prognosis	[26–28]
NOTCH1	10–15%	Chromosome 9	NF-κB signaling	Poor prognosis	[29–31]
ATM	10–12%	Chromosome 11	Aberrations in DNA repair mechanisms	Poor prognosis	[32–34]
SF3B1	5–10%	Chromosome 2	Splicing RNAm	Poor prognosis	[35,36]
MYD88	3%	Chromosome 3	NF-κB signaling	Good prognosis	[36,37]

3.2. Microenvironment

The advancement of tumors involves an intricate process governed by the dynamic interaction between tumor cells and the host immune system. The interaction between the modified functionalities of innate and adaptive immune factors plays a pivotal role in the initiation, progression, and response to treatment in CLL [38]. T cells have some anti-tumor activity, particularly Th1 cells that produce interferon gamma (IFN-γ). Furthermore, regulatory T cells (Treg) play a prominent role in tumor pathogenesis. In CLL patients, the number of Treg cells is increased, and they show signs of exhaustion in proliferation and cellular activity [39].

T cells are primarily responsible for cytokine production. Therefore, alterations in the balance of these molecules increase resistance to cell apoptosis or programmed cell death. The main cytokines affected in CLL patients are interleukin 2 (IL-2), interleukin 4 (IL-4), interleukin 6 (IL-6), interleukin 8 (IL-8), interleukin 9 (IL-9), and interleukin 10 (IL-10) [40]. The CLL implications of each of these are summarized in Table 2.

Table 2. Role of cytokines in CLL.

Cytokine	Action	Mechanism	Ref.
Il-2	Improves the function of CLL cells.	Promotes the differentiation and proliferation of CLL cells.	[41]
Il-4	Increases CLL cell survival and proliferation. Reduces apoptosis.	Activates JAK/STAT signaling pathway and enhances expression of antiapoptotic proteins.	[42]
Il-6	Increases CLL cell survival and proliferation.	Activates JAK/STAT signaling pathway and enhances expression of antiapoptotic proteins.	[43]
Il-8	Survival and chemoresistance of CLL cells.	Activates JAK/STAT signaling pathway.	[44]
Il-9	Stimulates growth and survival of CLL cells.	Activates the JAK/STAT pathway and the phosphatidylinositol phosphokinase subunit 3 (PI3K)/Akt/mTOR signaling pathway.	[45]
Il-10	Suppresses anti-tumor immunity.	Reduce the production of effector CD4 and CD8 T cells.	[46]
Il-17	Increases CLL cell survival and proliferation.	Activates the NF-κB pathway and increases the expression of antiapoptotic proteins.	[47]
TNF-α	Induces apoptosis.	Attaches to the TNF receptor found on CLL cells, activating caspases to induce programmed cell death.	[48]
IFN-γ	Inhibits proliferation.	Attaches to the IFN-γ receptor present on CLL cells, initiating the JAK-STAT pathway to hinder cell proliferation.	[49]

In CLL patients, a macrophage population acquires a pro-tumor phenotype driven by the CLL cells themselves through the secretion of soluble factors (e.g., IL-10, adenosine, and nicotinamide phosphoribosyl transferase) [50].

In these patients, dendritic cells exhibit dysfunctionality, characterized by changes in the cytokine profile, the absence of the maturation antigen CD83, and the co-stimulatory molecule CD80. Additionally, there is an incapacity to initiate appropriate type 1 T cell responses [49].

The tumor microenvironment of the lymphoid niche is highly hypoxic, and the cells are practically adapted to oxygen deprivation [51]. This stimulates the generation of energy through glycolysis by means of HIF1-α-mediated transcriptional control, tightly managing the expression of glycolytic enzymes as well as glucose and lactate transporters. This encourages a regulatory T-cell phenotype by increasing FOXP3 expression, along with PD-1, IL-10, and VEGFA, while reducing IFN-γ [52].

This metabolic adaptation is accompanied by increased production and release into the extracellular space of intermediates and cofactors such as nicotinamide adenine dinucleotide and adenosine triphosphate. High adenosine signaling is widely associated with immunosuppression in cancer through significantly decreased production of IL-10 and IL-6, negative modulation of T-cell and macrophage depletion markers, and reduced expansion of Treg [51,52].

4. Diagnosis, Risk Assessment, and Prognosis

The diagnostic criteria for CLL established by the World Health Organization (WHO), iwCLL, the National Comprehensive Cancer Network (NCCN), and the European Society for Medical Oncology (ESMO) are based on the morphology and immunophenotype of neoplastic B-cells. This includes the co-expression of CD19, CD5, and CD23, with weak CD20 and monoclonal surface immunoglobulin expression [53].

However, the current diagnostic criteria have certain limitations, particularly concerning the flexibility in the requirement for the presence or absence of each marker and the required expression level of each marker. According to the WHO definition, CLL/SLL cells typically co-express CD5 and CD23, and flow cytometry reveals that tumor cells express dim surface IgM/IgD, CD20, CD22, CD5, CD19, CD79a, CD23, CD43, and CD11c (weak). CD10 is negative, and FMC7 and CD79b are usually negative or weakly expressed in typical CLL. It is also acknowledged that some cases may exhibit an atypical immunophenotype [54].

The diagnosis of CLL necessitates the presence of $\geq 5 \times 10^9$/L B lymphocytes in the peripheral blood, persisting for a minimum of 3 months. Confirmation of the clonality of these B lymphocytes is crucial and can be achieved by demonstrating immunoglobulin light chain restriction through flow cytometry. Morphologically, leukemic cells identified in the blood smear exhibit characteristics such as small, mature lymphocytes with a narrow cytoplasmic border, a dense nucleus lacking evident nucleoli, and partially aggregated chromatin. Gumprecht nuclear shadows, also known as smudge cells, are commonly observed as cellular debris in association with CLL. A small proportion of larger or atypical cells, including prolymphocytes, may be present alongside morphologically typical CLL cells. A diagnosis of prolymphocytic leukemia is favored if ≥ 55% of prolymphocytes are detected. However, the diagnostic process is intricate and relies on morphological criteria, as no reliable immunological or genetic marker has been identified. A substantial presence of circulating prolymphocytes indicates a potentially more aggressive form of CLL [55].

CLL cells express the surface antigen CD5 in conjunction with B-cell antigens CD19, CD20, and CD23. Each clone of leukemia cells is restricted to the expression of either κ or λ immunoglobulin light chains. A recent standardization effort has affirmed that a panel consisting of CD19, CD5, CD20, CD23, κ, and λ is typically adequate for establishing the diagnosis. In ambiguous cases, markers such as CD43, CD79b, CD81, CD200, CD10, or ROR1 may be useful in refining the diagnosis [56].

The immunophenotype of CLL cells has been incorporated into a scoring system designed to aid in distinguishing between CLL and other B-cell leukemias during the differential diagnosis. The categorization of leukemic mature lymphoproliferative disorders (LPD) through flow cytometry has traditionally revolved around the Moreau score, which was introduced in 1997. The results of this study suggested that the SN8 antibody might be a useful marker to differentiate between CLL and non-CLL. The highest accuracy was found for SN8, followed by CD23 and CD5. Within the standard panel, CD5 and CD23, and to a lesser extent, CD22, emerged as the most reliably scored markers in CLL. However, these markers may also yield positive scores in non-CLL cases. Conversely, SmIg and, to a lesser degree, FMC7 stand out as markers with the lowest occurrence of false-positive scores in non-CLL scenarios [55].

In a recent study involving patients with LPD, it was observed that a significant proportion of individuals with LPD received different classifications in flow cytometry depending on the scores or diagnostic systems utilized. The analysis encompassed all published scores and diagnostic systems for CLL, revealing suboptimal concordance among them. Consequently, it concluded that relying on score-based flow cytometry assessment for LPD may not be ideal, especially in the current landscape where multiple scores are available without a consensus on their use or performance. Despite the substantial overlap in the markers considered and how they are evaluated, the study results imply that flow cytometric classification is somewhat variable, often hinging on dichotomous determinations of continuous variables. The findings suggest that, if employed, the most suitable scores or diagnostic systems for each flow cytometry unit are likely influenced by various technical factors (such as the availability of antibodies) and interpretive preferences (e.g., fluorescence intensity versus the percentage of positive cells). Exploring non-score-based systems, such as the "full phenotype" system, appears to be a worthwhile consideration. Finally, the study underscores the importance of evaluating the reproducibility of the integrated diagnosis of leukemic LPD, encompassing not only flow cytometry but also cytology, cytogenetics, and molecular biology [57].

Numerous additional tests, although not mandatory for confirming a CLL diagnosis, are essential in assessing the patient's prognosis and clinical condition. Table 3 delineates the diagnostic factors specified in different guidelines for diagnosing CLL.

Table 3. The amendments from iwCLL, ERIC, and ESMO about the diagnosis regime.

	Morphology and Immunophenotype	Test Genetic	Radiographic Imaging	Prognosis	Refs.
	Obligatory				
ESMO	Diagnosis is usually possible through immunophenotyping peripheral blood only (III, A). LN biopsy and/or bone marrow biopsy may be helpful if immunophenotyping is not conclusive for the diagnosis of CLL (IV, A).	Del(17p), *TP53*mut, and IGHV status should be assessed before treatment (III, A). In the early and asymptomatic stage is not recommended (V, D).	It is not recommended in asymptomatic patients. Recommended for pulmonary symptomatic patients. Recommended before treatment with the BCL2 inhibitor to assess the tumor load and risk of tumor lysis syndrome.	Binet and Rai staging systems are relevant for treatment indication (III, A)	[58]
iwCLL	Obligatory	Molecular cytogenetics (FISH) for del(13q), del(11q), del(17p), and add (12) in PB lymphocytes. (Desirable). Conventional karyotyping in PB lymphocytes (Desirable). *TP53* mutation (needed to establish a prognostic profile in addition to the clinical staging). IGHV mutational status (needed to establish a prognostic profile in addition to the clinical staging). Serum β_2-microglobulin (Desirable).	CT scan of chest, abdomen, and pelvis (Desirable) MRI and PET scans (NGI) Abdominal ultrasound (NGI)	Binet and Rai staging systems. CLL-IPI (Desirable).	[9]

Table 3. Cont.

	Morphology and Immunophenotype	Test Genetic	Radiographic Imaging	Prognosis	Refs.
ERIC	Obligatory	Strongly needed TP53 gene before starting the first and each subsequent line of treatment. Analyzing exons 4–10 is a minimal requirement with Sanger sequencing or NGS. Strongly needed to interpret IGHV mutational analysis before starting the first line of treatment. Alignment and determination of homology with PAGE or GeneScan.			[59,60]

CLL-IPI: CLL international prognostic index, NGI: not generally indicated, PAGE: Polyacrylamide gel electrophoresis, and PB: peripherical blood.

The diagnostic procedure depends on the primary set of findings, usually characterized by the key finding of lymphocytosis with or without accompanying lymphadenopathy. A time-dependent evaluation is shown in Figure 2.

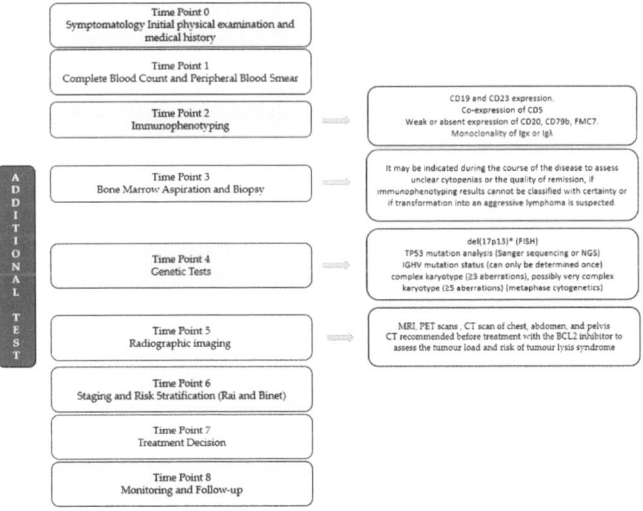

Figure 2. A time-dependent evaluation of diagnosis.

There are two widely accepted systems for use in both clinical practice and clinical trials: the Rai [61] and Binet [62] classifications. These two staging systems are simple, inexpensive, and based on standard physical examinations and laboratory tests. They do not require imaging techniques without considering imaging techniques. They provide information on tumor burden and the prognosis of patients. However, these scales do not identify patients with aggressive behavior, especially in the early stages, nor do they identify the possible response to a given treatment.

The Rai staging system categorizes low-risk disease as individuals with lymphocytosis and the presence of leukemic cells in the blood and/or marrow (lymphoid cells > 30%) —formerly classified as Rai stage 0. Intermediate-risk disease, previously designated as stage I or stage II, is characterized by lymphocytosis, enlarged lymph nodes in any location, and the presence of splenomegaly and/or hepatomegaly. Patients with these features who have anemia (hemoglobin (Hb) less than 11 g/dL) (formerly stage III) or thrombocytopenia (platelet count less than 100×10^9/L) (formerly stage IV) are considered high-risk disease patients [11,61].

Moreover, the Binet staging system relies on the enumeration of affected regions, characterized by the presence of enlarged lymph nodes exceeding 1 cm in diameter or organomegaly, along with the existence of anemia or thrombocytopenia. The implicated areas encompass (1) the head and neck, including Waldeyer's ring; (2) axillae; (3) groin, including superficial femoral; (4) a palpable spleen; and (5) a palpable (clinically enlarged) liver. Within the Binet staging system, stage A is defined by Hb $\geq$ 10 g/dL and platelets $\geq 100 \times 10^9$/L, with involvement of up to two of the aforementioned regions; stage B includes Hb $\geq$ 10 g/dL and platelets $\geq 100 \times 10^9$/L, with organomegaly exceeding that defined for stage A; and stage C is characterized by Hb less than 10 g/dL and/or a platelet count less than 100×10^9/L [62].

Due to recent advances in CLL treatment, these clinical staging systems have become insufficient to distinguish prognostic subgroups as they do not consider the aberrations in genetics or chromosomes discussed previously [11]. Consequently, the CLL international prognostic index (CLL-IPI) [63] was developed that combines clinical, biological, and genetic information [11,64–66]. This system employs five prognostic factors: TP53 deletion and/or mutation, variable immunoglobulin heavy chain mutational status, serum β2-microglobulin, clinical stage, and age.

According to the prognostic factor score, the patients will be classified as a risk group (low, intermediate, high, and very high risk) associated with a 5-year overall survival (OS) [63]. Its main limitation is that it has been validated in patients treated mainly with immunochemotherapy, its applicability has not yet been clearly demonstrated for new treatments directed at specific targets, and it can only be used in the prognostic evaluation of patients if the necessary molecular studies are available. Therefore, it is not a score that is used in clinical practice [30].

Despite the progress made with the implementation of the CLL-IPI index, factors such as tumor metabolism during leukemogenesis and the importance of nutritional status remain underrepresented [67]. Hypocholesterolemia has been reported in oncohematological disorders. Decreased levels of total cholesterol, HDL-C, and LDL-C were observed in patients with multiple myeloma [68], lymphoma [69], and, most recently, in patients with newly diagnosed CLL [70]. One study [67] developed a prognostic nomogram including these analytical parameters at the time of diagnosis as a significant predictive predictor. However, there is not enough evidence to incorporate it into clinical practice.

CLL has one of the strongest hereditary predispositions for hematologic malignancies. As many as 10% of individuals who develop the disease have a prior family history. Other risk factors that have been found are living on a farm or exposure to herbicides and pesticides, a medical history of atopic conditions, exposure to hepatitis C, and common infections [71].

Further mutations or chromosomal changes acquired throughout the course of the disease contribute to a more aggressive pathology that becomes resistant to treatment. Deletion of chromosome 13q del(13q) is observed in around 55% of cases, while the acquisition of chromosome 12 (trisomy 12) occurs in 10–20% of cases. Del(11q) is present in roughly 10% of cases and del(17p) in approximately 5–8% of cases, although these aberrations typically occur in the later stages of the disease [72].

Genetic mutations influence disease prognosis and response to treatment. Therefore, patients with mutated VIGCs are associated with a better prognosis [73]. Recurrent mutations in MYD88 have been tentatively linked to a positive prognosis, although the evidence is not definitive [40]. Conversely, individuals with del(17p) exhibited poorer survival, whereas those with del(13q) or trisomy 12 demonstrated more favorable outcomes. Patients harboring del(11q) displayed an intermediate survival rate. CLL patients with mutations in TP53, NOTCH1, SF3B1, ATM, or BIRC3 were associated with an unfavorable prognosis [28,30,33–36].

The prognostic and therapeutic implications of TP53mut alterations are noteworthy. Its presence, as well as that of del(17p), implies an adverse prognosis and a poor response to conventional CIT. The PFS and OS of patients with del(17p) and those with TP53mut in the absence of del(17p) are similar, and therefore it is mandatory to study both in patients requiring treatment, both first-line and relapsed. It is also relevant that the incidence of TP53 alterations increases progressively as the disease progresses. This phenomenon is mainly because chemotherapy-resistant subclones are not eliminated and progress years later. Patients who received FCR or BR have much higher rates of TP53mut at relapse than at baseline [74]. This increase is also observed in other alterations with a poor prognosis, such as NOTCH1, SF3B1, and BIRC3, although not as markedly [32,75].

Genomic aberrations at CLL diagnosis, such as TP53 disruption, trisomy 12, and NOTCH1 mutation, increase the risk of Richter transformation (RT). RT is identified by a shift in histopathology and biology from the original CLL. It is characterized as the emergence of an aggressive lymphoma in individuals previously diagnosed with or concurrently experiencing CLL [76]. Additional risk factors contributing to the development of RT include bulky lymphadenopathy or hepato-splenomegaly, elevated beta-2-microglobulin, low platelet count, advanced disease stage, prior CLL therapy involving a combination of purine analogs and alkylating agents, and a higher number of lines of therapy [76,77].

It is linked to an unfavorable prognosis, with a median survival of less than one year. Managing the condition is intricate, and currently, available therapeutic approaches yield limited success in achieving sustained responses. Initial treatment for RT typically involves anthracycline-based chemotherapy regimens like R-CHOP (rituximab, cyclophosphamide, doxorubicin, vincristine, and prednisone) or R-EPOCH (rituximab, etoposide, prednisolone, vincristine, cyclophosphamide, and doxorubicin), as well as platinum-containing regimens such as ESHAP (etoposide, methylprednisolone, cytarabine, and cisplatin) and DHAP (dexamethasone, cytarabine, and cisplatin). Over the last five years, several new therapeutic options have emerged as possible treatments for individuals with B-cell malignancies, and their effectiveness in managing patients with RT has been assessed. These encompass targeted small-molecule inhibitors, innovative monoclonal antibodies (mAb), and approaches centered on stimulating an anti-tumor immune response, notably chimeric antigen receptor (CAR-T) cell therapy and T-cell-engaging bispecific antibodies [78].

5. Selecting the Right Treatment: How to Treat CLL?

Currently, initiation of treatment in patients with CLL in the first-line and relapsed disease should only consider patients with active or symptomatic disease. Initiation of treatment is recommended if the patient meets one of the criteria described in iwCLL guidelines [5].

Asymptomatic patients with early-stage CLL (Rai 0, Binet A) have not demonstrated the benefit of early therapeutic interventions. Therefore, they are initially managed without pharmacological treatment.

When initiating treatment for CLL, the patient's age, the presence of alterations in renal, cardiac, pulmonary, hepatic, and immunological functions, and life expectancy should be considered. The Cumulative Illness Rating Scale (CIRS) is the most widely used in the different clinical trials of CLL when measuring comorbidities [79].

Although CLL predominantly affects older adults, risk stratification systems for CLL have not focused on geriatric domains, such as subjective and objective measures of function and cognition [80]. This patient profile is characterized by medical and psychosocial problems that affect their ability to tolerate treatment and contribute to negative outcomes and increased morbidity. The unfit patient is, therefore, defined as that fraction of patients with marked comorbidity that prevents them from tolerating CIT regimens [17]. Thus, a comprehensive geriatric assessment (CGA) can help to robustly characterize health status and represent a better measure of the health of elderly patients than a simple assessment of functional status or consideration of chronological age alone.

Although most studies have been reported in patients with solid tumors [81,82], studies demonstrate the importance of geriatric assessment in hematological malignancies [83–86]. Previous research on older adults undergoing chemotherapy for various hematologic malignancies has identified a correlation between the degree of geriatric impairments and OS. [80,85–88].

In "unfit" patients, in parallel to assessing the presence and type of comorbidities and the existence of concomitant treatments, it is important to evaluate the convenience of prescribing indefinite or time-limited treatment and the convenience of indefinite versus time-limited treatment. A finite treatment has the advantage of higher patient convenience, and it is usually associated with lower toxicity [17]. It is important to evaluate not only the treatment's effectiveness and safety but also drug accessibility, associated costs, and therapeutic objectives [89].

6. Treatment of CLL

6.1. Cytostatic Agents

Alkylating agents were the first therapeutic options for the treatment of CLL. Chlorambucil was the gold standard treatment until 1990 [90]. Despite the advantages of oral administration and its low cost, the overall response rate (ORR) oscillated between 35 and 65%. The limited efficacy combined with the side effects of prolonged use (cytopenia and myelodysplastic syndromes/acute leukemia) result in limited use of this treatment. A palliative prescription may be considered for elderly or unfit patients. The combination of chlorambucil with corticosteroids or other chemotherapy (CHOP) has not been shown to be superior to monotherapy [91].

Purine analogs were then introduced into CLL treatment, especially fludarabine, pentostatin, and cladribine. Fludarabine was notable for its superior ORR compared to other treatment regimens available at the time. However, fludarabine used as monotherapy did not demonstrate an increase in OS [92].

Bendamustine is an alkylating agent that is structurally intermediate between alkylating agents and purine analogs, with the advantage of lower hematological toxicity. It showed significantly superior efficacy to chlorambucil in the first line with significantly higher OR and PFS rates (29 vs. 4% and 68 vs. 39%, respectively). In relapsed or refractory (r/r) CLL, it demonstrated a superior OR rate to fludarabine (76 vs. 62%) and PFS (27 vs. 9%). The combination with mAb increases response rates [93].

6.2. Monoclonal Antibodies

The predominant choices involve antibodies targeting CD20. It is believed that this protein functions as a calcium channel within the cell membrane. Given its presence in most B-cell malignancies, the incorporation of these antibodies has enhanced the treatment outcomes for CLL [94].

Rituximab was the first chimeric mAb directed against an epitope of this molecule that demonstrated an antitumor effect in virtually all mature B neoplasms. This agent can induce direct tumor lysis by apoptosis and activation of antibody-dependent cytotoxicity (ADCC) and antibody-dependent cytotoxicity (CDC) mechanisms. Its efficacy as a monotherapy agent in CLL or maintenance therapy is limited. The response rate is lower than other types of lymphomas, probably related to the lower expression density in CLL. However, its association with the chemotherapy regimens used (fludarabine, pentostatin, and cyclophosphamide) resulted in a significant improvement in the treatment of CLL [79].

Obinutuzumab is a humanized and glycoengineered mAb, which resulted in higher affinity binding to a type II CD20 epitope and greater direct induction of cell death. The GAUGUIN trial (phase 1/2) evaluated obinutuzumab monotherapy in patients with r/r

CLL. It demonstrated that obinutuzumab was an active treatment. ORR was 62% (phase 1) and 30% (phase 2). Phase 2 median PFS was 10.7 months [95].

Ofatumumab is a humanized MoAct directed against a different CD20 epitope than rituximab, with a higher CDC lytic capacity and an ADCC similar to rituximab. In the randomized phase II trial of 201 patients with r/r CLL refractory to fludarabine and alemtuzumab or fludarabine/presence of mass greater than 5 cm, ofatunumab alone achieved an OR rate of 51% and 44%, respectively [96]. A clinical trial studied the efficacy and safety of ofatumumab versus ibrutinib. The OS rate was significantly higher for ibrutinib (hazard ratio for death in the ibrutinib group, 0.43; 95% CI, 0.24 to 0.79; $p = 0.005$), as was the response rate (42.6% vs. 4.1%, $p < 0.001$). As a result, this treatment is rarely used in clinical practice [97].

Ublituximab is another anti-CD 20, a chimeric antibody with a higher affinity for FcγRIIIa/CD16 receptors and a higher ADCC compared to rituximab. As a monotherapy agent, it induces up to a 50% response in patients with r/r CLL. This agent is currently under development in combination with BTKi, PI3K, and B-cell lymphoma gene 2 (BCL-2) [98].

Alemtuzumab is an anti-CD52 antigen that is recombinant and fully humanized. In monotherapy, response rates range from 33% to 53%, and the median duration of response falls within the range of 8.7 to 15.4 months. This applies specifically to patients with advanced CLL who were previously treated with alkylating agents and experienced failure or relapse after undergoing second-line treatment with fludarabine. It is also a particularly active drug in patients with high-risk genetic markers such as del17p/TP53mut. The main limitation is its profound immunosuppression, with a high rate of opportunistic infections that require a triple antibiotic, antifungal, and antiviral prophylaxis and close patient monitoring. Its marketing license was removed in 2012, and it can only be used on a compassionate use basis [99,100].

Otlertuzumab is a single-chain anti-CD37 Ac capable of inducing a 23% response rate in monotherapy. It has also been combined with bendamustine and compared in a phase II trial to bendamustine alone, with a significantly higher response rate (69 vs. 39%; $p = 0.02$) and median PFS (15.9 vs. 10.1 months; $p = 0.019$) [101].

6.3. Chemoimmunotherapy

CIT remains a viable choice for fit patients with low- and intermediate-risk CLL. The combination of FCR stands out as a well-established standard of care for patients eligible for treatment without the presence of del(17p) and/or TP53mut. Several clinical studies have explored the application of CIT in CLL patients. Table 4 summarizes the main studies carried out on this subject.

Table 4. Clinical studies of CIT use in CLL patients.

Clinical Study	Type of Study	Eligible Patients	Treatment	Endpoints	Conclusion	Ref.
FLAIR	Open label Randomized Phase III Controlled	Age between 18 and 75 years WHO performance status of 2 or lower Previously untreated CLL	Ibrutinib + rituximab (IR) vs. FCR	PFS	BR demonstrated a notable enhancement in PFS. It did not result in a significant improvement in OS.	[102]
CCL18	Multicenter Phase II Prospective Non-randomized	18 years old WHO performance status of 0 to 2 Life expectancy of at least 12 weeks Adequate renal and liver function	IR	Safety and efficacy of BR in previously untreated patients.	Apart from those with del(17p) who showed resistance to the treatment, the combination of BR is a safe and effective treatment for naïve CLL patients.	[103]
CCL10	Phase III Randomized Open label	Untreated fit patients with advanced CLL without del(17p)	FCR vs. BR	ORR	Smaller difference in median PFS between FCR and BR as well as no difference in OS.	[104]
ICLL-07-Filo	Phase II	≥18 years Binet stage C or Binet stage A and B with active disease. No prior treatment Absence of del(17p).	Obinutuzumab + ibrutinib followed by ibrutinib in patients achieving CR vs. FC-obinutuzumab in conjunction with ibrutinib.	PFS, OS, and minimal residual disease (MRD) in PB.	CIT with a set duration resulted in profound and lasting responses, leading to high survival rates. No distinctions were observed in the extent and persistence of MRD responses in PB based on the IGHV mutational status.	[105]

It should be noted that CIT has a limited, if any, role in treating CLL because this class of drugs is inferior to BTKi and venetoclax-based regimens in different clinical settings. It also causes an increased risk of therapy-related myeloid malignancy and infections. In the CLL13 study trial, which was performed with venetoclax plus anti-CD20 antibodies as a first-line treatment in fit patients, it can be appreciated that treatment with VO or VO-ibrutinib produced a significant PFS benefit in IGHVum patients but not in IGHVm patients. In these patients, improving the high efficacy of the FCR regimen in young, generally well-conditioned patients may be difficult. However, as a finite therapy, venetoclax has the benefit of a lower risk of toxicity and adverse events (AE) associated with treatment, as well as second malignancies or clonal selection. Hence, the use of FCR is less and less recommended, even though numerous clinical guidelines still state the contrary [106].

6.4. Agents Targeting the Signaling in CLL Cells and in Their Microenvironment

A detailed study of the pathophysiology of the disease has been key to the design of specific molecules targeting several tyrosine kinases involved in the main intracellular signaling pathways that are key to tumor cell survival and proliferation, including BTK and PI3K.

6.4.1. PI3K Inhibitors: Idelalisib, Duvelisib, and Umbralisib

Idelalisib is an irreversible inhibitor of the δ-subunit of the catalytic portion of PI3K, blocking the transmission of signals from BCR and reducing the phosphorylation of AKT. This results in reduced interaction with the cellular microenvironment. It is administered with rituximab. In the phase III trial comparing idelalisib + rituximab with placebo + rituximab, the response rate was 81 vs. 13% ($p < 0.001$), respectively, with a significantly higher OS at 12 months (92 vs. 80%; $p = 0.02$). This study showed that the drug was active in patients with 17p deletion and in patients with IGHVum. Drug toxicity severely limits its use, including high rates of myelosuppression, grade ≥ 3 transaminitis, and colitis [107].

Duvelisib is a dual PI3kδ and PI3kγ inhibitor. The phase Ib monotherapy trial demonstrated 74% ORR in patients with r/r CLL. Although its activity is remarkable, and the FDA has approved it for treating r/r CLLL, its development has also been limited by toxicity (mainly hematological and hepatic toxicity) and has not been approved by the EMA [108]. In 2022, the FDA issued a safety alert warning about the possible increased risk of death and severe side effects such as infections, diarrhea, inflammation of the intestines and lungs, skin reactions, and elevated levels of liver enzymes in the blood. As a result, this treatment is not reflected in CLL clinical guidelines [109].

Umbralisib is a PI3Kδ inhibitor with a markedly different chemical structure from the ones above. The phase I trial showed 85% OR in patients with r/r CLL with a significantly lower frequency of hepatotoxicity and colitis [110]. Recently, the UNITY study explored umbralisib in combination with ublituximab in treatment-naïve and r/r CLL and provided a median PFS of 32 versus 18 months after a median follow-up of 36 months [111].

6.4.2. BTK Inhibitors: Ibrutinib, Acalabrutinib, Zanubritinib, and Pirtobrutinib

Ibrutinib

This orally active, small-molecule BTKi triggers apoptosis in B-cell lymphomas and CLL cells. BTK participates in migration and tissue adhesion pathways. Its inhibition leads to a redistribution of neoplastic lymphocytes into the bloodstream, where they die via apoptosis. Patients generally respond to ibrutinib initially with a rapid reduction in lymph node size and transient peripheral blood lymphocytosis, which appears after 4–6 weeks and resolves spontaneously in 80% of cases within the first year of treatment [112]. Table 5 shows the main clinical studies carried out with this drug.

Table 5. Ibrutinib clinical studies in patients with CLL or SLL.

Clinical Study	Type of Study	Eligible Patients	Treatment	Endpoints	Conclusion	Refs.
RESONATE-2	Phase III, randomized, open label, multicenter.	CLL and small SLL patients (naïve or previously treated) and ineligible for purine analog therapy.	Ibrutinib vs. chlorambucil as first-line treatment	PFS, ORR, safety.	Ibrutinib demonstrated an extended OS. The extended RESONATE-2 data illustrate the advantages of initiating treatment with ibrutinib, even for patients exhibiting high risk.	[113,114]

Table 5. Cont.

Clinical Study	Type of Study	Eligible Patients	Treatment	Endpoints	Conclusion	Refs.
PCYC-1102	Phase Ib/II study.	Patients receiving single-agent ibrutinib in first-line or r/r CLL/SLL.	Ibrutinib	Frequency and severity of AE	Ibrutinib demonstrated prolonged responses and sustained tolerability in first-line r/r CLL/SLL. Individuals who had a history of ≥ 4 prior therapies and those with del(17p) exhibited a higher frequency of progression.	[115]
ILLUMINATE	Phase III, randomized, open label.	Untreated CLL/SLL patients. Aged ≥ 65 or <65 years. At least one of the following conditions: cumulative illness rating score > 6, creatinine clearance < 70 mL/min, del(17p), or TP53 mut.	Ibrutinib + obinutuzumab vs. chlorambucil + obinutuzumab as a first-line therapy	PFS	Ibrutinib + obinutuzumab for individuals with previously untreated CLL showed prolonged PFS compared to chlorambucil + Obinutuzumab.	[116]
E1912	Phase III, randomized.	CLL naïve patients aged 70 or less years.	Long-term efficacy ibrutinib + rituximab vs. FCR	PFS, OS	OS improvement in patients treated with ibrutinib + rituximab. This therapy provides better PFS compared to FCR in both IGHVm and IGHVum CLL patients.	[117]
ALLIANCE A041202	Phase III, randomized, open label.	Adults aged ≥ 65 years who had not received prior treatment for CLL.	BR vs. ibrutinib vs. ibrutinib + rituximab	PFS	Ibrutinib demonstrates superior PFS in older CLL patients compared to BR. However, the disparity in treatment duration complicates the comparison of AE.	[118,119]

In addition, we found a phase II study providing information on the first-line use of ibrutinib in patients with CLL and del 17p/TP53 mut. In this study, 51 patients with CLL with del17p or TP53mut treated first-line or r/r were treated with ibrutinib. A response was achieved in 97% of first-line patients, and in r/r patients, 80% had a response. OS at 24 months was 80% in first-line patients and 74% in r/r patients [120].

The tolerability profile is very favorable; diarrhea, rash, muscle pain, spasms, and infections tend to progressively disappear after 6–12 months of treatment. Medium-term AEs include hypertension and complete atrial fibrillation arrhythmia. These side effects are the main cause of long-term drug discontinuation [121]. This treatment achieves one of the best remission durations documented to date. One of his main problems is that it is an indefinite therapy.

Acalabrutinib

It is a highly selective irreversible covalent inhibitor of second-generation BTK with lower affinity for IL-2-inducible kinase (ITK) and epidermal growth factor receptor (EGFR). This lower affinity theoretically results in a reduction of the side effects of ibrutinib. It is indicated as monotherapy or in combination with obinutuzumab for treating adult patients with CLL who are previously untreated or have received at least one previous treatment [122]. Table 6 summarizes the clinical trials performed with acalabrutinib.

Table 6. Acalabrutinib clinical studies in patients with CLL or SLL.

Clinical Study	Type of Study	Eligible Patients	Treatment	Endpoint	Conclusion	Refs.
ELEVATE-TN	Phase III, randomized, controlled.	Untreated patients aged ≥ 65 years.	Acalabrutinib + obinutuzumab, acalabrutinib or obinutuzumab + chlorambucil	PFS	Acalabrutinib, or acalabrutinib + obinutuzumab, demonstrated a significant enhancement in PFS compared to obinutuzumab + chlorambucil. Consider acalabrutinib monotherapy or in combination with obinutuzumab as treatment in naïve patients.	[123]
ASCEND	Phase III, randomized, open label, multicenter.	Patients aged ≥ 18 years diagnosed with CLL who had undergone at least one systemic therapy before.	Acalabrutinib, Idelasib + rituximab (idR) or BR	PFS	Meaningful enhancement in PFS when comparing acalabrutinib monotherapy to IdR or BR treatment regimens. Acalabrutinib demonstrated tolerability and profile. These results support the use of acalabrutinib monotherapy as a treatment for patients with r/r CLL, including those presenting high risk.	[124,125]

Table 6. Cont.

Clinical Study	Type of Study	Eligible Patients	Treatment	Endpoint	Conclusion	Refs.
ELEVATE R/R	Phase III, randomized, international. multicenter, open label, non-inferiority.	Individuals who had undergone at least one previous therapy. ECOG ≤ 2 del(17) (p13.1) and/or del(11).	Acalabrutinib vs. ibrutinib	PFS	Acalabrutinib exhibited non-inferiority to ibrutinib in terms of PFS. There was a statistically significant reduction in the incidence of atrial fibrillation/flutter with acalabrutinib in patients with previously treated CLL. The incidence of hypertension was higher with ibrutinib.	[126]
MAJIC	Phase III, prospective, multicenter, randomized, open label.	Adults with naïve CLL/SLL meeting indication for treatment.	Acalabrutinib + venetoclax (AV) vs. VO	PFS	Evaluation to see if MRD-guided limited AV treatment is comparable to MRD-guided limited VO treatment in terms of PFS. The study is still in progress.	[127]

Zanubrutinib

It is a second-generation oral BTKi that irreversibly and covalently binds to the catalytic region of BTK, blocking its function. It proved to be more selective than ibrutinib against BTK in relation to other similar enzymes. Particularly remarkable is the selectivity of zanubrutinib for ITK and EGFR enzymes, resulting in less inhibition of T and NK cell function and greater antibody-dependent cytotoxicity for zanubrutinib [128].

However, for HER4, the difference between zanubrutinib and ibrutinib was marginal, and there were no significant differences with respect to three other kinases: BMX/ETK, BLK, and TXK [128]. As we can see in Table 7, there are several studies carried out with zanubrutinib.

Table 7. Zanubrutinib clinical studies in patients with CLL or SLL.

Clinical Study	Type of Study	Eligible Patients	Treatment	Endpoints	Conclusion	Ref.
SEQUOIA	Phase III, open-label, multicenter study	Previously untreated CLL or SLL ≥65 or ≥18 years ECOG 0-2	Zanubrutinib vs. BR	PFS	Zanubrutinib showed a notable improvement in PFS and safety profile compared to BR accompanied. These results lend support to zanubrutinib as a potential treatment option for untreated CLL and SLL.	[128]

Table 7. Cont.

Clinical Study	Type of Study	Eligible Patients	Treatment	Endpoints	Conclusion	Ref.
ALPINE	Head-to-head Phase III study	r/r CLL/SLL patients	Zanubrutinib vs. ibrutinib	ORR PFS OS	Zanubrutinib demonstrated superiority over ibrutinib in terms of PFS, OS, and safety profile. In patients with del17p, TP53mut, or both, those treated with zanubrutinib experienced PFS compared with ibrutinib.	[129]
NCT03206918	Phase II, single-arm, multicenter study	r/r CLL/SLL patients	Zanubrutinib	ORR PFS	Results showed that administering zanubrutinib twice daily led to a significant occurrence of lasting responses. Zanubrutinib presents the possibility of enhanced safety and tolerability compared to current treatment choices.	[130]

The most frequently observed AEs included infections, neutropenia, and diarrhea. In general, events leading to treatment discontinuation were less prevalent with zanubrutinib compared to ibrutinib [120,130].

Pirtobrutinib

It is a highly selective yet reversible BTKi, exhibiting efficacy in patients with the C481S mutation of BTK.

BRUIN TRIAL: Open-label phase I/II trial. This study focused on determining the maximum tolerated dose (phase I) and ORR (phase II) of pirtobrutinib. The trial included patients treated for CLL or SLL. Pirtobrutinib exhibited an ORR of 62% in these individuals. ORR remained consistent across different CLL subgroups, including those with previous covalent BTKi resistance (67%), covalent BTKi intolerance (52%), C481-mutant BTK disease (71%), and wild-type BTK (66%). These results suggest that reversible BTKi, such as pirtobrutinib, may provide an alternative for patients facing intolerance or resistance to traditional BTKi [131].

6.5. BCL-2 Inhibitors

Venetoclax: It is a BCL-2 inhibitor (BCL-2i) that binds directly to the BH3 binding site. It displaces proapoptotic proteins with BH3 domains and initiates mitochondrial outer membrane permeabilization, activating the caspase pathway and programmed cell death. Thus, venetoclax depletes dendritic cells and total lymphocytes while reducing interferon α production [132]. Table 8 lists the main studies with venetoclax alone or in combination with other drugs.

Table 8. Venetoclax clinical studies in patients with CLL.

Clinical Study	Type of Study	Eligible Patients	Treatment	Endpoints	Conclusion	Refs.
CCL14	Phase III, multicenter, randomized, open label.	Untreated CLL ≥18 years.	VO vs. chlorambucil + Obinutuzumab.	PFS	2 years post-treatment discontinuation, the combination of VO demonstrated a significant enhancement of PFS compared to chlorambucil + obinutuzumab. In cases where the use of BTKi is not feasible due to potential AE, VO remains a reasonable choice.	[133,134]
CAPTIVATE	Phase II, randomized.	Previously untreated CLL patients age < 70 years.	3 cycles of ibrutinib, followed by 12 cycles of ibrutinib or ibrutinib + venetoclax. Confirmed undetectable MRD (uMRD): placebo or ibrutinib. Not confirmed uMRD: ibrutinib or ibrutinib + venetoclax.	1-year disease-free survival (DFS), uMRD status, and safety	The 95% 1-year DFS rate observed in patients randomly assigned to the placebo group, with confirmed uMRD, indicates the potential viability of a fixed-duration treatment using this all-oral, once-daily, chemotherapy-free regimen as a first line.	[135]
MURANO	Phase III, open label, randomized.	Patients with r/r CLL.	Venetoclax + rituximb (VR) vs. BR in patients with r/r CLL.	PFS, safety, and MRD status	VR treatment provides a long-lasting clinical response and confers a survival benefit compared to BR therapy.	[136]
GLOW	Phase III.	Patients aged ≤ 70 years with previously untreated CLL without del(17p) or tp53mut.	Fixed duration treatment ibrutinib + venetoclax.	Complete response (CR) rate, uMRD, PFS, OS, and safety	In older patients and/or those with comorbidities, the first-line treatment for CLL with ibrutinib + venetoclax exhibited superior PFS and achieved deeper and more enduring responses compared to chlorambucil–obinutuzumab.	[137]

Table 8. *Cont.*

Clinical Study	Type of Study	Eligible Patients	Treatment	Endpoints	Conclusion	Refs.
CLL2-GIVe	Phase II, open label, multicenter.	Previously untreated patients with high-risk CLL and del(17p)/TP53 mut.	Triple combination of obinutuzumab + ibrutinib + venetoclax.	CR rate at cycle 15, PFS, and OS	After a median observation period of 38.4 months, the study found a 79.9% PFS and a 92.6% OS at 36 months. The research suggests that the CLL2-GIVe regimen is a hopeful fixed-duration first-line treatment for patients with high-risk CLL.	[138,139]

6.6. Lenalidomide

It is a 4-aminoglutamyl analog of thalidomide with activity against various hematological malignancies. It has been shown to be an immunomodulator that affects the immune system and has anti-angiogenic properties. In people with CLL, lenalidomide might interact with cancer cells, affecting how CLL cells and their surroundings interact. The effectiveness and safety of using lenalidomide as an ongoing treatment for CLL are still uncertain and debated in different studies [140]. The ORR of lenalidomide monotherapy ranged from 32% to 54% [141]. In a long-term study of 60 patients, an OS of 82% was observed. Thirty-five (58%) patients had a response lasting longer than 36 months (long-term responders [LTR]). The best long-term responses were 25 (71%) CR and 10 (29%) PR [142]. Other studies of lenalidomide in maintenance versus placebo after second-line therapy did not demonstrate a significant improvement in OS [143].

6.7. Other Therapies: Allogeneic Transplantation and CAR-T

New targeted therapies have led to a decline in the utilization of allogeneic hematopoietic stem cell transplantation (alloHCT) in CLL patients. This shift is attributed to the significant morbidity risk associated with alloHCT, which includes organ toxicity, as well as the potential for acute and chronic graft-versus-host disease. Nevertheless, this therapy still has an important role, particularly for eligible patients with high-risk genetics. Within the category of high-risk patients, two distinct groups can be identified: high-risk I, characterized by clinically resistant disease to CIT with TP53 aberrations but a positive response to signaling pathway inhibitors, and high-risk II, marked by disease resistance to both CIT and signaling pathway inhibitors. In cases where resistance to BTKi and/or BCL-2 is observed, alloHCT could be a viable alternative, especially when therapeutic options are limited [144].

When choosing a patient for alloHCT, factors such as the patient's functional status, age, comorbidities, donor availability, status of del17p and TP53mut, prior treatment history and response duration, the level of response to the current therapy, and the availability of alternative treatment options should also be considered [145]. The benefits of alloHCT in CLL have never been confirmed with a randomized controlled trial; large data sets from retrospective studies demonstrate that alloHCT achieves durable remissions in up to 30–50% of patients with heavily pretreated CLL [146,147]. There is a suggestion that alloHCT is linked to a reduced risk of relapse and enhanced survival. However, it is crucial to interpret these findings with caution as the studies were conducted before the emergence of BTKi and BCL-2i, and there is a potential risk of selection bias [148].

Another therapy that is under study for refractory patients is CAR-T. In one study, 24 patients diagnosed with CLL who had previously undergone ibrutinib treatment were administered anti-CD19 CAR-T cell therapy. Four weeks following the infusion of CAR-T cells, the ORR stood at 71% (17 out of 24). Among the 19 patients re-evaluated, the ORR four weeks post-infusion was 74% (CR, in 4/19, 21%; Partial Response (PR) in 10/19, 53%). Moreover, 88% of the patients (15 out of 17) who had marrow disease before CAR-T cell treatment exhibited no disease via flow cytometry after CAR-T cells, and in 7 patients (58%), no malignant IGH sequences were detected [149].

In the TRANSCEND-CLL004 study, individuals with r/r CLL received lisocel as monotherapy, delivered in equal proportions of CD8+ and CD4+ CAR-T cells (23 patients), or a combination of lyocell and ibrutinib to enhance engraftment by BTKi (19 patients). Both groups displayed an ORR exceeding 90%. Cytokine release syndrome occurred in 74% of patients (9% graded as 3), and neurological events were observed in 39% (22% graded as 3/4) [150].

7. Selection of First-Line Treatment of Symptomatic Patients according to Clinical Guidelines and Expert Consensus

7.1. Treatment of Patients with del(17p) and/or TP53 Mutation

Aberrations in TP53 have been acknowledged to impart an unfavorable prognosis concerning response rate, PFS, and OS, especially with CIT but also with novel agents. However, there has not been a randomized clinical trial specifically exploring patients exclusively with del(17p) and/or TP53-mutated CLL. There are several recommendations regarding the treatment of patients with del(17p) or TP53mut. They are summarized in Table 9.

Table 9. Treatment recommendations in patients with del17 or tp53mut according to the main clinical guidelines.

Guideline	Drugs	Additional Information	Ref.
Spanish group of CLL (SGCLL)	Acalabrutinib Zanubrutinib Ibrutinib Ibrutinib + Venetoclax VO	Treatments are placed in order of recommendation.	[151]
Canadian Guideline	BTKi Ibrutinib Acalabrutinib	Favor ACAL for the best side effect profile. Indefinite therapy.	[152]
	VO	Improved PFS compared to CIT (chemoimmunotherapy). Less durable remission compared to BTKi. Finite therapy.	

Table 9. Cont.

Guideline	Drugs	Additional Information	Ref.
Expert consensus on the management of CLL in Asia	BTKi Ibrutinib Acalabrutinib	Preferred first-line treatment of choice for patients with del17p or TP53 mutation. Patients who are intolerant to ibrutinib or who have relative contraindications to ibrutinib may still tolerate acalabrutinib. Second-generation BTKi, including acalabrutinib, may have a better safety profile than ibrutinib, especially in patients with high-risk disease characteristics.	[153]
	VO	BCL-2i can be considered in all CLL patients in need of therapy, including those with high-risk genomic features such as TP53 abnormalities.	
JAMA (Journal of the American Medical Association) First-line treatment	Indefinite treatment BTKi Acalabrutinib Ibrutinib Zanubrutinib	Second-generation BTKi (acalabrutinib and zanubrutinib) is preferred, given improved safety extrapolating from head-to-head trials in patients with relapse. Zanubrutinib had superior efficacy compared with ibrutinib.	[154]
	Fixed duration treatment VO	Consider continuation of venetoclax in patients with abnormal TP53, especially in patients with evidence of detectable disease at 12 months.	
ESMO	Ibrutinib or Acalabrutinib VO Venetoclax IdR	For the choice between VO versus ibrutinib or other BTKis, time-limited therapy would be preferred, but side effect profile and application mode must be considered.	[58]
German Society for Haematology and Medical Oncology (DGHO)	Acalabrutinib Zanubrutinib Ibrutinib	Continuous use of BTKi, mainly acalabrutinib or zanubrutinib, is preferred. If acalabrutinib or zanubrutinib are contraindicated or unavailable, ibrutinib (+/− obinutuzumab) remains a therapeutic option.	[155]
	VO		
	Ibrutinib + Venetoclax	Since August 2022, time-limited combination therapy (14 months) based on ibrutinib + venetoclax is also possible in the first line, which also includes patients with high-risk aberration. Based on the CAPTIVATE study.	

7.2. Treatment of Patients with No TP53 Aberrations or del 17p

Patients ought to be categorized based on the mutational status of the IGHV gene locus, distinguishing between mutated and unmutated variants. In instances where prospective stratification proves challenging, the analysis should involve a subgroup assessment of IGHVm and IGHVum patients.

7.2.1. Mutated IGHV

As shown in Table 10, the recommendations made by the different clinical guidelines are very similar, distinguishing between FIT and non-FIT patients and with differences in their therapeutic approach, which we will see below.

Table 10. Treatment recommendations in patients with no del17p or tp53 mut and IGHVm according to the main clinical guidelines.

Guideline	Type of Patient	Drugs	Additional Information	Ref.
SGCLL	Assess CIT scheme adapted to age and/or comorbidities (FCR/BR or Chlorambucil-O) when it is not possible to administer recommended treatment	Ibrutinib + Venetoclax VO	Treatments are placed in order of recommendation.	[151]
		Acalabrutinib Zanubrutinib		
		Ibrutinib		
Canadian Guideline	FIT patients	FCR	Longest remissions documented to date and possibility of cure. Finite therapy (only 6 months).	[152]
		VO	Highly effective therapy with very long remissions.	
		BTKi (Acalabrutinib)	Long remissions. Indefinite therapy (high cost).	
	UNFIT patients	VO	Preferred therapy. Finite therapy (only 12 months).	
		Acalabrutinib	Indefinite therapy. Very high cost.	
		CIT	Shorter remission than V-O. Finite duration therapy.	
Expert consensus on the management of CLL in Asia	FIT patients	BTKi	Fit patients < 65 years of age with IGHVm.	[153]
		CIT	Either FCR or other novel agents may be considered. Inform young patients about the risk of secondary malignancy and offer the option of CIT or novel agents (BTKi).	
	UNFIT patients	VO	Both BTKi and BCL-2i have good clinical data to support their use.	
		BTKi		
ESMO	FIT patients	CIT: FCR or BR (patients > 65 years)	CIT is an alternative treatment used only if there is a reason for not using targeted therapies or when they are not available.	[58]
	UNFIT patients	VO CIT: Chlorambucil + Obinutuzumab, Ibrutinib, or Acalabrutinib		

Table 10. Cont.

Guideline	Type of Patient	Drugs	Additional Information	Ref.
DGHO		VO	If the genetic risk profile is favorable time-limited therapy with VO (12 cycles) should be preferred. If there are severe cardiac comorbidities, VO is primarily recommended.	[155]
	Acalabrutinib +/− Obinutuzumab		If renal function is impaired or if all-oral therapy is desired, primary therapy with a second-generation BTKi.	
	Zanubrutinib			
	Ibrutinib +/− Obinutuzumab		Higher cardiotoxicity of ibrutinib compared to second-generation BTKi. However, in the case of renal failure, preference should be given a BTKi.	
	Ibrutinib + Venetoclax		Can be used in intermediate-risk patients (IGHVum) as a temporary therapy (15 cycles).	

7.2.2. Unmutated IGHV

Patients with the IGHVum gene have an inferior outcome to those with the mutated IGHV gene. Table 11 shows the recommendations according to the different clinical practice guidelines for the treatment of this group of patients.

Table 11. Treatment recommendations in patients with no del17p or tp53mut and IGHVum according to the main clinical guidelines.

Guideline	Type of Patient	Drugs	Additional Information	Ref.
SGCLL	Acalabrutinib Ibrutinib + Venetoclax VO Zanubrutinib Ibrutinib		Same level of recommendation. To be evaluated according to patient profile.	[151]
Canadian Guideline	FIT patients	Acalabrutinib	Better PFS (elevate R/R study) than Ibrutinib. Conflicting OS	[152]
		VO	Less PFS than BTKi	
	FCR Ineligible	Acalabrutinib	Improved PFS compared to CIT.	
		VO	Effective therapy expected to provide several years of treatment-free duration. Finite duration (12 months)	
		Acalabrutinib-Obinutuzumab	Improved OS compared to CIT.	
Expert consensus on the management of CLL in Asia	FIT patients	BTKi	Could be used in preference to CIT. Lower toxicity.	[153]
		CIT	Can be used as a first-line treatment option.	
	UNFIT patients	VO		
		BTKi	May be considered the preferred first-line treatment of choice for this patient.	
ESMO	FIT patients		Ibrutinib or CIT: FCR or BR (>65 years patients)	[58]
	UNFIT patients		VO, Ibrutinib–Acalabrutinib, CIT: Chlorambucil–Obinutuzumab	
DGHO	Acalabrutinib +/− Obinutuzumab Zanubrutinib Ibrutinib +/− Obinutuzumab		Some studies (ALLIANCE and ILLUMINATE) with BTKi showed reduced PFS in the IGHVum group. Due to the cardiovascular toxicity profile, therapy with ibrutinib is primarily not recommended unless patients are young, fit, and have no prior cardiac disease.	[155]
	VO		Temporary therapy (12 cycles). CCL14 showed a significant difference in PFS in patients with unmutated IGHV status. However, the result of the CLL17 study on whether VO is inferior to long-term treatment with BTKi (including non-mutated patients) is still pending.	
	Ibrutinib + Venetoclax		Data from the GLOW study show shorter PFS for IGHVum at short follow-up for this group compared to the subgroup with IGHVm.	

Table 11. Cont.

Guideline		Type of Patient			Drugs			Additional Information		Ref.
NCCN/iwCLL [13,156]	Front-line therapy	Acalabrutinib +/− obinutuzumab VO Zanubrutinib						These options are recommended across almost every subgroup of patients.		
	Clinical trial available	Yes			With no clear evidence of a functional cure, it is important to enroll patients in clinical trials when available.					
		No	Check IGHV status	Mutated	Check CLL FISH	Only del 13q+	Age < 65	Yes	Discuss/consider FCRx6. This regimen is not preferred in the current era of targeted therapies for CLL and SLL.	
								No	Check FISH/tp53 mutations.	
				Unmutated	Check CLL FISH/tp53 mutation.	del17+ or tp53mut	Acalabrutinib		Renal insufficiency. Extensive infections (except in cases of aspergillosis). Atrial fibrillation or hypertension. Need for anticoagulation. Preference for time-limited therapy.	
							Zanubrutinib			
						Others	Consider comorbidities.	VO (12 mo)		

According to JAMA, first-line treatment in patients with normal TP53, regardless of IGHV status, consists of either VO (a fixed-duration treatment) or covalent BTKi such as acalabrutinib, Zanubrutinib, or ibrutinib. Second-generation BTKi (acalabrutinib and zanubrutinib) is preferred, given improved safety. Also, zanubrutinib had superior efficacy compared to ibrutinib [154].

8. Rescue Treatment in Relapsed/Refractory Patients

The understanding of novel agent therapy is advancing with the progression of clinical trial data. This stems from the fact that a significant proportion of patients enrolled in registration trials that led to the approval of novel agents did not undergo prior novel agent treatments; however, robust retrospective analyses have provided significant guidance [157]. Individuals resistant to current therapies or those experiencing remission periods of less than 2 to 3 years, along with patients who relapse and exhibit evidence of del17p or TP53mut, face an unfavorable prognosis. Prior to selecting further treatment for any patient with r/r CLL, it is crucial to evaluate whether the treatment criteria outlined in the iwCLL 2018 guidelines are met [13].

Performing FISH to detect del17p and conducting tests for TP53mut is recommended before initiating the first-line treatment and at each subsequent treatment stage for r/r CLL patients. The mutational status of IGHV does not change during the disease, and repeat testing is not indicated. In the realm of r/r CLL patients, innovative treatments outperform conventional CIT regimens, resulting in markedly improved survival rates. The selection of therapeutic agents is contingent upon diverse factors, including age, functional capacity, comorbidities, organ functionality, and patient preferences [1]. Some factors have been identified as prognostic in CLL, at both treatment-free interval and OS level. Certain factors contributing to this include the presence of an IGHVum gene, cytogenetic abnormalities like a complex karyotype, del(17p), TP53mut, and others. The temporal aspect of disease progression also stands as a crucial prognostic element in relapsed CLL patients [15].

The early onset of disease progression, defined as occurring within 24 months of frontline therapy, is a recognized predictor of lower response rates to subsequent therapy and diminished survival. The context of relapse is also noteworthy, with disease recurrence following finite-limited therapy potentially treated using the same regimen, provided the initial therapy's response duration is satisfactory [158]. Patients experiencing disease progression after maintaining a response for at least 6 months are categorized as having relapsed CLL. On the other hand, those who show no response to treatment or relapse within 6 months of the last therapy dose are classified as having refractory CLL. The subsequent approach for both r/r cases depends on their prior treatment histories.

According to the recommendations of the SGCCL [151], iwCLL/NCNN [1,156], and DGHO [155] guidelines, treatment for those patients who have undergone prior CIT should be acalabrutinib, zanubrutinib, ibrutinib (only in cases where acalabrutinib and zanubrutinib are contraindicated), or VR. The SGCCL guideline [151] distinguishes between TP53mut/non-del(17p) patients (within these, those with IGHVm or IGHVum) and patients with TP53mut/del(17p). In all cases, treatment is as previously recommended according to the patient profile. DGHO guidelines [155] recommend stopping therapy after 24 months of treatment with late-relapsed VR.

On the other hand, those patients who have received a previous BTKi and have not responded to it should be treated with others such as acalabrutinib or zanubrutinib (in case the patient does not present resistance to BTKi), VO for 24 months [1,156], or VR (stop after 24 months of treatment) [151,155]. Those patients experiencing intolerance or early relapse (less than 24–36 months of treatment) or those patients with late relapse who have del(17p)/TP53mut and have been treated with a prior BCL-2i are recommended to be treated with acalabrutinib, Zanubrutinib, or in those who do not respond to these treatments, clinical trials, or cell therapy [151]. Ibrutinib is recommended when acalabrutinib and zanubrutinib are contraindicated [155], and VO can be used (for 24 months) [1,156]. Patients with non-del(17p)/TP53mut late relapse who have IGHVm or IGHVum can be treated with either VR, acalabrutinib, Zanubrutinib, or ibrutinib according to clinical practice guidelines.

If the patient has been doubly refractory (which means not responding to BCL-2i and BTKi), guidelines recommend including the patient in clinical trials and using cell therapy (CAR-T) or idR in exceptional cases according to the safety profile. For frail patients, supportive care is the preferred option [151,155,156].

JAMA guidelines consider that if the patient is intolerant or the disease progresses to first-line treatment, there are several options. Patients previously treated with BTKi who are intolerant to the treatment can be treated with other BTKi or with VR (in those with rapidly progressive disease, inpatient care with rapid dose escalation should be considered). If the patient is treated with a BTKi and experiments with disease progression after it, the treatment should be VR (considering rapid dose escalation in those with rapidly progressive disease) or a non-covalent BTKi inhibitor such as pirtobrutinib (when available) [154].

Patients previously treated with venetoclax who experienced progression while receiving treatment or early after discontinuation can be treated with acalabrutinib, Zanubrutinib, or ibrutinib (second-generation BTKi are preferred, given improved safety based on clinical trials). Also, non-covalent BTKi inhibitors such as pirtobrutinib can be used when available. If the patient experiences a late progression after discontinuation, they can be treated with acalabrutinib, zanubrutinib, ibrutinib, or pirtobrutinib, and retreatment with venetoclax can be considered [154,159].

Finally, if the disease progresses after BTKi or venetoclax, either noncovalent BTKi (pirtobrutinib) or PIK3 inhibitors (idR or durvalumab) can be used. Pirtobrutinib is preferred over PIK3 inhibitors, as its efficacy has been shown in a clinical trial, including after receipt of BTKi and venetoclax. At least, cellular immunotherapy should be considered. CAR-T therapy is recommended when available in patients with controlled disease (while responsive to treatment) and alloHCT if there is no access to CAR-T or after CAR-T [154].

ESMO guidelines consider that first-line therapy should only be used in symptomatic patients. Patients with relapsed and asymptomatic CLL can be followed without therapy. If CLL is in remission, stopping BTKi or venetoclax can be considered and does not need an immediate alternative. If CLL progresses rapidly, therapy should be changed immediately. If a symptomatic relapse or non-response appears within 3 years after a fixed-duration therapy regimen, it should be changed regardless of the type or first-line treatment (contrary to the most recent guidelines that consider previous treatments) [58].

Treatment should be either VR for 24 months, ibrutinib/acalabrutinib, or other BTKis (if available) as continuous therapy. Alternative options include PIK3 inhibitors such as idelalisib in combination with rituximab or CIT unless a TP53 mutation or del(17p) is found and no other treatment options with inhibitors or cellular therapy are available, and it is not recommended because it increases toxicity rates and the risk of secondary neoplasm. When a progression is observed on BCR inhibitor (BCRi) therapy after prior CIT, venetoclax-based therapy is preferred because it has been observed that changing to a different CIT or BCRi does not induce long-lasting remissions. Patients may be re-exposed to the same treatment regimen when there is a long-lasting remission (more than 36 months) from prior therapy [58].

There are several studies, such as CLARITY [160], in which a phase II trial was conducted, investigating the combination of ibrutinib and venetoclax in individuals with r/r CLL. The primary objective was the elimination of MRD after 12 months of concurrent therapy. Key secondary objectives included evaluating responses according to iwCLL criteria, ensuring safety, and assessing PFS and OS. The combination of ibrutinib and venetoclax demonstrated good tolerability in patients with r/r CLL. A notable proportion of patients achieved MRD eradication, leading to the discontinuation of therapy in some cases.

The PFS and OS rates were encouraging for individuals with r/r CLL [161]. Venetoclax response rates ranging from 71% to 79% have been observed among patients in subgroups with an adverse prognosis, such as those with fludarabine resistance, del(17p), or IGHVum. The 15-month PFS for the 400 mg dose groups was 69%. In another trial in patients with r/r del(17p) CLL, an OR was achieved by independent review in 85 patients (79.4%) [162].

There is a lack of data from randomized clinical trials directly comparing novel agents. Nevertheless, indications propose that individuals experiencing late relapse (beyond 2 years) following fixed-duration therapies may derive benefits from identical retreatment. In contrast, those with short-lived remissions or progressive disease under continuous drug intake may find a favorable outcome with a class switch. The treatment of patients previously exposed to both covalent BTKi and BCL-2 remains an unresolved medical challenge. Early clinical trials indicate the promising efficacy of novel drugs, especially noncovalent BTKi, in addressing the therapeutic needs of this challenging subgroup [163].

9. Treatment Resistance

The emergence of resistance to treatment is related to the progression of subclones with clear proliferative advantages. Subclones that are not eliminated via chemotherapy can lead to disease progression years later. Therefore, in patients treated with CIT, the acquisition of TP53 mutations or deletions is not uncommon [74].

On the other hand, the acquisition of mutations at the BTK or BCL-2 level is a cause of resistance to ibrutinib and venetoclax, respectively. Concerning BTKi, the mechanism of resistance is similar among the covalent BTK inhibitors. Switching between drugs in this category after disease progression should be avoided. When treatment is deemed necessary, clinical trials have demonstrated the effective use of acalabrutinib or zanubrutinib in patients intolerant of ibrutinib. Additionally, zanubrutinib can be employed in patients intolerant of either ibrutinib or acalabrutinib. The preference for zanubrutinib and acalabrutinib over ibrutinib is supported by their favorable safety profiles, and zanubrutinib exhibits superior efficacy compared to ibrutinib. Findings from the E1912 study indicate that the median time between discontinuing ibrutinib due to AE and initiating new therapy is 25 months [160].

In very pre-treated patients, acquired resistance to ibrutinib can emerge, primarily mediated through the mutation of BTK cysteine-481—the amino acid that ibrutinib irreversibly reacts with—to serine.

This mutation blocks the covalent binding of ibrutinib, resulting in the inability of ibrutinib to exert its therapeutic effect. This same resistance pattern has also been observed with acalabrutinib and zanubrutinib, although the incidence of resistance associated with these drugs requires further investigation [164]. Non-covalent BTK inhibitors were developed to improve pharmacological properties and maintain potency against BTK C481 mutations. However, BTK L528W-mediated resistance mechanisms have recently been observed for pirtobrutinib [165]. BTK L528W also leads to a decrease in the pharmacological potency of zanubrutinib [166].

Progression to ibrutinib treatment has also been observed in patients with del 8p. The presence of mutations in PLCG2 (R665WW and L845F mutations) leads to autonomous BCR activity [167]. The BCL-2 G101V mutation diminishes the binding strength of venetoclax to BCL-2 by 180-fold. This selective reduction in affinity contributes to resistance to therapy [168].

10. Where Are We Going in the Therapeutic Approach to CLL?

Selecting therapy is a challenging task that requires evaluating the patient regarding all aspects that could interfere, such as other diseases and patient preferences. Also, side effects, comedications, and economic aspects should be considered. Updated NCCN guidelines and the recent iwCLL algorithm recommend second-generation BTKis, such as zanubrutinib and acalabrutinib, for the treatment of naïve patients and r/r CLL regardless of patient fitness due to their increased selectivity and favorable drug toxicity profiles [156].

Fixed-duration chemo-free therapies in CLL, which can induce a complete response, are becoming more important in treating CLL. The CIT approach has a marginal role in r/r CLL nowadays, and therapies such as venetoclax and antiCD20 mAbs are alternatives that must be discussed in each patient, considering advantages and disadvantages. Offering the best treatment option is a challenge nowadays and requires a deep knowledge of the growing evidence [169].

Some studies show that despite advances in CLL treatment regarding efficacy and tolerability, premature treatment discontinuation is frequent in all types of therapies. The feasibility of the fixed-duration treatment regimen is nowadays a question unsolved. Targeted therapies have typically been used continuously until disease progression. This poses problems for patients, such as economic expense or intolerance to the drug, which can lead to dose reductions or even a lack of treatment adherence, sometimes leading to treatment abandonment. Patients with increasing comorbidities (advanced age or health problems) may be especially prone to lower tolerability of long-term drugs, so fixed-duration treatment may be a very good option for them. This can be seen in the MURANO [135] study, where it was seen that 70% of patients maintained the achieved level of uMRD, and among patients who achieved uMRD, 98% of patients did not progress. It is important for prescribers to consider the problem of sustainability. That is why the option of using fixed-duration treatments represents an opportunity to provide access to treatments that are sustainable for the national health system, and in cases where there is no evidence of benefits from a certain treatment over another potentially equally effective and tolerable one, it could help the prescribers as an important factor to consider. Additional studies are needed to evaluate the efficacy of these fixed-duration therapies and the impact of treatment discontinuation rates [170].

Ongoing investigations into triple therapy are yielding exceptionally promising outcomes. Time-limited triple therapy demonstrates elevated rates of achieving undetectable minimal residual disease and maintaining remissions in individuals with high-risk CLL. The occurrence of AE is early in the induction therapy phase and diminishes as treatment progresses. The CLL2-GIVe study assesses the response and tolerability of the triple combination comprising obinutuzumab, ibrutinib, and venetoclax (GIVe regimen) in forty-one previously untreated high-risk CLL patients with del(17p) and/or TP53 mutation. The 36-month PFS was 79.9%, and the 36-month OS was 92.6% [138]. Time-limited triple therapy with obinutuzumab, venetoclax, and acalabrutinib was evaluated in 37 patients with previously untreated CLL. The primary endpoint was complete remission with uMRD in the bone marrow at cycle 16, day 1. The results showed that 86% of participants had a complete remission with uMRD in the peripheral blood and bone marrow [171]. In a trial with zanubrutinib, venetoclax, and obinutuzumab in 39 previously untreated CLL patients, 89% of them had undetectable MRD in both blood and bone marrow (median follow-up 25.8 months, IQR 24.0–27.3). After median surveillance after treatment of 15.8 months (IQR 13.0–18.6), 31 (94%) of 33 patients had undetectable MRD [172]. The existing data on targeted therapies face several limitations. Firstly, the comparison between triplet combinations with sequential single novel agent therapies is lacking. Although combination regimens have generally been well-tolerated, they do exhibit a level of toxicity higher than that of single agents. Therefore, it is imperative to identify those who benefit most from combination therapy and those who would be better served by less toxic sequential monotherapies. When considering doublet versus triplet regimens, it is essential to acknowledge that the individual contributions of drugs in combination regimens, especially CD20 mAbs, remain unclear [173].

11. Take-Home Message

What is success in CLL? The goal in CLL, as in any cancer, remains to prolong the quality of life and overall survival while offering the least possible toxicity. To achieve this, it is necessary to specify what we bring to the table in terms of efficacy and safety with combination treatments. While the current data suggest that the combinations have a present and a bright future, it is necessary to do so from the point of view of the heterogeneity of CLL patients, taking into account the age, the life perspectives of the patients, and the fact that it is a chronic and incurable disease, resulting in the treatment target and the toxicities to be assumed being very different. Therefore, knowing the chronic nature of hemopathy, treatment must be individualized according to three fundamental pillars (or three vertices of a triangle): the patient (age, frailty, comorbidities, concomitant medication, hospital accessibility, and preferences), the disease (genetic status, risk markers, acquired resistances, and expected efficacy obtained with the treatment), and the physician (accessibility and approval of treatments in your environment, experience with treatments, training,...). We must also bear in mind that strategies guided by minimal residual disease are a vital part of today's CLL clinical trials, although we need to know what impact they really have on different patients since the treatment objective is not the same in someone aged 77 who is going to relapse at 83 as in someone we are treating at 40, and yet we do know that the toxicity of continuing indefinite treatments increases over time. It is clear that the paradigm of CLL treatment is changing; we have gone from treating patients with aggressive chemotherapy to being able to predict a targeted treatment with less toxicity, which is even giving us the option of being able to stop treatment in certain patients with what this entails in terms of improved quality of life, improved adherence to treatment, less toxicity in the long term, greater sustainability of the health system, and better health outcomes. All this must be carried out through a multidisciplinary approach (hematologist, hospital pharmacist, and nursing) in order to offer personalized and specialized care and to be able to offer the patient adequate and individualized treatment.

12. Conclusions

Thanks to new therapeutic targets, the current panorama is moving towards more sustainable, personalized treatments with less risk of toxicity for patients, trying to adapt the therapy to the profile of the patient to whom it is directed. This requires the help of a multidisciplinary team working together to achieve the best outcome for the patient and the health system. The increased progressive knowledge of the disease through genetic techniques and its consequent therapeutic implications allow us to better predict the disease, anticipate diseases of more or less risk, detect resistance mutations, or follow up on minimal residual disease. The development of new treatment strategies, such as fixed-duration chemo-free and time-limited triple therapy, represents a new paradigm in the treatment of the disease, offering benefits at the level of acquired resistance, costs, accumulated adverse effects, and probably at the emotional level (offering treatment-free and disease-free periods), so we believe that in the coming years, they will oppose continuous therapies until disease progression.

Author Contributions: Conceptualization, C.A.-P.; methodology, M.D.M.S.S. and C.A.-P.; investigation, M.D.M.S.S., A.M.R., J.M.P.P., M.Á.R.-G., J.E.P.-J. and A.J.M.; writing—original draft preparation, C.A.-P., M.D.M.S.S., A.M.R., J.M.P.P., M.Á.R.-G., J.E.P.-J. and A.J.M.; writing—review and editing, C.A.-P.; supervision, C.A.-P.; funding acquisition, A.J.M. All authors have read and agreed to the published version of the manuscript.

Funding: This research received no external funding.

Institutional Review Board Statement: Not applicable.

Informed Consent Statement: Not applicable.

Data Availability Statement: Not applicable.

Conflicts of Interest: The authors declare no conflicts of interest.

References

1. Hampel, P.J.; Parikh, S.A. Chronic lymphocytic leukemia treatment algorithm 2022. *Blood Cancer J.* **2022**, *12*, 161. [CrossRef] [PubMed]
2. Mukkamalla, S.K.R.; Taneja, A.; Malipeddi, D.; Master, S.R. *Chronic Lymphocytic Leukemia*; StatPearls Publishing: Treasure Island, FL, USA, 2020. Available online: https://pubmed.ncbi.nlm.nih.gov/29261864/ (accessed on 15 July 2023).
3. Reinart, N.; Nguyen, P.H.; Boucas, J.; Rosen, N.; Kvasnicka, H.M.; Heukamp, L.; Rudolph, C.; Ristovska, V.; Velmans, T.; Mueller, C.; et al. Delayed development of chronic lymphocytic leukemia in the absence of macrophage migration inhibitory factor. *Blood* **2013**, *121*, 812–821. [CrossRef] [PubMed]
4. The Surveillance E, and End Results (SEER) Program of the National Cancer Institute. Cancer Stat Facts: Leukemia—Chronic LymphocyticLeukemia (CLL). 2021. Available online: https://seer.cancer.gov/statfacts/html/clyl.html (accessed on 15 July 2023).
5. Hallek, M.; Cheson, B.D.; Catovsky, D.; Caligaris-Cappio, F.; Dighiero, G.; Döhner, H.; Hillmen, P.; Keating, M.; Montserrat, E.; Chiorazzi, N.; et al. iwCLL guidelines for diagnosis, indications for treatment, response assessment, and supportive management of CLL. *Blood* **2018**, *131*, 2745–2760. [CrossRef] [PubMed]
6. Siegel, R.L.; Miller, K.D.; Jemal, A. Cancer statistics. *CA Cancer J. Clin.* **2019**, *69*, 7–34. [CrossRef] [PubMed]
7. Kay, N.E.; Hampel, P.J.; Van Dyke, D.L.; Parikh, S.A. CLL update 2022: A continuing evolution in care. *Blood Rev.* **2022**, *54*, 100930. [CrossRef] [PubMed]
8. Hallek, M.; Al-Sawaf, O. Chronic lymphocytic leukemia: 2022 update on diagnostic and therapeutic procedures. *Am. J. Hematol.* **2021**, *96*, 1679–1705. [CrossRef] [PubMed]
9. Chiorazzi, N.; Chen, S.S.; Rai, K.R. Chronic Lymphocytic Leukemia. *Cold Spring Harb. Perspect. Med.* **2021**, *11*, a035220. [CrossRef]
10. Fabbri, G.; Dalla-Favera, R. The molecular pathogenesis of chronic lymphocytic leukaemia. *Nat. Rev. Cancer* **2016**, *16*, 145–162. [CrossRef]
11. Swerdlow, S.H.; Campo, E.; Pileri, S.A.; Harris, N.L.; Stein, H.; Siebert, R.; Advani, R.; Ghielmini, M.; Salles, G.A.; Zelenetz, A.D.; et al. The 2016 revision of the World Health Organization classification of lymphoid neoplasms. *Blood* **2016**, *127*, 2375–2390. [CrossRef]
12. Seifert, M.; Sellmann, L.; Bloehdorn, J.; Wein, F.; Stilgenbauer, S.; Dürig, J.; Küppers, R. Cellular origin and pathophysiology of chronic lymphocytic leukemia. *J. Exp. Med.* **2012**, *209*, 2183–2198. [CrossRef]
13. Knisbacher, B.A.; Lin, Z.; Hahn, C.K.; Nadeu, F.; Duran-Ferrer, M.; Stevenson, K.E.; Tausch, E.; Delgado, J.; Barbera-Mourelle, A.; Taylor-Weiner, A.; et al. Molecular map of chronic lymphocytic leukemia and its impact on outcome. *Nat. Genet.* **2022**, *54*, 1664–1667. [CrossRef] [PubMed]
14. Puente, X.S.; Beà, S.; Valdés-Mas, R.; Villamor, N.; Gutiérrez-Abril, J.; Martín-Subero, J.I.; Munar, M.; Rubio-Pérez, C.; Jares, P.; Aymerich, M. Non-coding recurrent mutations in chronic lymphocytic leukaemia. *Nature* **2015**, *526*, 519–524. [CrossRef]
15. Kulis, M.; Martin-Subero, J.I. Integrative epigenomics in chronic lymphocytic leukaemia: Biological insights and clinical applications. *Br. J. Haematol.* **2023**, *200*, 280–290. [CrossRef] [PubMed]
16. Zenz, T.; Vollmer, D.; Trbusek, M.; Smardova, J.; Benner, A.; Soussi, T.; Helfrich, H.; Heuberger, M.; Hoth, P.; Fuge, M.; et al. TP53 mutation profile in chronic lymphocytic leukemia: Evidence for a disease specific profile from a comprehensive analysis of 268 mutations. *Leukemia* **2010**, *24*, 2072–2079. [CrossRef] [PubMed]
17. Duffy, M.J.; Synnott, N.C.; Crown, J. Mutant p53 as a target for cancer treatment. *Eur. J. Cancer* **2017**, *83*, 258–265. [CrossRef]
18. Norbury, C.J.; Zhivotovsky, B. DNA damage-induced apoptosis. *Oncogene* **2004**, *23*, 2797–2808. [CrossRef]
19. Buccheri, V.; Barreto, W.G.; Fogliatto, L.M.; Capra, M.; Marchiani, M.; Rocha, V. Prognostic and therapeutic stratification in CLL: Focus on 17p deletion and p53 mutation. *Ann. Hematol.* **2018**, *97*, 2269–2278. [CrossRef]
20. Tate, J.G.; Bamford, S.; Jubb, H.C.; Sondka, Z.; Beare, D.M.; Bindal, N.; Boutselakis, H.; Cole, C.G.; Creatore, C.; Dawson, E.; et al. COSMIC: The catalogue of somatic mutations in cancer. *Nucleic Acids Res.* **2018**, *45*, D777. [CrossRef]
21. Nguyen-Khac, F. "Double-Hit" Chronic Lymphocytic Leukemia, Involving the *TP53* and *MYC* Genes. *Front. Oncol.* **2022**, *11*, 826245. [CrossRef]

22. Maher, N.; Mouhssine, S.; Matti, B.F.; Alwan, A.F.; Gaidano, G. Treatment Refractoriness in Chronic Lymphocytic Leukemia: Old and New Molecular Biomarkers. *Int. J. Mol. Sci.* **2023**, *24*, 10374. [CrossRef]
23. Mansouri, L.; Thorvaldsdottir, B.; Sutton, L.A.; Karakatsoulis, G.; Meggendorfer, M.; Parker, H.; Nadeu, F.; Brieghel, C.; Laidou, S.; Moia, R.; et al. Different prognostic impact of recurrent gene mutations in chronic lymphocytic leukemia depending on IGHV gene somatic hypermutation status: A study by ERIC in HARMONY. *Leukemia* **2023**, *37*, 339–347. [CrossRef] [PubMed]
24. Al Jamal, I.; Parquet, M.; Guiyedi, K.; Aoufouchi, S.; Le Guillou, M.; Rizzo, D.; Pollet, J.; Dupont, M.; Boulin, M.; Faumont, N.; et al. IgH 3'RR recombination uncovers a non-germinal center imprint and c-MYC-dependent IgH rearrangement in unmutated chronic lymphocytic leukemia. *Haematologica*, 2023; advance online publication. [CrossRef]
25. Medina, A.; Ramírez, A.; Hérnandez, J.A.; Loscertales, J.; Serna, J.; Andreu, R.; Yáñez, L.; Terol, M.J.; González, M.; Delgado, J.; et al. Guia Nacional de Leucemia Linfática Crónica y Linfoma Linfocítico. 2020. Available online: https://www.sehh.es/images/stories/recursos/2020/05/18/Guia-Clinica-LLC-abril-2020.pdf (accessed on 25 July 2023).
26. Lau, R.; Niu, M.Y.; Pratt, M.A. cIAP2 represses IKKα/β-mediated activation of MDM2 to prevent p53 degradation. *Cell Cycle* **2012**, *11*, 4009–4019. [CrossRef] [PubMed]
27. Nadeu, F.; Delgado, J.; Royo, C.; Baumann, T.; Stankovic, T.; Pinyol, M.; Jares, P.; Navarro, A.; Martín-García, D.; Beà, S.; et al. Clinical impact of clonal and subclonal TP53, SF3B1, BIRC3, NOTCH1, and ATM mutations in chronic lymphocytic leukemia. *Blood* **2016**, *127*, 2122–2130. [CrossRef] [PubMed]
28. Sadria, R.; Motamed, N.; Saberi Anvar, M.; Mehrabani Yeganeh, H.; Poopak, B. Prognostic correlation of NOTCH1 and SF3B1 mutations with chromosomal abnormalities in chronic lymphocytic leukemia patients. *Cancer Rep.* **2023**, *6*, e1757. [CrossRef] [PubMed]
29. Rosati, E.; Baldoni, S.; De Falco, F.; Del Papa, B.; Dorillo, E.; Rompietti, C.; Albi, E.; Falzetti, F.; Di Ianni, M.; Sportoletti, P. NOTCH1 Aberrations in Chronic Lymphocytic Leukemia. *Front. Oncol.* **2018**, *8*, 229. [CrossRef]
30. Rossi, D.; Rasi, S.; Spina, V.; Fangazio, M.; Monti, S.; Greco, M.; Ciardullo, C.; Famà, R.; Cresta, S.; Bruscaggin, A.; et al. Different impact of NOTCH1 and SF3B1 mutations on the risk of chronic lymphocytic leukemia transformation to Richter syndrome. *Br. J. Haematol.* **2012**, *158*, 426–429. [CrossRef]
31. Rio-Machin, A. ATM serine/threonine kinase germline mutations in chronic lymphocytic leukaemia come in different flavours. *Br. J. Haematol.* **2022**, *199*, 307–309. [CrossRef]
32. Tiao, G.; Improgo, M.R.; Kasar, S.; Poh, W.; Kamburov, A.; Landau, D.A.; Tausch, E.; Taylor-Weiner, A.; Cibulskis, C.; Bahl, S.; et al. Rare germline variants in ATM are associated with chronic lymphocytic leukemia. *Leukemia* **2017**, *31*, 2244–2247. [CrossRef]
33. Puente, X.S.; Pinyol, M.; Quesada, V.; Conde, L.; Ordóñez, G.R.; Villamor, N.; Escaramis, G.; Jares, P.; Beà, S.; González-Díaz, M.; et al. Whole-genome sequencing identifies recurrent mutations in chronic lymphocytic leukaemia. *Nature* **2011**, *475*, 101–105. [CrossRef]
34. Quesada, V.; Conde, L.; Villamor, N.; Ordóñez, G.R.; Jares, P.; Bassaganyas, L.; Ramsay, A.J.; Beà, S.; Pinyol, M.; Martínez-Trillos, A.; et al. Exome sequencing identifies recurrent mutations of the splicing factor SF3B1 gene in chronic lymphocytic leukemia. *Nat. Genet.* **2011**, *44*, 47–52. [CrossRef]
35. Martínez-Trillos, A.; Pinyol, M.; Navarro, A.; Aymerich, M.; Jares, P.; Juan, M.; Rozman, M.; Colomer, D.; Delgado, J.; Giné, E.; et al. Mutations in TLR/MYD88 pathway identify a subset of young chronic lymphocytic leukemia patients with favorable outcome. *Blood* **2014**, *123*, 3790–3796. [CrossRef]
36. Baliakas, P.; Hadzidimitriou, A.; Agathangelidis, A.; Rossi, D.; Sutton, L.A.; Kminkova, J.; Scarfo, L.; Pospisilova, S.; Gaidano, G.; Stamatopoulos, K.; et al. Prognostic relevance of MYD88 mutations in CLL: The jury is still out. *Blood* **2015**, *126*, 1043–1044. [CrossRef]
37. Bosch, F.; Dalla-Favera, R. Chronic lymphocytic leukaemia: From genetics to treatment. *Nat. Rev. Clin. Oncol.* **2019**, *16*, 684–701. [CrossRef]
38. Mhibik, M.; Wiestner, A.; Sun, C. Harnessing the effects of BTKi on T cells for effective immunotherapy against CLL. *Int. J. Mol. Sci.* **2019**, *21*, 68. [CrossRef]
39. Idris, S.Z.; Hassan, N.; Lee, L.J.; Md Noor, S.; Osman, R.; Abdul-Jalil, M.; Nordin, A.J.; Abdullah, M. Increased regulatory T cells in acute lymphoblastic leukaemia patients. *Hematology* **2016**, *21*, 206–212. [CrossRef]
40. Andreescu, M.; Berbec, N.; Tanase, A.D. Assessment of Impact of Human Leukocyte Antigen-Type and Cytokine-Type Responses on Outcomes after Targeted Therapy Currently Used to Treat Chronic Lymphocytic Leukemia. *J. Clin. Med.* **2023**, *12*, 2731. [CrossRef]
41. Huang, R.; Tsuda, H.; Takatsuki, K. Interleukin-2 prevents programmed cell death in chronic lymphocytic leukemia cells. *Int. J. Hematol.* **1993**, *58*, 83–92.
42. Coscia, M.; Pantaleoni, F.; Riganti, C.; Vitale, C.; Rigoni, M.; Peola, S.; Castella, B.; Foglietta, M.; Griggio, V.; Drandi, D. IGHV unmutated CLL B cells are more prone to spontaneous apoptosis and subject to environmental prosurvival signals than mutated CLL B cells. *Leukemia* **2011**, *25*, 828–837. [CrossRef]
43. Wang, H.Q.; Jia, L.; Li, Y.T.; Farren, T.; Agrawal, S.G.; Liu, F.T. Increased autocrine interleukin-6 production is significantly associated with worse clinical outcome in patients with chronic lymphocytic leukemia. *J. Cell. Physiol.* **2019**, *234*, 13994–14006. [CrossRef]
44. Arruga, F.; Gyau, B.B.; Iannello, A.; Vitale, N.; Vaisitti, T.; Deaglio, S. Immune Response Dysfunction in Chronic Lymphocytic Leukemia: Dissecting Molecular Mechanisms and Microenvironmental Conditions. *Int. J. Mol. Sci.* **2020**, *21*, 1825. [CrossRef]

45. Jaffe, E.S.; Harris, N.L.; Stein, H.; Isaacson, P.G. Classification of lymphoid neoplasms: The microscope as a tool for disease discovery. *Blood J. Am. Soc. Hematol.* **2008**, *112*, 4384–4399. [CrossRef]
46. Alhakeem, S.S.; McKenna, M.K.; Oben, K.Z.; Noothi, S.K.; Rivas, J.R.; Hildebrandt, G.C.; Fleischman, R.A.; Rangnekar, V.M.; Muthusamy, N.; Bondada, S. Chronic Lymphocytic Leukemia-Derived IL-10 Suppresses Antitumor Immunity. *J. Immunol.* **2018**, *200*, 4180–4189. [CrossRef]
47. Jadidi-Niaragh, F.; Ghalamfarsa, G.; Memarian, A.; Asgarian-Omran, H.; Razavi, S.M.; Sarrafnejad, A.; Shokri, F. Downregulation of IL-17-producing T cells is associated with regulatory T cell expansion and disease progression in chronic lymphocytic leukemia. *Tumour Biol.* **2013**, *34*, 929–940. [CrossRef]
48. Foa, R.; Massaia, M.; Cardona, S.; Tos, A.G.; Bianchi, A.; Attisano, C.; Guarini, A.; di Celle, P.F.; Fierro, M.T. Production of tumor necrosis factor-alpha by B-cell chronic lymphocytic leukemia cells: A possible regulatory role of TNF in the progression of the disease. *Blood* **1990**, *76*, 393–400. [CrossRef]
49. Mo, X.D.; Zhang, X.H.; Xu, L.P.; Wang, Y.; Yan, C.H.; Chen, H.; Chen, Y.H.; Han, W.; Wang, F.R.; Wang, J.Z. IFN-α is effective for treatment of minimal residual disease in patients with acute leukemia after allogeneic hematopoietic stem cell transplantation: Results of a registry study. *Biol. Blood Marrow Transplant.* **2017**, *23*, 1303–1310. [CrossRef]
50. Tsukada, N.; Burger, J.A.; Zvaifler, N.J.; Kipps, T.J. Distinctive features of "nurselike" cells that differentiate in the context of chronic lymphocytic leukemia. *Blood* **2002**, *99*, 1030–1037. [CrossRef]
51. Petrova, V.; Annicchiarico-Petruzzelli, M.; Melino, G.; Amelio, I. The hypoxic tumour microenvironment. *Oncogenesis* **2018**, *7*, 10. [CrossRef]
52. Serra, S.; Vaisitti, T.; Audrito, V.; Bologna, C.; Buonincontri, R.; Chen, S.S.; Arruga, F.; Brusa, D.; Coscia, M.; Jaksic, O.; et al. Adenosine signaling mediates hypoxic responses in the chronic lymphocytic leukemia microenvironment. *Blood Adv.* **2016**, *1*, 47–61. [CrossRef]
53. Swerdlow, S.H.; Campo, E.; Harris, N.L.; Jaffe, E.S.; Pileri, S.A.; Stein, H.; Thiele, J.; Vardiman, J.W. *WHO Classification of Tumours of Haematopoietic and Lymphoid Tissues*; WHO Press: Geneve, Switzerland, 2008.
54. Hallek, M.; Cheson, B.D.; Catovsky, D.; Caligaris-Cappio, F.; Dighiero, G.; Dohner, H.; Hillmen, P.; Keating, M.J.; Montserrat, E.; Rai, K.R.; et al. Guidelines for the diagnosis and treatment of chronic lymphocytic leukemia: A report from the International Workshop on Chronic Lymphocytic Leukemia updating the National Cancer InstituteWorking Group 1996 guidelines. *Blood* **2008**, *111*, 5446–5456. [CrossRef]
55. Moreau, E.J.; Matutes, E.; A'Hern, R.P.; Morilla, A.M.; Morilla, R.M.; Owusu-Ankomah, K.A.; Seon, B.K.; Catovsky, D. Improvement of the chronic lymphocytic leukemia scoring system with the monoclonal antibody SN8 (CD79b). *Am. J. Clin. Pathol.* **1997**, *108*, 378–382. [CrossRef]
56. Rosenquist, R.; Niemann, C.U.; Kern, W.; Westerman, D.; Trneny, M.; Mulligan, S.; Doubek, M.; Pospisilova, S.; Hillmen, P.; Oscier, D.; et al. Reproducible diagnosis of chronic lymphocytic leukemia by flow cytometry: An European Research Initiative on CLL (ERIC) & European Society for Clinical Cell Analysis (ESCCA) Harmonisation project. *Cytom. B Clin. Cytom.* **2018**, *94*, 121–128.
57. Sorigue, M.; Raya, M.; Vergara, S.; Junca, J. Concordance between flow cytometry CLL scores. *Int. J. Lab. Hematol.* **2021**, *43*, 743–751. [CrossRef]
58. Eichhorst, B.; Robak, T.; Montserrat, E.; Ghia, P.; Niemann, C.U.; Kater, A.P.; Gregor, M.; Cymbalista, F.; Buske, C.; Hillmen, P.; et al. Chronic lymphocytic leukaemia: ESMO Clinical Practice Guidelines for diagnosis, treatment and follow-up. *Ann. Oncol.* **2021**, *32*, 23–33. [CrossRef]
59. Malcikova, J.; Tausch, E.; Rossi, D.; Sutton, L.A.; Soussi, T.; Zenz, T.; Kater, A.P.; Niemann, C.U.; Gonzalez, D.; Davi, F.; et al. ERIC recommendations for TP53 mutation analysis in chronic lymphocytic leukemia-update on methodological approaches and results interpretation. *Leukemia* **2018**, *32*, 1070–1080. [CrossRef]
60. Ghia, P.; Stamatopoulos, K.; Belessi, C.; Moreno, C.; Stilgenbauer, S.; Stevenson, F.; Davi, F.; Rosenquist, R. European Research Initiative on CLL. ERIC recommendations on IGHV gene mutational status analysis in chronic lymphocytic leukemia. *Leukemia* **2007**, *21*, 1–3. [CrossRef]
61. Rai, K.R.; Sawitsky, A.; Cronkite, E.P.; Chanana, A.D.; Levy, R.N.; Pasternack, B.S. Clinical staging of chronic lymphocytic leukemia. *Blood* **1975**, *46*, 219–234. [CrossRef]
62. Binet, J.L.; Auquier, A.; Dighiero, G.; Chastang, C.; Piguet, H.; Goasguen, J.; Vaugier, G.; Potron, G.; Colona, P.; Oberling, F.; et al. A new prognostic classification of chronic lymphocytic leukemia derived from a multivariate survival analysis. *Cancer* **1981**, *48*, 198–204. [CrossRef]
63. Pflug, N.; Bahlo, J.; Shanafelt, T.D.; Eichhorst, B.F.; Bergmann, M.A.; Elter, T.; Bauer, K.; Malchau, G.; Rabe, K.G.; Stilgenbauer, S.; et al. Development of a comprehensive prognostic index for patients with chronic lymphocytic leukemia. *Blood* **2014**, *124*, 49–62. [CrossRef]
64. International CLL IPI Working Group. An international prognostic index for patients with chronic lymphocytic leukaemia (CLL-IPI): A meta-analysis of individual patient data. *Lancet Oncol.* **2016**, *17*, 779–790. [CrossRef]
65. Cortese, D.; Sutton, L.A.; Cahill, N.; Smedby, K.E.; Geisler, C.; Gunnarsson, R.; Juliusson, G.; Mansouri, L.; Rosenquist, R. On the way towards a 'CLL prognostic index': Focus on TP53, BIRC3, SF3B1, NOTCH1 and MYD88 in a population-based cohort. *Leukemia* **2014**, *28*, 710–713. [CrossRef]
66. Shanafelt, T.D.; Jenkins, G.; Call, T.G.; Zent, C.S.; Slager, S.; Bowen, D.A.; Schwager, S.; Hanson, C.A.; Jelinek, D.F.; Kay, N.E. Validation of a new prognostic index for patients with chronic lymphocytic leukemia. *Cancer* **2009**, *115*, 363–372. [CrossRef]

67. Wierda, W.G.; O'Brien, S.; Wang, X.; Faderl, S.; Ferrajoli, A.; Do, K.A.; Cortes, J.; Thomas, D.; Garcia-Manero, G.; Koller, C.; et al. Prognostic nomogram and index for overall survival in previously untreated patients with chronic lymphocytic leukemia. *Blood* **2007**, *109*, 4679–4685. [CrossRef]
68. Gao, R.; Du, K.; Liang, J.; Xia, Y.; Wu, J.; Li, Y.; Pan, B.; Wang, L.; Li, J.; Xu, W. Low Serum Cholesterol Level Is a Significant Prognostic Factor That Improves CLL-IPI in Chronic Lymphocytic Leukaemia. *Int. J. Mol. Sci.* **2023**, *24*, 7396. [CrossRef]
69. Yavasoglu, I.; Tombuloglu, M.; Kadikoylu, G.; Donmez, A.; Cagirgan, S.; Bolaman, Z. Cholesterol levels in patients with multiple myeloma. *Ann. Hematol.* **2008**, *87*, 223–228. [CrossRef]
70. Lim, U.; Gayles, T.; Katki, H.A.; Stolzenberg-Solomon, R.; Weinstein, S.J.; Pietinen, P.; Taylor, P.R.; Virtamo, J.; Albanes, D. Serum high-density lipoprotein cholesterol and risk of non-hodgkin lymphoma. *Cancer Res.* **2007**, *67*, 5569–5574. [CrossRef]
71. Yavasoglu, I.; Sargin, G.; Yilmaz, F.; Altindag, S.; Akgun, G.; Tombak, A.; Toka, B.; Dal, S.; Ozbas, H.; Cetin, G.; et al. Cholesterol Levels in Patients with Chronic Lymphocytic Leukemia. *J. Natl. Med. Assoc.* **2017**, *109*, 23–27. [CrossRef]
72. Tresckow, J.V.; Eichhorst, B.; Bahlo, J.; Hallek, M. The Treatment of Chronic Lymphatic Leukemia. *Dtsch. Arztebl. Int.* **2019**, *116*, 41–46. [CrossRef]
73. Hallek, M.; Shanafelt, T.D.; Eichhorst, B. Chronic lymphocytic leukaemia. *Lancet* **2018**, *391*, 1524–1537. [CrossRef]
74. Rasi, S.; Khiabanian, H.; Ciardullo, C.; Terzi-di-Bergamo, L.; Monti, S.; Spina, V.; Bruscaggin, A.; Cerri, M.; Deambrogi, C.; Martuscelli, L.; et al. Clinical impact of small subclones harboring NOTCH1, SF3B1 or BIRC3 mutations in chronic lymphocytic leukemia. *Haematologica* **2016**, *101*, 135–138. [CrossRef]
75. Huang, Y.J.; Kuo, M.C.; Chang, H.; Wang, P.N.; Wu, J.H.; Huang, Y.M.; Ma, M.C.; Tang, T.C.; Kuo, C.Y.; Shih, L.Y. Distinct immunoglobulin heavy chain variable region gene repertoire and lower frequency of del(11q) in Taiwanese patients with chronic lymphocytic leukaemia. *Br. J. Haematol.* **2019**, *187*, 82–92. [CrossRef]
76. Kittai, A.S.; Lunning, M.; Danilov, A.V. Relevance of Prognostic Fac- tors in the Era of Targeted Therapies in CLL. *Curr. Hematol. Malig. Rep.* **2019**, *14*, 302–309. [CrossRef] [PubMed]
77. Tadmor, T.; Levy, I. Richter Transformation in Chronic Lymphocytic Leukemia: Update in the Era of Novel Agents. *Cancers* **2021**, *13*, 5141. [CrossRef] [PubMed]
78. Abrisqueta, P.; Nadeu, F.; Bosch-Schips, J.; Iacoboni, G.; Serna, A.; Cabirta, A.; Yáñez, L.; Quintanilla-Martínez, L.; Bosch, F. From genetics to therapy: Unraveling the complexities of Richter transformation in chronic lymphocytic leukemia. *Cancer Treat. Rev.* **2023**, *120*, 102619. [CrossRef] [PubMed]
79. Rossi, D.; Cerri, M.; Capello, D.; Deambrogi, C.; Rossi, F.M.; Zucchetto, A.; De Paoli, L.; Cresta, S.; Rasi, S.; Spina, V.; et al. Biological and clinical risk factors of chronic lymphocytic leukaemia transformation to Richter syndrome. *Br. J. Haematol.* **2008**, *142*, 202–215. [CrossRef] [PubMed]
80. Hallek, M. Chronic lymphocytic leukemia: 2020 update on diagnosis, risk stratification and treatment. *Am. J. Hematol.* **2019**, *94*, 1266–1287. [CrossRef] [PubMed]
81. Johnson, P.C.; Woyach, J.A.; Ulrich, A.; Marcotte, V.; Nipp, R.D.; Lage, D.E.; Nelson, A.M.; Newcomb, R.A.; Rice, J.; Lavoie, M.W.; et al. Geriatric assessment measures are predictive of outcomes in chronic lymphocytic leukemia. *J. Geriatr. Oncol.* **2023**, *14*, 101538. [CrossRef] [PubMed]
82. Hurria, A.; Togawa, K.; Mohile, S.G.; Owusu, C.; Klepin, H.D.; Gross, C.P.; Lichtman, S.M.; Gajra, A.; Bhatia, S.; Katheria, V.; et al. Predicting chemotherapy toxicity in older adults with cancer: A prospective multicenter study. *J. Clin. Oncol. Off. J. Am. Soc. Clin. Oncol.* **2011**, *29*, 3457–3465. [CrossRef]
83. Giantin, V.; Valentini, E.; Iasevoli, M.; Falci, C.; Siviero, P.; De Luca, E.; Maggi, S.; Martella, B.; Orrù, G.; Crepaldi, G.; et al. Does the Multidimensional Prognostic Index (MPI), based on a Comprehensive Geriatric Assessment (CGA), ¿predict mortality in cancer patients? Results of a prospective observational trial. *J. Geriatr. Oncol.* **2013**, *4*, 208–217. [CrossRef]
84. Goede, V.; Bahlo, J.; Chataline, V.; Eichhorst, B.; Dürig, J.; Stilgenbauer, S.; Kolb, G.; Honecker, F.; Wedding, U.; Hallek, M. Evaluation of geriatric assessment in patients with chronic lymphocytic leukemia: Results of the CLL9 trial of the German CLL study group. *Leuk. Lymphoma* **2016**, *57*, 789–796. [CrossRef]
85. Molica, S.; Giannarelli, D.; Levato, L.; Mirabelli, R.; Levato, D.; Lentini, M.; Piro, E. A simple score based on geriatric assessment predicts survival in elderly newly diagnosed chronic lymphocytic leukemia patients. *Leuk. Lymphoma* **2019**, *60*, 845–847. [CrossRef]
86. Huang, L.W.; Sheng, Y.; Andreadis, C.; Logan, A.C.; Mannis, G.N.; Smith, C.C.; Gaensler, K.M.L.; Martin, T.G.; Damon, L.E.; Steinman, M.A.; et al. Functional Status as Measured by Geriatric Assessment Predicts Inferior Survival in Older Allogeneic Hematopoietic Cell Transplantation Recipients. *Biol. Blood Marrow Transplant.* **2020**, *26*, 189–196. [CrossRef] [PubMed]
87. Liu, M.A.; DuMontier, C.; Murillo, A.; Hshieh, T.T.; Bean, J.F.; Soiffer, R.J.; Stone, R.M.; Abel, G.A.; Driver, J.A. Gait speed, grip strength, and clinical outcomes in older patients with hematologic malignancies. *Blood* **2019**, *134*, 374–382. [CrossRef] [PubMed]
88. Klepin, H.D.; Geiger, A.M.; Tooze, J.A.; Kritchevsky, S.B.; Williamson, J.D.; Pardee, T.S.; Ellis, L.R.; Powell, B.L. Geriatric assessment predicts survival for older adults receiving induction chemotherapy for acute myelogenous leukemia. *Blood* **2013**, *121*, 4287–4294. [CrossRef] [PubMed]
89. Arguello-Tomas, M.; Albiol, N.; Moreno, C. Frontline therapy in Chronic Lymphocytic Leukemia. *Acta Haematol.* **2023**. [CrossRef] [PubMed]
90. Scheepers, E.R.M.; Vondeling, A.M.; Thielen, N.; van der Griend, R.; Stauder, R.; Hamaker, M.E. Geriatric assessment in older patients with a hematologic malignancy: A systematic review. *Haematologica* **2020**, *105*, 1484–1493. [CrossRef] [PubMed]

91. CLL Trialists Collaborative Group. Chemotherapeutic options in chronic lymphocytic leukemia. *J. Natl. Cancer Inst.* **1999**, *91*, 861–868. [CrossRef]
92. Gribben, J.G.; O'Brien, S. Update on therapy of chronic lymphocytic leukemia. *J. Clin. Oncol.* **2011**, *29*, 544–550. [CrossRef]
93. CLL Trialists' Collaborative Group. Systematic review of purine analog treatment for chronic lymphocytic leukemia: Lessons for future trials. *Haematologica* **2012**, *97*, 428–436. [CrossRef]
94. Niederle, N.; Megdenberg, D.; Balleisen, L.; Heit, W.; Knauf, W.; Weiß, J.; Freier, W.; Hinke, A.; Ibach, S.; Eimermacher, H. Bendamustine compared to fludarabine as second-line treatment in chronic lymphocytic leukemia. *Ann. Hematol.* **2013**, *92*, 653–660. [CrossRef]
95. Bauer, K.; Rancea, M.; Roloff, V.; Elter, T.; Hallek, M.; Engert, A.; Skoetz, N. Rituximab, ofatumumab and other monoclonal anti-CD20 antibodies for chronic lymphocytic leukaemia. *Cochrane Database Syst. Rev.* **2012**, *11*, CD008079. [CrossRef]
96. Cartron, G.; de Guibert, S.; Dilhuydy, M.S.; Morschhauser, F.; Leblond, V.; Dupuis, J.; Mahe, B.; Bouabdallah, R.; Lei, G.; Wenger, M.; et al. Obinutuzumab (GA101) in relapsed/refractory chronic lymphocytic leukemia: Final data from the phase 1/2 GAUGUIN study. *Blood* **2014**, *124*, 2196–2202. [CrossRef]
97. Byrd, J.C.; Brown, J.R.; O'Brien, S.; Barrientos, J.C.; Kay, N.E.; Reddy, N.M.; Coutre, S.; Tam, C.S.; Mulligan, S.P.; Jaeger, U.; et al. Ibrutinib versus ofatumumab in previously treated chronic lymphoid leukemia. *N. Engl. J. Med.* **2014**, *371*, 213–223. [CrossRef]
98. Wierda, W.G.; Kipps, T.J.; Mayer, J.; Stilgenbauer, S.; Williams, C.D.; Hellmann, A.; Robak, T.; Furman, R.R.; Hillmen, P.; Trneny, M.; et al. Ofatumumab as single-agent CD20 immunotherapy in fludarabine-refractory chronic lymphocytic leukemia. *J. Clin. Oncol.* **2010**, *28*, 1749–1755. [CrossRef]
99. Sawas, A.; Farber, C.M.; Schreeder, M.T.; Khalil, M.Y.; Mahadevan, D.; Deng, C.; Amengual, J.E.; Nikolinakos, P.G.; Kolesar, J.M.; Kuhn, J.G.; et al. A phase 1/2 trial of ublituximab, a novel anti-CD20 monoclonal antibody, in patients with B-cell non-Hodgkin lymphoma or chronic lymphocytic leukaemia previously exposed to rituximab. *Br. J. Haematol.* **2017**, *177*, 243–253. [CrossRef]
100. Osterborg, A.; Dyer, M.J.; Bunjes, D.; Pangalis, G.A.; Bastion, Y.; Catovsky, D.; Mellstedt, H. Phase II multicenter study of human CD52 antibody in previously treated chronic lymphocytic leukemia. European Study Group of CAMPATH-1H Treatment in Chronic Lymphocytic Leukemia. *J. Clin. Oncol.* **1997**, *15*, 1567–1574. [CrossRef]
101. Keating, M.J.; Flinn, I.; Jain, V.; Binet, J.L.; Hillmen, P.; Byrd, J.; Albitar, M.; Brettman, L.; Santabarbara, P.; Wacker, B.; et al. Therapeutic role of alemtuzumab (Campath-1H) in patients who have failed fludarabine: Results of a large international study. *Blood* **2002**, *99*, 3554–3561. [CrossRef]
102. Hillmen, P.; Pitchford, A.; Bloor, A.; Broom, A.; Young, M.; Kennedy, B.; Walewska, R.; Furtado, M.; Preston, G.; Neilson, J.R.; et al. Ibrutinib and rituximab versus fludarabine, cyclophosphamide, and rituximab for patients with previously untreated chronic lymphocytic leukaemia (FLAIR): Interim analysis of a multicentre, open label, randomised, phase 3 trial. *Lancet Oncol.* **2023**, *24*, 535–552. [CrossRef]
103. Fischer, K.; Bahlo, J.; Fink, A.M.; Goede, V.; Herling, C.D.; Cramer, P.; Langerbeins, P.; von Tresckow, J.; Engelke, A.; Maurer, C.; et al. Long-term remissions after FCR chemoimmunotherapy in previously untreated patients with CLL: Updated results of the CLL8 trial. *Blood* **2016**, *127*, 208–215. [CrossRef]
104. Kutsch, N.; Bahlo, J.; Robrecht, S.; Franklin, J.; Zhang, C.; Maurer, C.; De Silva, N.; Lange, E.; Weide, R.; Kiehl, M.G.; et al. Long Term Follow-up Data and Health-Related Quality of Life in Frontline Therapy of Fit Patients Treated with FCR Versus BR (CLL10 Trial of the GCLLSG). *Hemasphere* **2020**, *4*, e336. [CrossRef]
105. Michallet, A.S.; Letestu, R.; Le Garff-Tavernier, M.; Campos, L.; Ticchioni, M.; Dilhuydy, M.S.; Morisset, S.; Rouille, V.; Mahé, B.; Laribi, K.; et al. Bruno A fixed-duration immunochemotherapy approach in CLL: 5.5-year results from the phase 2 ICLL-07 FILO trial. *Blood Adv.* **2023**, *7*, 3936–3945. [CrossRef] [PubMed]
106. Von Tresckow, J.; Niemann, C.; Arnon, P.K.; Jasmin, B.; Moritz, F.; Anna-Maria, F.; Michael, G.; Thornton, P.; Tamar Tadmor, T.; Fischer, K.; et al. The GAIA (CLL13) trial: An international intergroup phase III study for frontline therapy in chronic lymphocytic leukemia (CLL). *J. Clin. Oncol.* **2018**, *36* (Suppl. S15), TPS7582.
107. Robak, T.; Hellmann, A.; Kloczko, J.; Loscertales, J.; Lech-Maranda, E.; Pagel, J.M.; Mato, A.; Byrd, J.C.; Awan, F.T.; Hebart, H.; et al. Randomized phase 2 study of otlertuzumab and bendamustine versus bendamustine in patients with relapsed chronic lymphocytic leukaemia. *Br. J. Haematol.* **2017**, *176*, 618–628. [CrossRef]
108. Furman, R.R.; Sharman, J.P.; Coutre, S.E.; Cheson, B.D.; Pagel, J.M.; Hillmen, P.; Barrientos, J.C.; Zelenetz, A.D.; Kipps, T.J.; Flinn, I.; et al. Idelalisib and Rituximab in Relapsed Chronic Lymphocytic Leukemia. *N. Engl. J. Med.* **2014**, *370*, 997–1007. [CrossRef]
109. FDA. Copiktra (Duvelisib): Drug Safety Communication—FDA Warns about Possible Increased Risk of Death and Serious Side Effects. 2022. Available online: https://www.fda.gov/safety/medical-product-safety-information/copiktra-duvelisib-drug-safety-communication-fda-warns-about-possible-increased-risk-death-and (accessed on 30 September 2023).
110. Flinn, I.W.; O'Brien, S.; Kahl, B.; Patel, M.; Oki, Y.; Foss, F.F.; Porcu, P.; Jones, J.; Burger, J.A.; Jain, N.; et al. Duvelisib, a novel oral dual inhibitor of PI3K-δ, γ, is clinically active in advanced hematologic malignancies. *Blood* **2018**, *131*, 877–887. [CrossRef]
111. Davids, M.S.; Kim, H.T.; Nicotra, A.; Savell, A.; Francoeur, K.; Hellman, J.M.; Bazemore, J.; Miskin, H.P.; Sportelli, P.; Stampleman, L.; et al. Umbralisib in combination with ibrutinib in patients with relapsed or refractory chronic lymphocytic leukaemia or mantle cell lymphoma: A multicentre phase 1-1b study. *Lancet Haematol.* **2019**, *6*, 38–47. [CrossRef]
112. Gribben, J.G.; Jurczak, W.; Jacobs, R.W.; Grosicki, S.; Giannopoulos, K.; Wrobel, T.; Zafar, S.F.; Cultrera, J.L.; Kambhampati, S.; Danilov, A.; et al. Umbralisib plus ublituximab (U2) is superior to obinutuzumab plus chlorambucil (O+Chl) in patients with

treatment Naïve (TN) and relapsed/refractory (R/R) chronic lymphocytic leukemia (CLL): Results from the phase 3 Unity-CLL study. *Blood* **2020**, *136*, 37–39. [CrossRef]
113. Gribben, J.G.; Bosch, F.; Cymbalista, F.; Geisler, C.H.; Ghia, P.; Hillmen, P.; Moreno, C.; Stilgenbauer, S. Optimising outcomes for patients with chronic lympho- cytic leukaemia on ibrutinib therapy: European recommendations for clinical practice. *Br. J. Haematol.* **2018**, *180*, 666–679. [CrossRef]
114. Barr, P.M.; Owen, C.; Robak, T.; Tedeschi, A.; Bairey, O.; Burger, J.A.; Hillmen, P.; Coutre, S.E.; Dearden, C.; Grosicki, S.; et al. Up to 8-year follow-up from RESONATE-2: First-line ibrutinib treatment for patients with chronic lymphocytic leukemia. *Blood Adv.* **2022**, *6*, 3440–3450. [CrossRef]
115. Byrd, J.C.; Furman, R.R.; Coutre, S.E.; Flinn, I.W.; Burger, J.A.; Blum, K.; Sharman, J.P.; Wierda, W.; Zhao, W.; Heerema, N.A.; et al. Ibrutinib Treatment for First-Line and Relapsed/Refractory Chronic Lymphocytic Leukemia: Final Analysis of the Pivotal Phase Ib/II PCYC-1102 Study. *Clin. Cancer Res.* **2020**, *26*, 3918–3927. [CrossRef]
116. Moreno, C.; Greil, R.; Demirkan, F.; Tedeschi, A.; Anz, B.; Larratt, L.; Simkovic, M.; Novak, J.; Strugov, V.; Gill, D.; et al. First-line treatment of chronic lymphocytic leukemia with ibrutinib plus obinutuzumab *versus* chlorambucil plus obinutuzumab: Final analysis of the randomized, phase III iLLUMINATE trial. *Haematologica* **2022**, *107*, 2108–2120. [CrossRef]
117. Shanafelt, T.D.; Wang, X.V.; Hanson, C.A.; Paietta, E.M.; O'Brien, S.; Barrientos, J.; Jelinek, D.F.; Braggio, E.; Leis, J.F.; Zhang, C.C.; et al. Long-term outcomes for ibrutinib-rituximab and chemoimmunotherapy in CLL: Updated results of the E1912 trial. *Blood* **2022**, *140*, 112–120. [CrossRef] [PubMed]
118. Ruppert, A.S.; Booth, A.M.; Ding, W.; Bartlett, N.L.; Brander, D.M.; Coutre, S.; Brown, J.R.; Nattam, S.; Larson, R.A.; Erba, H.; et al. Adverse event burden in older patients with CLL receiving bendamustine plus rituximab or ibrutinib regimens: Alliance A041202. *Leukemia* **2021**, *35*, 2854–2861. [CrossRef] [PubMed]
119. O'Brien, S.; Furman, R.R.; Coutre, S.E.; Sharman, J.P.; Burger, J.A.; Blum, K.A.; Grant, B.; Richards, D.A.; Coleman, M.; Wierda, W.; et al. Ibrutinib as initial therapy for elderly patients with chronic lymphocytic leukaemia or small lymphocytic lymphoma: An open-label, multicentre, phase 1b/2 trial. *Lancet Oncol.* **2014**, *15*, 48–58. [CrossRef] [PubMed]
120. Farooqui, M.Z.; Valdez, J.; Martyr, S.; Aue, G.; Saba, N.; Niemann, C.U.; Herman, S.E.; Tian, X.; Marti, G.; Soto, S.; et al. Ibrutinib for previously untreated and relapsed or refractory chronic lymphocytic leukaemia with TP53 aberrations: A phase 2, single-arm trial. *Lancet Oncol.* **2015**, *16*, 169–176. [CrossRef] [PubMed]
121. Burger, J.A.; O'Brien, S. Evolution of CLL treatment—From chemoimmunotherapy to targeted and individualized therapy. *Nat. Rev. Clin. Oncol.* **2018**, *15*, 510–527. [CrossRef]
122. Delgado, J.; Josephson, F.; Camarero, J.; Garcia-Ochoa, B.; Lopez-Anglada, L.; Prieto-Fernandez, C.; van Hennik, P.B.; Papadouli, I.; Gisselbrecht, C.; Enzmann, H.; et al. EMA Review of Acalabrutinib for the Treatment of Adult Patients with Chronic Lymphocytic Leukemia. *Oncologist* **2021**, *26*, 242–249. [CrossRef]
123. Sharman, J.P.; Egyed, M.; Jurczak, W.; Skarbnik, A.; Pagel, J.M.; Flinn, I.W.; Kamdar, M.; Munir, T.; Walewska, R.; Corbett, G.; et al. Acalabrutinib with or without obinutuzumab versus chlorambucil and obinutuzmab for treatment-naive chronic lymphocytic leukaemia (ELEVATE TN): A randomised, controlled, phase 3 trial. *Lancet* **2020**, *395*, 1278–1291. [CrossRef]
124. Ghia, P.; Pluta, A.; Wach, M.; Lysak, D.; Šimkovič, M.; Kriachok, I.; Illés, Á.; de la Serna, J.; Dolan, S.; Campbell, P.; et al. Acalabrutinib Versus Investigator's Choice in Relapsed/Refractory Chronic Lymphocytic Leukemia: Final ASCEND Trial Results. *Hemasphere* **2022**, *6*, e801. [CrossRef]
125. Ghia, P.; Pluta, A.; Wach, M.; Lysak, D.; Kozak, T.; Simkovic, M.; Kaplan, P.; Kraychok, I.; Illes, A.; de la Serna, J.; et al. ASCEND: Phase III, Randomized Trial of Acalabrutinib Versus Idelalisib Plus Rituximab or Bendamustine Plus Rituximab in Relapsedor Refractory Chronic Lymphocytic Leukemia. *J. Clin. Oncol.* **2020**, *38*, 2849–2861. [CrossRef]
126. Seymour, J.F.; Byrd, J.C.; Ghia, P.; Kater, A.P.; Chanan-Khan, A.; Furman, R.R.; O'Brien, S.; Brown, J.R.; Munir, T.; Mato, A.; et al. Detailed safety profile of acalabrutinib vs ibrutinib in previously treated chronic lymphocytic leukemia in the ELEVATE-RR trial. *Blood* **2023**, *142*, 687–699. [CrossRef]
127. Ryan, C.E.; Davids, M.S.; Hermann, R.; Shahkarami, M.; Biondo, J.; Abhyankar, S.; Alhasani, H.; Sharman, J.P.; Mato, A.R.; Roeker, L.E. MAJIC: A phase III trial of acalabrutinib + venetoclax versus venetoclax + obinutuzumab in previously untreated chronic lymphocytic leukemia or small lymphocytic lymphoma. *Future Oncol.* **2022**, *18*, 3689–3699. [CrossRef]
128. Tam, C.S.; Giannopoulos, K.; Jurczak, W.; Šimkovič, M.; Shadman, M.; Österborg, A.; Laurenti, L.; Walker, P.; Opat, S.; Chan, H.; et al. SEQUOIA: Results of a Phase 3 Randomized Study of Zanubrutinib versus Bendamustine + Rituximab (BR) in Patients with Treatment-Naïve (TN) Chronic Lymphocytic Leukemia/Small Lymphocytic Lymphoma (CLL/SLL). *Blood* **2021**, *138*, 396. [CrossRef]
129. Hillmen, P.; Brown, J.R.; Eichhorst, B.F.; Lamanna, N.; O'Brien, S.M.; Qiu, L.; Salmi, T.; Hilger, J.; Wu, K.; Cohen, A.; et al. ALPINE: Zanubrutinib versus ibrutinib in relapsed/refractory chronic lymphocytic leukemia/small lymphocytic lymphoma. *Future Oncol.* **2020**, *16*, 517–523. [CrossRef]
130. Xu, W.; Yang, S.; Zhou, K.; Pan, L.; Li, Z.; Zhou, J.; Gao, S.; Zhou, D.; Hu, J.; Feng, R.; et al. Treatment of relapsed/refractory chronic lymphocytic leukemia/small lymphocytic lymphoma with the BTK inhibitor zanubrutinib: Phase 2, single-arm, multicenter study. *J. Hematol. Oncol.* **2020**, *13*, 48. [CrossRef]
131. Mato, A.R.; Shah, N.N.; Jurczak, W.; Cheah, C.Y.; Pagel, J.M.; Woyach, J.A.; Fakhri, B.; Eyre, T.A.; Lamanna, N.; Patel, M.R.; et al. Pirtobrutinib in relapsed or refractory B-cell malignancies (BRUIN): A phase 1/2 study. *Lancet* **2021**, *397*, 892–901. [CrossRef]

132. Souers, A.J.; Leverson, J.D.; Boghaert, E.R.; Ackler, S.L.; Catron, N.D.; Chen, J.; Dayton, B.D.; Ding, H.; Enschede, S.H.; Fairbrother, W.J.; et al. ABT-199, a potent and selective BCL-2 inhibitor, achieves antitumor activity while sparing platelets. *Nat. Med.* **2013**, *19*, 202–208. [CrossRef]
133. Al-Sawaf, O.; Zhang, C.; Tandon, M.; Sinha, A.; Fink, A.M.; Robrecht, S.; Samoylova, O.; Liberati, A.M.; Pinilla-Ibarz, J.; Opat, S.; et al. Venetoclax plus obinutuzumab versus chlorambucil plus obinutuzumab for previously untreated chronic lymphocytic leukaemia (CLL14): Follow-up results from a multicentre, open-label, randomised, phase 3 trial. *Lancet Oncol.* **2020**, *21*, 1188–1200. [CrossRef]
134. Fischer, K.; Al-Sawaf, O.; Bahlo, J.; Fink, A.-M.; Tandon, M.; Dixon, M.; Robrecht, S.; Warburton, S.; Humphrey, K.; Samoylova, O.; et al. Venetoclax and Obinutuzumab in Patients with CLL and Coexisting Conditions. *N. Engl. J. Med.* **2019**, *380*, 2225–2236. [CrossRef]
135. Wierda, W.G.; Allan, J.N.; Siddiqi, T.; Kipps, T.J.; Opat, S.; Tedeschi, A.; Badoux, X.C.; Kuss, B.J.; Jackson, S.; Moreno, C.; et al. Ibrutinib Plus Venetoclax for First-Line Treatment of Chronic Lymphocytic Leukemia: Primary Analysis Results from the Minimal Residual Disease Cohort of the Randomized Phase II CAPTIVATE Study. *J. Clin. Oncol.* **2021**, *39*, 3853–3865. [CrossRef] [PubMed]
136. Kater, A.P.; Seymour, J.F.; Hillmen, P.; Eichhorst, B.; Langerak, A.W.; Owen, C.; Verdugo, M.; Wu, J.; Punnoose, E.A.; Jiang, Y.; et al. Fixed Duration of Venetoclax-Rituximab in Relapsed/Refractory Chronic Lymphocytic Leukemia Eradicates Minimal Residual Disease and Prolongs Survival: Post-Treatment Follow-Up of the MURANO Phase III Study. *J. Clin. Oncol.* **2019**, *37*, 269–277. [CrossRef] [PubMed]
137. Tam, C.S.; Allan, J.N.; Siddiqi, T.; Kipps, T.J.; Jacobs, R.W.; Opat, S.; Barr, P.M.; Tedeschi, A.; Trentin, L.; Bannerji, R.; et al. Fixed-duration ibrutinib plus venetoclax for first-line treatment of CLL: Primary analysis of the CAPTIVATE FD cohort. *Blood* **2022**, *139*, 3278–3289. [CrossRef] [PubMed]
138. Huber, H.; Tausch, E.; Schneider, C.; Edenhofer, S.; von Tresckow, J.; Robrecht, S.; Giza, A.; Zhang, C.; Fürstenau, M.; Dreger, P.; et al. Final analysis of the CLL2-GIVe trial: Obinutuzumab, ibrutinib, and venetoclax for untreated CLL with del(17p)/TP53mut. *Blood* **2023**, *142*, 961–972. [CrossRef]
139. Eichhorst, B.; Niemann, C.U.; Kater, A.P.; Fürstenau, M.; von Tresckow, J.; Zhang, C.; Robrecht, S.; Gregor, M.; Juliusson, G.; Thornton, P.; et al. First-Line Venetoclax Combinations in Chronic Lymphocytic Leukemia. *N. Engl. J. Med.* **2023**, *388*, 1739–1754. [CrossRef]
140. Acebes-Huerta, A.; Huergo-Zapico, L.; Gonzalez-Rodriguez, A.P.; Fernandez-Guizan, A.; Payer, A.R.; López-Soto, A.; Gonzalez, S. Lenalidomide induces immunomodulation in chronic lymphocytic leukemia and enhances antitumor immune responses mediated by NK and CD4 T cells. *Biomed. Res. Int.* **2014**, *2014*, 265840. [CrossRef]
141. Chanan-Khan, A.; Miller, K.C.; Musial, L.; Lawrence, D.; Padmanabhan, S.; Takeshita, K.; Porter, C.W.; Goodrich, D.W.; Bernstein, Z.P.; Wallace, P.; et al. Clinical efficacy of lenalidomide in patients with relapsed or refractory chronic lymphocytic leukemia: Results of a phase II study. *J. Clin. Oncol.* **2006**, *24*, 5343–5349. [CrossRef]
142. Ferrajoli, A.; Lee, B.N.; Schlette, E.J.; O'Brien, S.M.; Gao, H.; Wen, S.; Wierda, W.G.; Estrov, Z.; Faderl, S.; Cohen, E.N.; et al. Lenalidomide induces com- plete and partial remissions in patients with relapsed and refractory chronic lymphocytic leukemia. *Blood* **2008**, *111*, 5291–5297. [CrossRef]
143. Chanan-Khan, A.A.; Zaritskey, A.; Egyed, M.; Vokurka, S.; Semochkin, S.; Schuh, A.; Kassis, J.; Simpson, D.; Zhang, J.; Purse, B.; et al. Lenalidomide mainte- nance therapy in previously treated chronic lymphocytic leukaemia (CONTINUUM): A randomised, double-blind, placebo-controlled, phase 3 trial. *Lancet Haematol.* **2017**, *4*, e534–e543. [CrossRef]
144. Katz, O.B.; Yehudai-Ofir, D.; Zuckerman, T. Cellular therapy in chronic lymphocytic leukemia: Have we advanced in the last decade? *Acta Haematol.* **2023**, *146*, 1. [CrossRef]
145. Kharfan-Dabaja, M.A.; Kumar, A.; Hamadani, M.; Stilgenbauer, S.; Ghia, P.; Anasetti, C.; Dreger, P.; Montserrat, E.; Perales, M.A.; Alyea, E.P.; et al. Clinical practice recommendations for use of allogeneic hematopoietic cell transplantation in chronic lymphocytic leukemia on behalf of the guidelines committee of the American society for blood and marrow transplantation. *Biol. Blood Marrow Transplant.* **2016**, *22*, 2117–2125. [CrossRef]
146. van Gelder, M.; de Wreede, L.C.; Bornhäuser, M.; Niederwieser, D.; Karas, M.; Anderson, N.S.; Gramatzki, M.; Dreger, P.; Michallet, M.; Petersen, E.; et al. Long-term survival of patients with CLL after allogeneic transplantation: A report from the European society for blood and marrow transplantation. *Bone Marrow Transplant.* **2017**, *52*, 372–380. [CrossRef]
147. Andersen, N.S.; Bornhäuser, M.; Gramatzki, M.; Dreger, P.; Vitek, A.; Karas, M.; Michallet, M.; Moreno, C.; van Gelder, M.; Henseler, A.; et al. Reduced intensity conditioning regimens including alkylating chemotherapy do not alter survival outcomes after allogeneic hematopoietic cell transplantation in chronic lymphocytic leukemia compared to low-intensity non-myeloablative conditioning. *J. Cancer Res. Clin. Oncol.* **2019**, *145*, 2823–2834. [CrossRef]
148. Poon, M.L.; Fox, P.S.; Samuels, B.I.; O'Brien, S.; Jabbour, E.; Hsu, Y.; Gulbis, A.; Korbling, M.; Champlin, R.; Abruzzo, L.V.; et al. Allogeneic stem cell transplant in patients with chronic lymphocytic leukemia with 17p deletion: Consult-transplant versus consult- no-transplant analysis. *Leuk. Lymphoma* **2015**, *56*, 711–715. [CrossRef]
149. Turtle, C.J.; Hay, K.A.; Hanafi, L.A.; Li, D.; Cherian, S.; Chen, X.; Wood, B.; Lozanski, A.; Byrd, J.C.; Heimfeld, S.; et al. Durable molecular remissions in chronic lymphocytic leukemia treated with CD19-specific chimeric antigen receptor-modified T cells after failure of Ibrutinib. *J. Clin. Oncol.* **2017**, *35*, 3010–3020. [CrossRef]
150. Wierda, W.G.; Dorritie, K.A.; Munoz, J.; Stephens, D.M.; Solomon, S.R.; Gillenwater, H.H.; Gong, L.; Yang, L.; Ogasawara, K.; Thorpe, B.S.; et al. Transcend CLL 004: Phase 1 cohort of lisocabtagene maraleucel (lisocel) in combination with ibrutinib for

patients with relapsed/refractory (R/R) chronic lymphocytic leukemia/small lymphocytic lymphoma (CLL/SLL). *Blood* **2020**, *136*, 39–40. [CrossRef]
151. Grupo Español de Leucemia Linfocítica Crónica (GELLLC). Guías de Tratamiento LLC. 2023. Available online: https://www.gellc.es/images/pdf/GUIA_GELLC_04_2023.pdf (accessed on 28 September 2023).
152. Owen, C.; Banerji, V.; Johnson, N.; Gerrie, A.; Aw, A.; Chen, C.; Robinson, S. Canadian evidence-based guideline for frontline treatment of chronic lymphocytic leukemia: 2022 update. *Leuk. Res.* **2023**, *125*, 107016. [CrossRef]
153. Tse, E.; Kwong, Y.L.; Goh, Y.T.; Bee, P.C.; Ng, S.C.; Tan, D.; Caguioa, P.; Nghia, H.; Dumagay, T.; Norasetthada, L.; et al. Expert consensus on the management of chronic lymphocytic leukaemia in Asia. *Clin. Exp. Med.* **2023**, *23*, 2895–2907. [CrossRef]
154. Shadman, M. Diagnosis and Treatment of Chronic Lymphocytic Leukemia: A Review. *JAMA* **2023**, *329*, 918–932. [CrossRef]
155. Wendtner, C.M.; Al-Sawaf, O.; Binder, M.; Dreger, P.; Eichhorst, B.; Gregor, M.; Greil, R.; Hallek, M.; Holtkamp, U.; Knauf, W.U.; et al. Chronische Lymphatische Leukämie. 2023. Available online: https://www.onkopedia.com/de/onkopedia/guidelines/chronische-lymphatische-leukaemie-cll/@@guideline/html/index.html#ID0ECWAE (accessed on 28 September 2023).
156. Wierda, W.G.; Brown, J.; Abramson, J.S.; Awan, F.; Bilgrami, S.F.; Bociek, G.; Brander, D.; Chanan-Khan, A.A.; Coutre, S.E.; Davis, R.S.; et al. NCCN Guidelines® Insights: Chronic Lymphocytic Leukemia/Small Lymphocytic Lymphoma, Version 3.2022. *J. Natl. Compr. Cancer Netw.* **2022**, *20*, 622–634. [CrossRef]
157. Islam, P. Current Treatment Options in Relapsed and Refractory Chronic Lymphocytic Leukemia/Small Lymphocytic Lymphoma: A Review. *Curr. Treat. Options Oncol.* **2023**, *24*, 1259–1273. [CrossRef]
158. Odetola, O.; Ma, S. Relapsed/Refractory Chronic Lymphocytic Leukemia (CLL). *Curr. Hematol. Malig. Rep.* **2023**, *18*, 130–143. [CrossRef]
159. Brown, J.R.; Eichhorst, B.; Hillmen, P.; Jurczak, W.; Kaźmierczak, M.; Lamanna, N.; O'Brien, S.M.; Tam, C.S.; Qiu, L.; Zhou, K.; et al. Zanubrutinib or Ibrutinib in Relapsed or Refractory Chronic Lymphocytic Leukemia. *N. Engl. J. Med.* **2023**, *388*, 319–332. [CrossRef] [PubMed]
160. Hillmen, P.; Rawstron, A.C.; Brock, K.; Muñoz-Vicente, S.; Yates, F.J.; Bishop, R.; Boucher, R.; MacDonald, D.; Fegan, C.; McCaig, A.; et al. Ibrutinib Plus Venetoclax in Relapsed/Refractory Chronic Lymphocytic Leukemia: The CLARITY Study. *J. Clin. Oncol.* **2019**, *37*, 2722–2729, Erratum in *J. Clin. Oncol.* **2020**, *38*, 1644. [CrossRef] [PubMed]
161. Roberts, A.W.; Davids, M.S.; Pagel, J.M.; Kahl, B.S.; Puvvada, S.D.; Gerecitano, J.F.; Kipps, T.J.; Anderson, M.A.; Brown, J.R.; Gressick, L.; et al. Targeting BCL-2 with Venetoclax in relapsed chronic lymphocytic leukemia. *N. Engl. J. Med.* **2016**, *374*, 311–322. [CrossRef] [PubMed]
162. Stilgenbauer, S.; Eichhorst, B.; Schetelig, J.; Coutre, S.; Seymour, J.F.; Munir, T.; Puvvada, S.D.; Wendtner, C.M.; Roberts, A.W.; Jurczak, W.; et al. Venetoclax in relapsed or refractory chronic lymphocytic leukaemia with 17p deletion: A multicentre, open-label, phase 2 study. *Lancet Oncol.* **2016**, *17*, 768–778. [CrossRef] [PubMed]
163. Taghiloo, S.; Asgarian-Omran, H. Current Approaches of Immune Checkpoint Therapy in Chronic Lymphocytic Leukemia. *Curr. Treat. Options Oncol.* **2023**, *24*, 1408–1438. [CrossRef] [PubMed]
164. Reiff, S.D.; Muhowski, E.M.; Guinn, D.; Lehman, A.; Fabian, C.A.; Cheney, C.; Mantel, R.; Smith, L.; Johnson, A.J.; Young, W.B.; et al. Noncovalent inhibition of C481S Bruton tyrosine kinase by GDC-0853: A new treatment strategy for ibrutinib-resistant CLL. *Blood* **2018**, *132*, 1039–1049. [CrossRef]
165. Wang, E.; Mi, X.; Thompson, M.C.; Montoya, S.; Notti, R.Q.; Afaghani, J.; Durham, B.H.; Penson, A.; Witkowski, M.T.; Lu, S.X.; et al. Mechanisms of Resistance to Noncovalent Bruton's Tyrosine Kinase Inhibitors. *N. Engl. J. Med.* **2022**, *386*, 735–743. [CrossRef]
166. Nakhoda, S.; Vistarop, A.; Wang, Y.L. Resistance to Bruton tyrosine kinase inhibition in chronic lymphocytic leukaemia and non-Hodgkin lymphoma. *Br. J. Haematol.* **2023**, *200*, 137–149. [CrossRef]
167. Burger, J.A.; Landau, D.A.; Taylor-Weiner, A.; Bozic, I.; Zhang, H.; Sarosiek, K.; Wang, L.; Stewart, C.; Fan, J.; Hoellenriegel, J.; et al. Clonal evolution in patients with chronic lymphocytic leukaemia developing resistance to BTK inhibition. *Nat. Commun.* **2016**, *7*, 11589. [CrossRef]
168. Birkinshaw, R.W.; Gong, J.N.; Luo, C.S.; Lio, D.; White, C.A.; Anderson, M.A.; Blombery, P.; Lessene, G.; Majewski, I.J.; Thijssen, R.; et al. Structures of BCL-2 in complex with venetoclax reveal the molecular basis of resistance mutations. *Nat. Commun.* **2019**, *10*, 2385. [CrossRef]
169. Cuneo, A.; Foà, R. Relapsed/Refractory Chronic Lymphocytic Leukemia: Chemoimmunotherapy, Treatment until Progression with Mechanism-Driven Agents or Finite-Duration Therapy? *Mediterr. J. Hematol. Infect. Dis.* **2019**, *11*, e2019024. [CrossRef] [PubMed]
170. Shadman, M.; Manzoor, B.S.; Sail, K.; Tuncer, H.H.; Allan, J.N.; Ujjani, C.; Emechebe, N.; Kamalakar, R.; Coombs, C.C.; Leslie, L.; et al. Treatment Discontinuation Patterns for Patients with Chronic Lymphocytic Leukemia in Real-World Settings: Results from a Multi-Center International Study. *Clin. Lymphoma Myeloma Leuk.* **2023**, *23*, 515–526. [CrossRef] [PubMed]
171. Davids, M.S.; Lampson, B.L.; Tyekucheva, S.; Wang, Z.; Lowney, J.; Pazienza, S.; Montegaard, J.; Patterson, V.; Weinstcok, M.; Crombie, J.L.; et al. Acalabrutinib, venetoclax, and Obinutuzumab as frontline treatment for chronic lymphocytic leukaemia: A single-arm, open-label, phase 2 study. *Lancet Oncol.* **2021**, *22*, 1391–1402. [CrossRef]

172. Soumerai, J.D.; Mato, A.R.; Dogan, A.; Seshan, V.E.; Joffe, E.; Flaherty, K.; Carter, J.; Hochberg, E.; Barnes, J.A.; Hamilton, A.M.; et al. Zanubrutinib, Obinutuzumab, and venetoclax with minimal residual disease-driven discontinuation in previously untreated patients with chronic lymphocytic leukaemia or small lymphocytic lymphoma: A multicentre, single-arm, phase 2 trial. *Lancet Haematol.* **2021**, *8*, E879–E890. [CrossRef]
173. Karr, M.; Roeker, L. A History of Targeted Therapy Development and Progress in Novel-Novel Combinations for Chronic Lymphocytic Leukemia (CLL). *Cancers* **2023**, *15*, 1018. [CrossRef]

Disclaimer/Publisher's Note: The statements, opinions and data contained in all publications are solely those of the individual author(s) and contributor(s) and not of MDPI and/or the editor(s). MDPI and/or the editor(s) disclaim responsibility for any injury to people or property resulting from any ideas, methods, instructions or products referred to in the content.

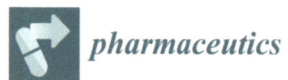

Article

Exploring Metabolic Pathways of Anamorelin, a Selective Agonist of the Growth Hormone Secretagogue Receptor, via Molecular Networking

Young Beom Kwak [1,2,†], Jeong In Seo [2,†] and Hye Hyun Yoo [2,*]

1 Korea Racing Authority, Gwachon 13822, Republic of Korea; kwakyoungbeom1301@gmail.com
2 Institute of Pharmaceutical Science and Technology, College of Pharmacy, Hanyang University, Ansan 15588, Republic of Korea; seojeongin@hanyang.ac.kr
* Correspondence: yoohh@hanyang.ac.kr; Tel.: +82-10-400-5804
† These authors contributed equally to this work.

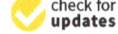

Citation: Kwak, Y.B.; Seo, J.I.; Yoo, H.H. Exploring Metabolic Pathways of Anamorelin, a Selective Agonist of the Growth Hormone Secretagogue Receptor, via Molecular Networking. *Pharmaceutics* 2023, *15*, 2700. https://doi.org/10.3390/pharmaceutics15122700

Academic Editors: Cristina Manuela Drăgoi, Alina Crenguța Nicolae and Ion-Bogdan Dumitrescu

Received: 10 October 2023
Revised: 23 November 2023
Accepted: 26 November 2023
Published: 29 November 2023

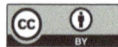

Copyright: © 2023 by the authors. Licensee MDPI, Basel, Switzerland. This article is an open access article distributed under the terms and conditions of the Creative Commons Attribution (CC BY) license (https://creativecommons.org/licenses/by/4.0/).

Abstract: In this study, we delineated the poorly characterized metabolism of anamorelin, a growth hormone secretagogue receptor agonist, in vitro using human liver microsomes (HLM), based on classical molecular networking (MN) and feature-based molecular networking (FBMN) from the Global Natural Products Social Molecular Networking platform. Following the in vitro HLM reaction, the MN analysis showed 11 neighboring nodes whose information propagated from the node corresponding to anamorelin. The FBMN analysis described the separation of six nodes that the MN analysis could not achieve. In addition, the similarity among neighboring nodes could be discerned via their respective metabolic pathways. Collectively, 18 metabolites (M1–M12) were successfully identified, suggesting that the metabolic pathways involved were demethylation, hydroxylation, dealkylation, desaturation, and *N*-oxidation, whereas 6 metabolites (M13a*-b*, M14a*-b*, and M15a*-b*) remained unidentified. Furthermore, the major metabolites detected in HLM, M1 and M7, were dissimilar from those observed in the CYP3A4 isozyme assay, which is recognized to be markedly inhibited by anamorelin. Specifically, M7, M8, and M9 were identified as the major metabolites in the CYP3A4 isozyme assay. Therefore, a thorough investigation of metabolism is imperative for future in vivo studies. These findings may offer prospective therapeutic opportunities for anamorelin.

Keywords: anamorelin; metabolism; molecular networking; LC-MS/MS; GHSR agonist

1. Introduction

Anamorelin is a ghrelin receptor agonist that stimulates the growth hormone secretagogue receptor (GHSR), that has been developed for treating anorexia and weight loss. It is also known as ONO-7643, RC-1291, or ST-1291 [1–5]. Anamorelin has shown promising outcomes in clinical trials targeting the anorexia and weight loss associated with advanced pancreatic cancer. However, it failed to receive marketing approval in Phase 3 clinical trials [1,6]. Despite the previous setback, investigations on similar drugs are ongoing, and further research on anamorelin is exploring methods to surmount past limitations regarding its use as a treatment by appraising its pros, cons, and side effects. In this regard, revealing anamorelin's metabolic mechanism in detail could offer insights into its advantages and disadvantages [7,8]. This is because studying metabolic mechanisms can facilitate the identification of and improvement in the therapeutic effects of drugs, thereby discovering and developing their potential applications in treating other diseases. However, at present, publicly reported data on the metabolism of anamorelin are unavailable.

Molecular network analysis is a computational strategy that can be used to visualize and interpret complex data resulting from MS analysis using the Global Natural Products Social Molecular Networking (GNPS) Platform (https://gnps.ucsd.edu/ProteoSAFe/static/gnps-splash.jsp (accessed on 23 November 2023)). Classical molecular networking

(MN) can identify potential similarities between all MS/MS spectra in a dataset and propagate annotations to unknown but structurally related molecules [9]. More specifically, MN analysis utilizes the similarity of the fragmentation patterns of molecules to determine their correlation [10]. Thus, it could facilitate the workflow of drug metabolism research compared with traditional methods. Consequently, there has been a notable increase in the number of studies adopting the MN approach in recent times [9,11]. Feature-based molecular networking (FBMN) is an advanced version of MN. The advantage of FBMN over MN is its utilization of a well-established MS processing software for data pre-processing, allowing for the incorporation of not only MS information, such as isotope patterns, but also chromatographic characteristics, such as retention times, peak width, and resolution. This incorporation enables compounds with similar MS^2 spectra but different retention times to be distinctively included in the network. Additionally, the relative intensity information of the spectrum is semi-quantified and displayed on the node, providing researchers with additional molecular information [12].

In the present study, our goal was to comprehensively delineate the largely unexplored metabolic profile of anamorelin to enhance its potential clinical success. To achieve this, we identified anamorelin metabolites using human liver microsomes (HLM) in vitro. Additionally, the structural information obtained was validated through additional experiments (the flavin-containing monooxygenases (FMO) incubation assay and utilization of an atmospheric pressure chemical ionization (APCI) source).

2. Materials and Methods

2.1. Materials

Anamorelin was provided by Toronto Research Chemical, Inc. (North York, ON, Canada). Pooled HLM, c-DNA-expressing CYP3A4, and three human flavin-containing monooxygenases (FMO) isoforms (FMO1, FMO3, and FMO5) were obtained from BD Gentest Corp. (Woburn, MA, USA). Glucose 6-phosphate (G6P), β-$NADP^+$, glucose 6-phosphate dehydrogenase (G6Pd), and ammonium formate were obtained from Sigma Chemical Co. (St. Louis, MO, USA). All chemicals were analytical grade and were used as received. HPLC-grade acetonitrile (ACN) and distilled water (DW) were purchased from J.T. Baker (Phillipsburg, NJ, USA). Formic acid was purchased from Junsei Chemical Co. (Chou-ku, Japan).

2.2. Microsomal and cDNA-Expressed Recombinant CYP Isozyme Incubation Assay

In vitro metabolites of anamorelin were investigated using 1 mg/mL of microsomal protein in 0.1 M potassium phosphate buffer (pH 7.4) at 37 °C for 2 h. The reaction was initiated by adding an NADPH-generating system (NGS) containing 10 mg/mL β-$NADP^+$, 0.1 M G6P, and 1 unit/mL of G6Pd to the reaction mixture. After incubation, the reaction was terminated by the addition of ice-cold ACN. The mixture was kept on ice followed by centrifugation for 5 min at 13,200 rpm. An aliquot (10 μL) of the supernatant was used for ultra-high-performance liquid chromatography (UHPLC) Q-Orbitrap analysis. All experiments were performed in duplicate.

Additionally, the anamorelin metabolism pathway was investigated using a cDNA-expressed recombinant CYP3A4 isozyme. Incubation was performed under the same conditions described above in the presence of recombinant CYP3A4.

2.3. LC/MS/MS Analysis of Anamorelin

The UHPLC Q-Orbitrap system consisted of a Thermo Ultimate 3000 UHPLC (Thermo Fisher Scientific, Bremen, Germany) and a Q-Exactive™ mass spectrometer (Thermo Fisher Scientific, Bremen, Germany). The column used for separation was a Phenomenex Luna Omega™ 1.6 μm column (2.1 × 100 mm). The column temperature was maintained at 50 °C using a thermostatically controlled column oven. The mobile phase consisted of 5 mM ammonium formate (pH 3.0) in DW (Solvent A) and 0.1% formic acid in ACN (Solvent B). A gradient program was used for liquid chromatographic separation at a flow rate of 0.25 mL/min. For anamorelin and metabolite analysis, solvent B was 0% as the initial condition (t = 0 min), held for 5 min, and then increased to 70% from t = 5 min to t = 23 min; solvent B was returned to 0% from t = 23.0 min to t = 23.1 min, and stabilized until t = 25 min before the next injection. The column eluent was introduced directly into the mass spectrometer. UHPLC was coupled with the MS via a heated ESI source (HESI-II) operated in the positive ionization mode. For drug metabolite detection, the positive ESI mode was used. The ionization voltage was set at 3.5 kV. Mass calibration was performed, and the HESI-II source was used with heating (413 °C). The acquisition modes employed were each full scan and parallel reaction monitoring (PRM). The full scan acquisition range was set to m/z 150–800 Da for the positive mode, with a mass resolution of 70,000 (FWHM) and automatic gain control (AGC) of 3×10^6. A mass resolution of 17,250 (FWHM) for the PRM mode was used with an isolation window of 0.8 amu. For MN analysis, the data-dependent MS^2 ($ddMS^2$) mode was applied to trigger the fragmentation with a normalized collision energy (NCE) of 40 eV. The 12 highest parent ions at each scan point of MS were selected as the target precursor ions for further MS^2 fragmentation. The acquisition range was set to m/z 150–600 Da for the positive mode, with a mass resolution of 35,000 (FWHM) and automatic gain control (AGC) of 2×10^4.

2.4. MN and FBMN Analyses for Metabolite Screening

For MN generation, the raw data files obtained from the $ddMS^2$ analysis were converted from .raw to .mzXML format using MSConvert (http://proteowizard.sourceforge.net (accessed on 23 November 2023)). The .mzXML file was uploaded to the Global Natural Product Social Molecular Networking (GNPS) web-based platform through WinSCP (version 5.15.3) and analyzed using GNPS (http://gnps.ucsd.edu (accessed on 23 November 2023)). The FBMN was created according to the workflow of the GNPS platform [12]. The mzXML input file was pre-processed and converted into output files (.mgf and _quant.csv) that included the peak isolation sample information and strengths of MS and MS^2 matched using the MZmine 2 (version MZmine 2.53) software. The output file was uploaded to the GNPS platform. For both MN and FBMN analyses in the GNPS platform, the base parameters were set to m/z 0.02 for the mass tolerance of the precursor and fragment ions. The minimum cluster size was set to 2. Links were also made between nodes when the cosine value was greater than 0.50 and the minimum number of common fragment ions matched by the MS/MS spectrum was 3. The MN and FBMN data were visualized and annotated using the Cytoscape 3.7.2 software (San Diego, CA, USA). Figure 1 outlines the sequential steps comprising the workflow for each molecular networking analysis.

2.5. FMO Incubation Assay

For the identification of the N-oxide metabolite, anamorelin was incubated with 0.5 mg/mL FMO isoforms (FMO1, FMO3, and FMO5) at 37 °C for 2 h. The reaction was initiated with NGS containing 10 mg/mL β-NADP$^+$, 0.1 M G6P, and 1 unit/mL of G6Pd in the reaction mixture. After incubation, the reaction was terminated by the addition of ice-cold ACN. The mixture was kept on ice followed by centrifugation for 5 min at 13,200 rpm. An aliquot (10 µL) of the supernatant was used for UHPLC Q-Orbitrap analysis. All experiments were performed in duplicate.

2.6. APCI/MS Analysis

Atmospheric pressure chemical ionization (APCI) analysis was performed to confirm the presence of additional N-oxide metabolites. The instrument and column separation conditions were identical to those in the method described above. The operating conditions for positive mode APCI/MS were as follows: mass resolution (FWHM), 35,000; sheath gas flow rate, 31; auxiliary gas flow rate, 31; sweep gas flow rate, 0 (arbitrary units); discharge current, 4.97 µA; capillary temperature, 320 °C; S-lens RF level, 40; and automatic gain control, 5×10^6.

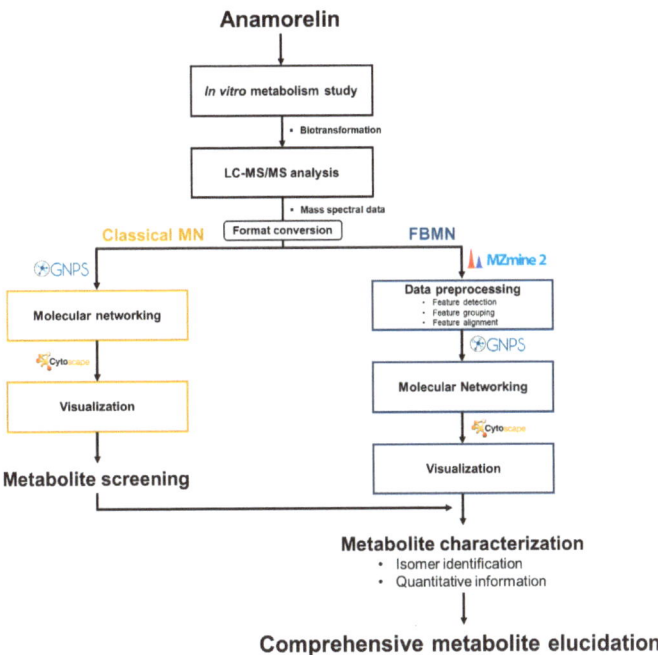

Figure 1. Molecular networking analysis flow chart.

3. Results

3.1. Anamorelin Metabolite Screening with Molecular Networking

To screen for anamorelin metabolites, we utilized MN analysis with ddMS^2 data on the GNPS platform. Within the resulting networks, our initial search focused on identifying a network containing the parent drug's node. This approach was based on the expectation that metabolites would likely share structural similarities and could thus be integrated into the same network as the parent drug [13]. Therefore, we identified the parent node with an m/z value of 547.3389 in a distinct network that was connected to 11 additional nodes ranging from 260.191 to 591.331 through our initial MN analysis of anamorelin metabolites (Figure 2A). However, during the manual inspection of the extracted ion chromatograms (EICs) for each node we observed several extra peaks eluted at different times, which could indicate the presence of isomers. To obtain a more accurate understanding of the metabolite landscape for anamorelin, we performed FBMN analysis, which enabled us to distinguish overlapping nodes. As a result, in the FBMN analysis, six nodes (563.336, 579.333, 549.318, 561.322, 575.339, 591.331) in the MN analysis were clearly separated into their respective nodes (Figure 2B).

3.2. Anamorelin Metabolite Structural Elucidation

The FBMN analysis yielded 18 metabolites (M1-M12) and 6 unknown compounds (M13a*-b*, M14a*-b*, and M15a*-b*), including anamorelin. To gain insight into the metabolic pathways of anamorelin, we examined the structures of each metabolite by analyzing their chromatographic characteristics and mass spectrum information, further comparing them to those of anamorelin (Table S1, Figure 3). M1 ($C_{30}H_{41}N_6O_3$; 533.3235) exhibited a 14 amu decrease from the parent compound (anamorelin; $C_{31}H_{43}N_6O_3$; m/z 547.3391), indicating demethylation. M2 ($C_{30}H_{39}N_6O_3$; 531.3078), with a 16 amu decrease from the parent, suggested both demethylation and desaturation. The product ion of each metabolite, m/z 262 ($C_{15}H_{24}N_3O$) for M1 and m/z 260 ($C_{15}H_{22}N_3O$) for M2, respectively, was 14 and 16 amu smaller than that of the parent (m/z 276), signifying the loss of the methyl group (-14 amu) and di-hydrogen (-2 amu) from the di-methylamine group of anamorelin. M3a-b ($C_{31}H_{43}N_6O_4$;

m/z 563.334) were attributed to the hydroxylation of the parent. The m/z 148 in the MS^2 of M3a originated from the oxidation of the indole nitrogen. M4a-c ($C_{31}H_{43}N_6O_5$; 579.3289) were metabolites with di-hydroxylation (+32 amu) of anamorelin. M5a ($C_{30}H_{41}N_6O_4$; m/z 549.3183) were demethylated metabolites (−14 amu) of M3a, in which demethylation occurred in the dimethylamine group, as indicated by the presence of m/z 262 in MS^2. M5b-c ($C_{30}H_{41}N_6O_4$; m/z 549.3183) were demethylated metabolites (−14 amu) of M3b, in which demethylation occurred in the dimethylamine group, as indicated by the presence of m/z 262 in MS^2. M6 ($C_{31}H_{41}N_6O_4$; m/z 561.3184) was determined as hydroxylation (+16 amu) and desaturation (−2 amu). M7 ($C_{16}H_{26}N_3O$; m/z 276.207) was indicated as an N-dealkylated metabolite (−271 amu). Meanwhile, M8 ($C_{15}H_{24}N_3O$, m/z 262.1914) and M9 ($C_{15}H_{22}N_3O$, m/z 260.1757) exhibited m/z values that were 14 and 16 amu lower than M7, respectively. The metabolic patterns observed in M8 and M9 were similar to those of M1 and M2 from the parent compound, suggesting that demethylation, with and without desaturation steps at the dimethylamine group, occurred after N-dealkylation. Interestingly, we observed that M10 ($C_{31}H_{43}N_6O_4$; m/z 563.334) was eluted later than anamorelin on the chromatograms and 16 amu higher than the parent, which might indicate an N-oxidized metabolite. Additionally, M11a-b ($C_{31}H_{43}N_6O_5$; m/z 579.3289) exhibited m/z values that were 28 amu higher than the parent. M12 ($C_{30}H_{41}N_6O_4$; m/z 549.3183) exhibited m/z values that were 2 amu higher than the parent. M13a*-b* ($C_{32}H_{43}N_6O_4$; m/z 575.3345) and M14a*-b* ($C_{32}H_{43}N_6O_5$; m/z 591.3274) displayed increased CO and CO$_2$ elemental compositions compared to the parent. M15a*-b* exhibited demethylation, accompanied by the addition of CO (Figure 4). But the interpretation of this observation was unclear. Methylation is not expected to occur during phase I biotransformation with NADPH fortification. The methylation of nitrogen-containing compounds in liver microsomes has been reported in several studies, but its applicability to this study is limited [14,15]. The asterisks used in compounds M13a*-b*, M14a*-b*, and M15a*-b* indicate substances whose biotransformation status under the in vitro microsomal system of anamorelin was unclear. Finally, the structurally characterized metabolites (M1–M12) were semi-quantitatively compared by measuring the area on the chromatogram, and as a result, M1 and M7 were found to be the major metabolites in HLM in vitro (Figure 5).

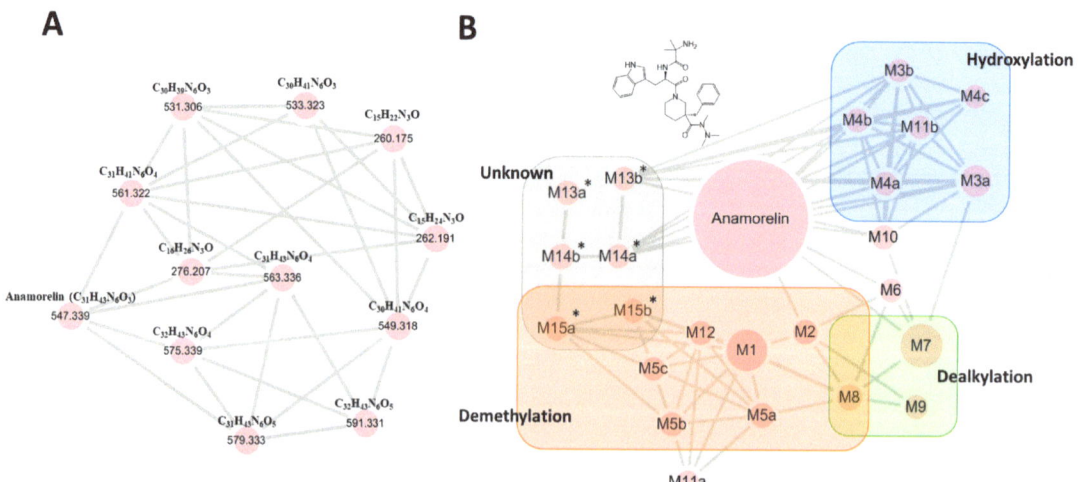

Figure 2. Molecular networking maps. (**A**) MN and (**B**) FBMN results of anamorelin and its metabolites generated from human liver microsome reaction for 2 h. The molecular networking result can be visualized directly on GNPS via the following links: https://gnps.ucsd.edu/ProteoSAFe/result.jsp?view=network_displayer&componentindex=15&highlight_node=1281&task=53b690a71dec466aa9a777916e8c0113#%257B%257D and

https://gnps.ucsd.edu/ProteoSAFe/result.jsp?view=network_displayer&highlight_node=60096&componentindex=1&task=7fabfeb68f9c4fb2bb3e36bbfe8133a1#%257B%257D, accessed on 23 November 2023.

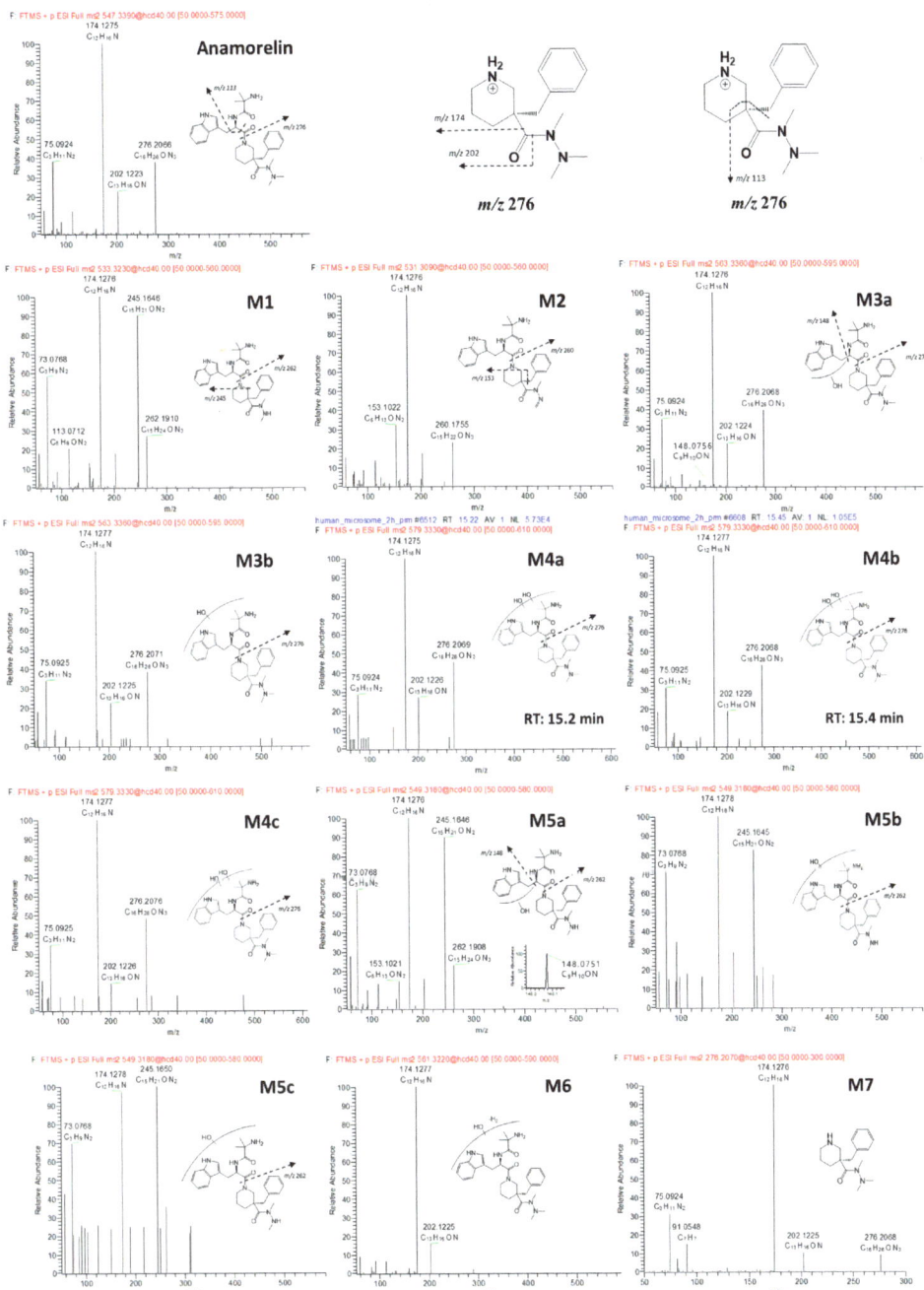

Figure 3. *Cont.*

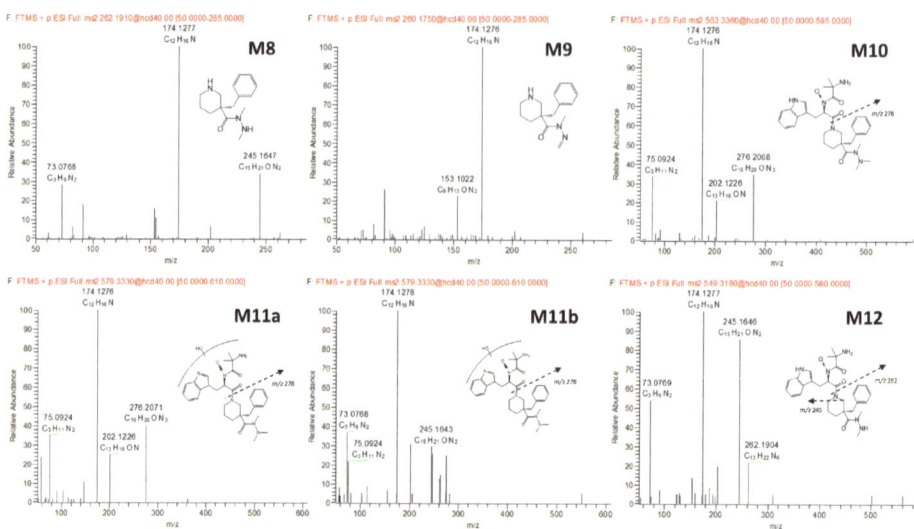

Figure 3. Representative MS/MS spectra and the proposed structure of each anamorelin metabolite generated from human liver microsome reaction for 2 h.

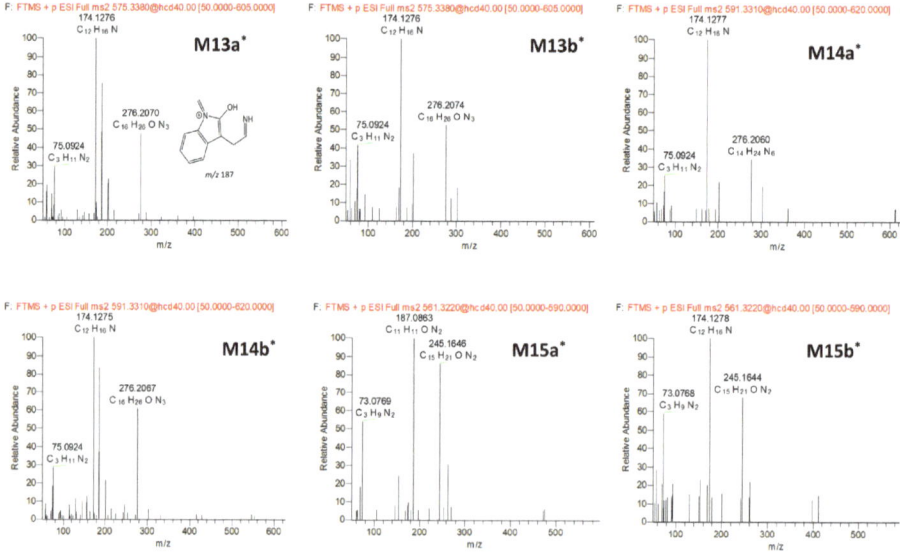

Figure 4. MS/MS spectra and the predicted structure of each unknown compound generated from human liver microsome reaction for 2 h.

3.3. Confirmation of N-Oxide Metabolites and Identification of CYP3A4-Mediated Metabolites

Our structural analysis led us to predict M10 as an N-oxide metabolite due to the later retention time (Figure 5) and higher m/z value (+16 amu) compared to the parent. Additionally, we suspected that M11a-b and M12 were metabolites generated through N-oxidation-mediated metabolism. However, the complexity of the metabolic process in HLM made it challenging to confidently determine the presence of N-oxidized metabolites. Therefore, we conducted an additional assay to verify the formation of N-oxidated metabolites using FMO [16,17]. As a result of the FMO incubation assay using three isozymes

(FMO1, FMO3, and FMO5), M10 was produced in all FMOs tested (Figure 6A). To further investigate the multistep metabolism mediated by both FMO and CYP, we modified our LC-MS system by replacing the ESI source with an APCI source. By utilizing an APCI source, we were able to identify metabolites derived from N-oxidation as an intermediate reaction via thermal deoxygenation during thermal energy activation in the vaporizer (Figure 6B) [18]. This method confirmed that M11a-b and M12 were the hydroxylated and demethylated metabolites generated after N-oxidation by FMO.

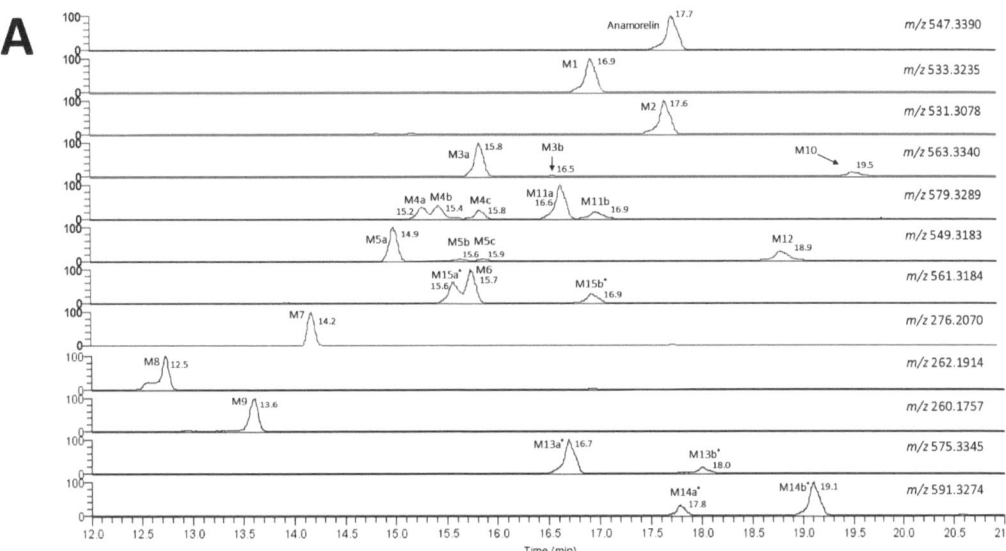

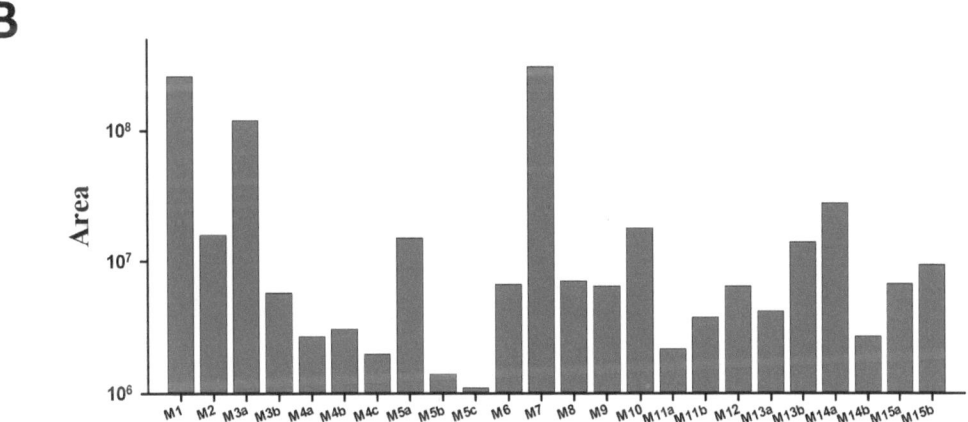

Figure 5. Chromatographic profiles of anamorelin metabolites. (**A**) Extracted ion chromatograms and (**B**) peak areas of anamorelin and its metabolites generated from human liver microsome reaction for 2 h.

A recent study reported that anamorelin is metabolized by CYP3A4, predominantly present in the liver. Furthermore, CYP3A4 inhibitors have been reported to increase the AUC of anamorelin. However, this study does not provide detailed information regarding the metabolic process of anamorelin [19–21]. To compare the metabolite profiles observed in the HLM metabolism study, we conducted additional experiments using the CYP3A4 isozyme. Our findings revealed that CYP3A4 primarily produced N-alkylated metabolites

(Figure 7), specifically M7, M8, and M9, despite M1 and M7 being identified as the major metabolites in HLM.

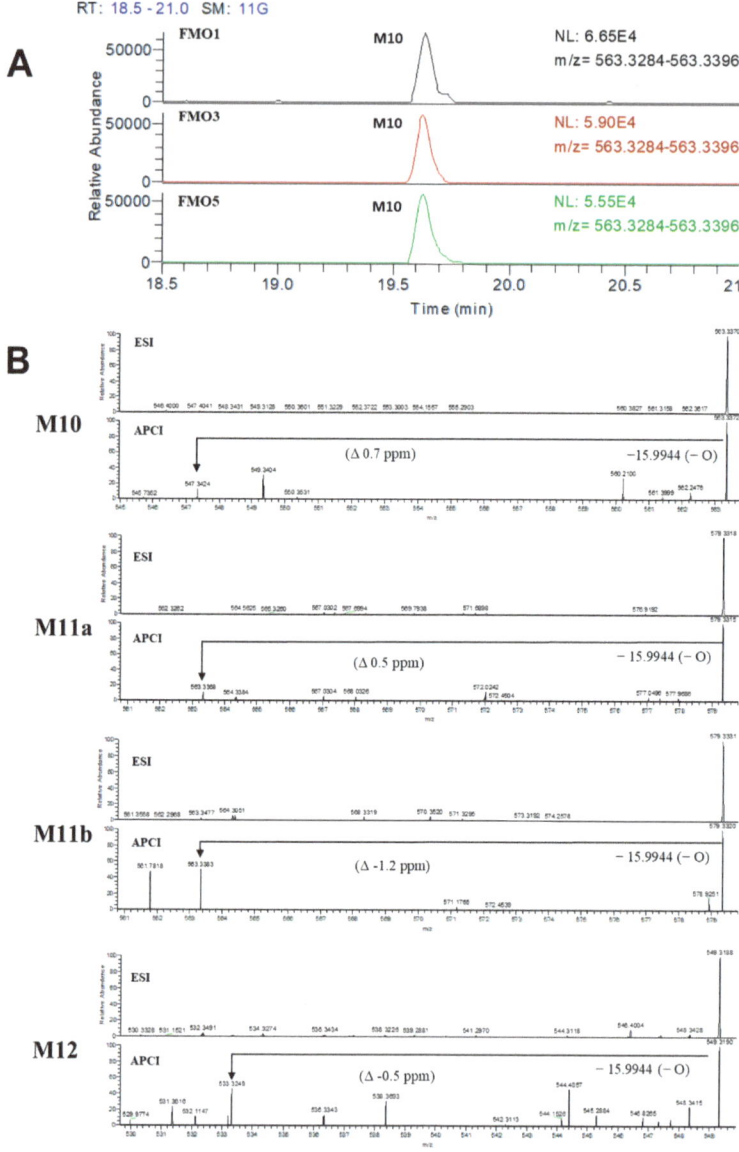

Figure 6. (**A**) M10 formation in the FMO incubation assay. (**B**) MS/MS spectra of M10, M11a, M11b, and M12 in ESI (top) and the thermal deoxygenation observed in the APCI (bottom) MS spectra.

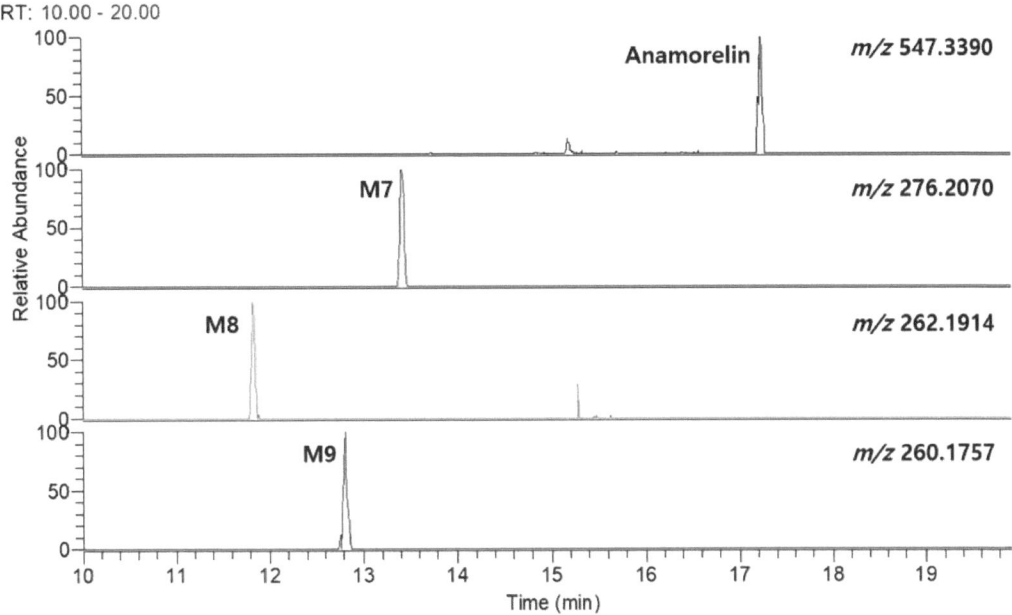

Figure 7. Extracted ion chromatograms of anamorelin and its metabolites generated from the incubation with cDNA-expressed recombinant CYP3A4 isozyme for 2 h.

4. Discussion

Drug metabolism profiling has traditionally been a challenging task due to the numerous possible metabolic pathways and the vast datasets that require manual inspection, making it time-consuming and expensive. This increases the likelihood that critical metabolites undergoing unusual pathways may be overlooked, leading to misinterpretations during the early preclinical stage. To address these challenges, molecular networking has emerged as a promising tool by providing a network of structurally relevant molecules in a semi-automatic fashion.

Initially, we employed MN analysis to quickly obtain snapshots of the novel anamorelin metabolites, as it has easy accessibility and a simple workflow that does not require data pre-processing. The MN analysis enabled us to identify 11 anamorelin metabolites (Figure 2). However, during our validation process, by checking the profile on the chromatograms, we observed multiple peaks in the same EIC, indicating the presence of overlapping nodes due to the isomers. This prompted us to use FBMN to unravel the metabolites of anamorelin in a more reliable manner. FBMN has several advantages over MN, including its ability to distinguish compounds that generate similar MS^2 spectra by incorporating their chromatographic separation, enhancing spectral annotation, and providing semi-quantitative information that aids the metabolomic statistical evaluation by reflecting peak abundance [12]. Through FBMN analysis, we were able to separate six nodes (563.336→M3a-b, M10; 579.333→M4a-c, M11a-b; 549.318→M5a-c; M12; 575.339→M13a*-b*; 591.331→M14a*-b*; 561.322→M6, M15a*-b*) that could not be achieved using MN analysis (Figure 2).

Based on the findings obtained from the FBMN analysis and by investigating fragmentation patterns, it was suggested that anamorelin undergoes hydroxylation, demethylation, and dealkylation in HLM (Figure 2B). Furthermore, the distinct chromatographic behavior of M10, M11a-b, and M12, in contrast to M3a-b, M4a-c, and M5a-c, respectively, suggested the involvement of additional metabolic mechanisms in their formation (Figure 5). Subsequent FMO incubation assays and the utilization of the APCI source showed that the N-oxidation through FMO was responsible for the generation of the terminal (M10) or N-oxidation-mediated metabolites (M11a-b and M12), as depicted in Figure 6. Overall, these findings allowed for the complete elucidation of the metabolic pathways of anamorelin in HLM, as summarized in Figure 8.

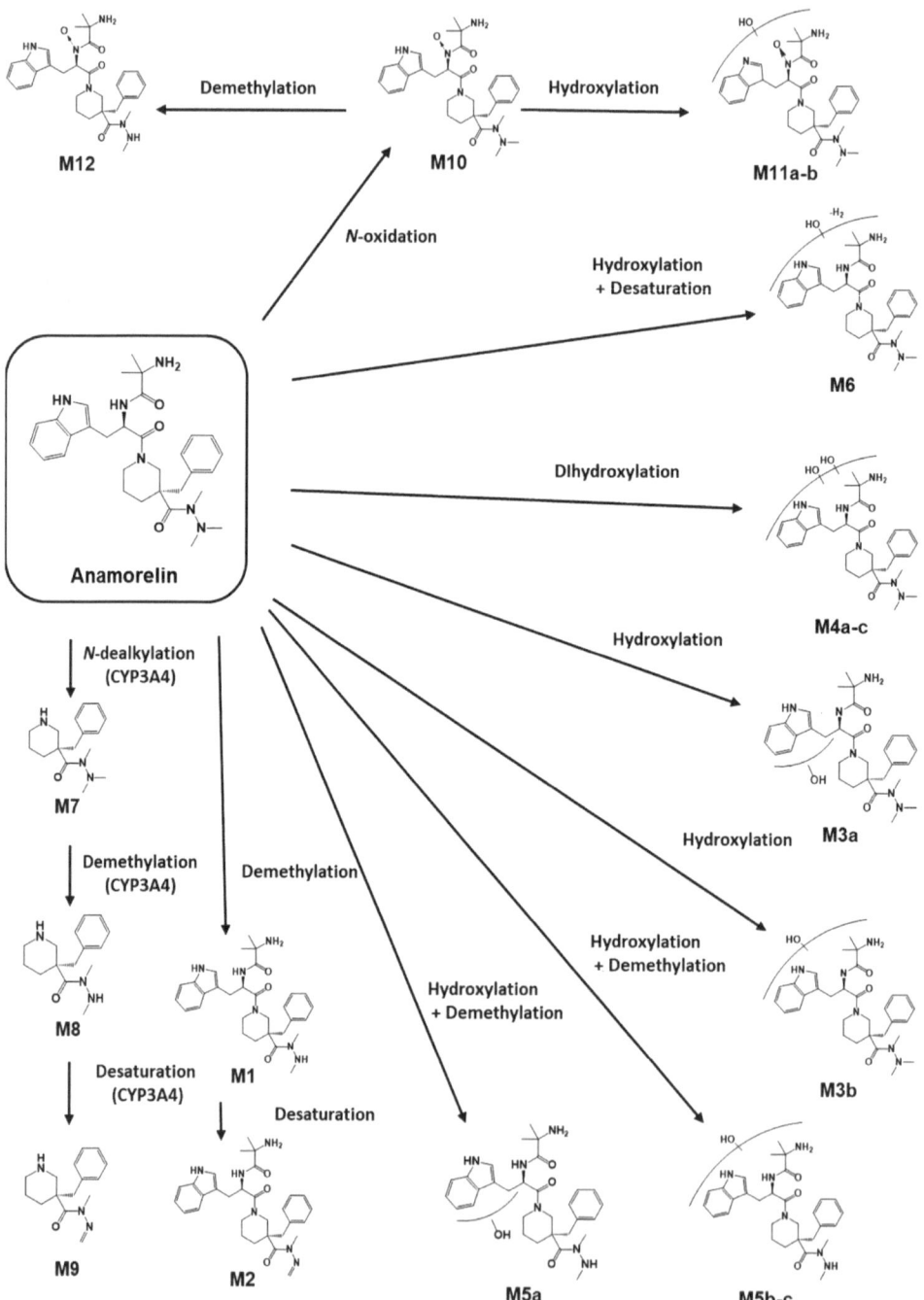

Figure 8. Postulated metabolic pathways of anamorelin in human liver microsomes.

Comprehending metabolic processes at the molecular level is paramount for the success of drug discovery and development [22]. This understanding plays a pivotal role in enhancing the stability, in vivo half-life, and the risk–benefit ratio of potential drug candidates [23]. Moreover, to mitigate the risk of expensive setbacks in the clinical stages stemming from insufficiently characterized drug metabolism, a thorough investigation of metabolic profiles is of utmost importance. This is because drug metabolism can lead to the generation of metabolites with markedly distinct physicochemical and pharmacological attributes compared to the parent drug, and these metabolites are associated with the drug's effectiveness and safety [24,25]. Hence, our in-depth insights into the metabolites of anamorelin would be valuable for reevaluating and reformulating it, with the aim of investigating new therapeutic applications. Additionally, the present method, employing molecular networking for metabolite identification, has the potential for broader adoption in other drug metabolism studies. This method offers the benefit of accelerating the process while providing a near-complete coverage of metabolite formation.

Anamorelin has been conventionally recognized to predominantly undergo hepatic metabolism mediated by CYP3A4 [19,20]. In a recent study, experimental validation was conducted in healthy human volunteers, demonstrating that the concomitant administration of a CYP3A4 inhibitor or inducer can result in a marked alteration of anamorelin's pharmacokinetic properties (i.e., maximum plasma concentration (C_{max}) and area under the plasma concentration–time curve ($AUC_{0-\infty}$)) [21]. However, our investigation uncovered a discrepancy in the metabolite profiles of anamorelin between HLM and CYP3A4 isozymes. Specifically, we observed that only N-alkylation-mediated metabolites (M7, M8, and M9) were detectable in the CYP3A4 isozyme assay (Figure 7). This contrasts with the results obtained from HLM, which indicated that demethylation (M1) could be a primary metabolic pathway, along with N-dealkylation (M7), while other metabolites were still exhibiting significant peak intensities (Figure 5). These findings are in line with a prior report suggesting that demethylation plays a significant role in the metabolism of anamorelin [26]. Furthermore, given the diverse nature of CYP enzymes [27], it is plausible to hypothesize that other CYP isozymes may be involved in anamorelin's metabolism. This raises important concerns regarding potential CYP-mediated drug–drug interactions, which could contribute to the reported adverse event of anamorelin, cardiac toxicity, due to its narrow therapeutic window characterized by non-linear pharmacokinetic profiles [26]. To mitigate potential adverse events from uncertainties, it is advisable not to rely solely on CYP3A4 as the target enzyme for studying anamorelin's metabolism, as this approach may have limitations. Future investigations should be conducted to comprehensively explore other CYP isozymes that might be closely associated with anamorelin's metabolism. Consequently, it is prudent to consider various metabolic pathways to achieve a thorough understanding of the therapeutic efficacy and safety of anamorelin.

5. Conclusions

In this study, we conducted a comprehensive investigation of the in vitro metabolism of anamorelin using HLM and analyzed the results using MN and FBMN approaches. Through these methods, we identified 18 metabolites (M1–M12) and 6 unknown compounds (M13a*-b*, M14a*-b*, and M15a*-b*) that were produced from anamorelin. Our analysis revealed that M1 and M7 were the primary metabolites, and we classified the metabolic pathways of anamorelin in HLM as hydroxylation, demethylation, and dealkylation. We also used the FMO incubation assay and thermal deoxygenation in the APCI source to investigate the complex nature of FMO-mediated metabolism. Our results indicated that hydroxylation and demethylation may occur after N-oxidation. Additionally, our CYP3A4 isozyme assay suggested that M7, M8, and M9 may also be the major forms of anamorelin metabolites in vivo, in addition to M1. Overall, these findings provide new insights into the metabolism of anamorelin and its potential as a novel therapeutic agent.

Supplementary Materials: The following supporting information can be downloaded at: https://www.mdpi.com/article/10.3390/pharmaceutics15122700/s1, Table S1. Accurate mass data of anamorelin and its metabolites in HLM. The table summarizes expected biotransformation based on retention time (RT) and characteristic fragment ions.

Author Contributions: Conceptualization, Y.B.K., J.I.S. and H.H.Y.; investigation, Y.B.K.; data curation, Y.B.K.; writing—original draft preparation, Y.B.K. and J.I.S.; writing—review and editing, Y.B.K., J.I.S. and H.H.Y.; project administration and supervision, H.H.Y. All authors have read and agreed to the published version of the manuscript.

Funding: This research was supported by the Horse Industry Research Center of the Korea Racing Authority and National Research Foundation of Korea (NRF) grants funded by the Ministry of Education (2021R1A2C1010428 and RS-2023-00217123).

Institutional Review Board Statement: Not applicable.

Informed Consent Statement: Not applicable.

Data Availability Statement: Data are contained within the article and Supplementary Materials.

Conflicts of Interest: The authors declare no conflict of interest.

References

1. Ishida, J.; Saitoh, M.; Ebner, N.; Springer, J.; Anker, S.D.; von Haehling, S. Growth Hormone Secretagogues: History, Mechanism of Action, and Clinical Development. *JCSM Rapid Commun.* **2020**, *3*, 25–37. [CrossRef]
2. Garcia, J.M.; Boccia, R.V.; Graham, C.D.; Yan, Y.; Duus, E.M.; Allen, S.; Friend, J. Anamorelin for Patients with Cancer Cachexia: An Integrated Analysis of Two Phase 2, Randomised, Placebo-Controlled, Double-Blind Trials. *Lancet Oncol.* **2015**, *16*, 108–116. [CrossRef] [PubMed]
3. Garcia, J.M.; Polvino, W.J. Pharmacodynamic Hormonal Effects of Anamorelin, a Novel Oral Ghrelin Mimetic and Growth Hormone Secretagogue in Healthy Volunteers. *Growth Horm. IGF Res.* **2009**, *19*, 267–273. [CrossRef] [PubMed]
4. Graf, S.A.; Garcia, J.M. Anamorelin Hydrochloride in the Treatment of Cancer Anorexia-Cachexia Syndrome: Design, Development, and Potential Place in Therapy. *Drug Des. Dev. Ther.* **2017**, *11*, 2325–2331. [CrossRef] [PubMed]
5. Wakabayashi, H.; Arai, H.; Inui, A. The Regulatory Approval of Anamorelin for Treatment of Cachexia in Patients with Non-Small Cell Lung Cancer, Gastric Cancer, Pancreatic Cancer, and Colorectal Cancer in Japan: Facts and Numbers. *J. Cachexia Sarcopenia Muscle* **2021**, *12*, 14–16. [CrossRef]
6. Temel, J.S.; Abernethy, A.P.; Currow, D.C.; Friend, J.; Duus, E.M.; Yan, Y.; Fearon, K.C. Anamorelin in Patients with Non-Small-Cell Lung Cancer and Cachexia (ROMANA 1 and ROMANA 2): Results from Two Randomised, Double-Blind, Phase 3 Trials. *Lancet Oncol.* **2016**, *17*, 519–531. [CrossRef] [PubMed]
7. Garcia, J.M. What Is next after Anamorelin? *Curr. Opin. Support. Palliat. Care* **2017**, *11*, 266. [CrossRef]
8. Ahmad, S.S.; Ahmad, K.; Shaikh, S.; You, H.J.; Lee, E.-Y.; Ali, S.; Lee, E.J.; Choi, I. Molecular Mechanisms and Current Treatment Options for Cancer Cachexia. *Cancers* **2022**, *14*, 2107. [CrossRef]
9. Vincenti, F.; Montesano, C.; Di Ottavio, F.; Gregori, A.; Compagnone, D.; Sergi, M.; Dorrestein, P. Molecular Networking: A Useful Tool for the Identification of New Psychoactive Substances in Seizures by LC–HRMS. *Front. Chem.* **2020**, *8*, 572952. [CrossRef]
10. Quinn, R.A.; Nothias, L.-F.; Vining, O.; Meehan, M.; Esquenazi, E.; Dorrestein, P.C. Molecular Networking As a Drug Discovery, Drug Metabolism, and Precision Medicine Strategy. *Trends Pharmacol. Sci.* **2017**, *38*, 143–154. [CrossRef]
11. Yu, J.S.; Seo, H.; Kim, G.B.; Hong, J.; Yoo, H.H. MS-Based Molecular Networking of Designer Drugs as an Approach for the Detection of Unknown Derivatives for Forensic and Doping Applications: A Case of NBOMe Derivatives. *Anal. Chem.* **2019**, *91*, 5483–5488. [CrossRef] [PubMed]
12. Nothias, L.-F.; Petras, D.; Schmid, R.; Dührkop, K.; Rainer, J.; Sarvepalli, A.; Protsyuk, I.; Ernst, M.; Tsugawa, H.; Fleischauer, M.; et al. Feature-Based Molecular Networking in the GNPS Analysis Environment. *Nat. Methods* **2020**, *17*, 905–908. [CrossRef] [PubMed]
13. Le Daré, B.; Ferron, P.-J.; Allard, P.-M.; Clément, B.; Morel, I.; Gicquel, T. New Insights into Quetiapine Metabolism Using Molecular Networking. *Sci. Rep.* **2020**, *10*, 19921. [CrossRef]
14. Rousu, T.; Tolonen, A. Characterization of Cyanide-Trapped Methylated Metabonates Formed during Reactive Drug Metabolite Screening in Vitro. *Rapid Commun. Mass Spectrom.* **2011**, *25*, 1382–1390. [CrossRef]
15. Li, C.; Surapaneni, S.; Zeng, Q.; Marquez, B.; Chow, D.; Kumar, G. Identification of a Novel in Vitro Metabonate from Liver Microsomal Incubations. *Drug Metab. Dispos.* **2006**, *34*, 901–905. [CrossRef] [PubMed]
16. Lee, S.K.; Kang, M.J.; Jin, C.; In, M.K.; Kim, D.-H.; Yoo, H.H. Flavin-Containing Monooxygenase 1-Catalysed N,N-Dimethylamphetamine N-Oxidation. *Xenobiotica* **2009**, *39*, 680–686. [CrossRef] [PubMed]
17. Kwak, Y.B.; Choi, M.S. Identification of a Metabolite for the Detection of the Hydrophilic Drug Diisopropylamine for Doping Control. *J. Pharm. Biomed. Anal.* **2023**, *234*, 115576. [CrossRef]

18. Kim, I.S.; Rehman, S.U.; Choi, M.S.; Jang, M.; Yang, W.; Kim, E.; Yoo, H.H. Characterization of in Vitro Metabolites of Methylenedioxypyrovalerone (MDPV): An N-Oxide Metabolite Formation Mediated by Flavin Monooxygenase. *J. Pharm. Biomed. Anal.* **2016**, *131*, 160–166. [CrossRef]
19. Okidono, Y.; Osada, J.; Otsu, K.; Kowase, S.; Aoki, H.; Yumoto, K. Two Cases of Wide QRS Complex Tachycardia Caused by Anamorelin. *J. Cardiol. Cases* **2022**, *26*, 212–216. [CrossRef]
20. Prommer, E. Oncology Update: Anamorelin. *Palliat. Care* **2017**, *10*, 1178224217726336. [CrossRef]
21. Duus, E.; Matson, M.A.; Bernareggi, A. Effects of Strong Cytochrome P450 (CYP)3A4 Inducers/Inhibitors on the Pharmacokinetic (PK) Profile of Anamorelin in Healthy Volunteers. *J. Clin. Oncol.* **2018**, *36*, e22180. [CrossRef]
22. Zhang, Z.; Zhu, M.; Tang, W. Metabolite Identification and Profiling in Drug Design: Current Practice and Future Directions. *Curr. Pharm. Des.* **2009**, *15*, 2220–2235. [CrossRef]
23. Kirchmair, J.; Göller, A.H.; Lang, D.; Kunze, J.; Testa, B.; Wilson, I.D.; Glen, R.C.; Schneider, G. Predicting Drug Metabolism: Experiment and/or Computation? *Nat. Rev. Drug Discov.* **2015**, *14*, 387–404. [CrossRef]
24. Testa, B. Drug Metabolism for the Perplexed Medicinal Chemist. *Chem. Biodivers.* **2009**, *6*, 2055–2070. [CrossRef]
25. Kirchmair, J.; Howlett, A.; Peironcely, J.E.; Murrell, D.S.; Williamson, M.J.; Adams, S.E.; Hankemeier, T.; van Buren, L.; Duchateau, G.; Klaffke, W.; et al. How Do Metabolites Differ from Their Parent Molecules and How Are They Excreted? *J. Chem. Inf. Model.* **2013**, *53*, 354–367. [CrossRef]
26. European Medicine Agency. Assessment Report–Aldumiz. Available online: https://www.ema.europa.eu/en/documents/assessment-report/adlumiz-epar-refusal-public-assessment-report_en.pdf (accessed on 8 November 2023).
27. Esteves, F.; Rueff, J.; Kranendonk, M. The Central Role of Cytochrome P450 in Xenobiotic Metabolism—A Brief Review on a Fascinating Enzyme Family. *J. Xenobiotics* **2021**, *11*, 94–114. [CrossRef] [PubMed]

Disclaimer/Publisher's Note: The statements, opinions and data contained in all publications are solely those of the individual author(s) and contributor(s) and not of MDPI and/or the editor(s). MDPI and/or the editor(s) disclaim responsibility for any injury to people or property resulting from any ideas, methods, instructions or products referred to in the content.

Article

Selegiline Modulates Lipid Metabolism by Activating AMPK Pathways of Epididymal White Adipose Tissues in HFD-Fed Obese Mice

Hye-Young Joung [1,†], Jung-Mi Oh [1,2,†], Min-Suk Song [3], Young-Bae Kwon [4] and Sungkun Chun [1,2,*]

1. Department of Physiology, Jeonbuk National University Medical School, Jeonju 54907, Republic of Korea; hyjyj007@hanmail.net (H.-Y.J.); biojmi@jbnu.ac.kr (J.-M.O.)
2. Research Institute for Endocrine Sciences, Jeonbuk National University Medical School, Jeonju 54907, Republic of Korea
3. Department of Microbiology, Chungbuk National University College of Medicine and Medical Research Institute, Cheongju 28644, Republic of Korea; songminsuk@chungbuk.ac.kr
4. Department of Pharmacology, Jeonbuk National University Medical School, Jeonju 54907, Republic of Korea; 1972y@jbnu.ac.kr
* Correspondence: sungkun.chun@jbnu.ac.kr; Tel.: +82-63-270-4290
† These authors contributed equally to this work.

Abstract: Obesity, as a major cause of many chronic diseases such as diabetes, cardiovascular disease, and cancer, is among the most serious health problems. Increased monoamine oxidase (MAO) activity has been observed in the adipose tissue of obese humans and animals. Although previous studies have already demonstrated the potential of MAO-B inhibitors as a treatment for this condition, the mechanism of their effect has been insufficiently elucidated. In this study, we investigated the anti-obesity effect of selegiline, a selective MAO-B inhibitor, using in vivo animal models. The effect was evaluated through an assessment of body energy homeostasis, glucose tolerance tests, and biochemical analysis. Pharmacological inhibition of MAO-B by selegiline was observed to reduce body weight and fat accumulation, and improved glucose metabolism without a corresponding change in food intake, in HFD-fed obese mice. We also observed that both the expression of adipogenenic markers, including C/EBPα and FABP4, and lipogenic markers such as pACC were significantly reduced in epididymal white adipose tissues (eWATs). Conversely, increased expression of lipolytic markers such as ATGL and pHSL and AMPK phosphorylation were noted. Treating obese mice with selegiline significantly increased expression levels of UCP1 and promoted eWAT browning, indicating increased energy expenditure. These results suggest that selegiline, by inhibiting MAO-B activity, is a potential anti-obesity treatment.

Keywords: selegiline; anti-obesity; adipogenesis; lipogenesis; lipolysis; eWAT browning

1. Introduction

Obesity is a major risk factor for metabolic diseases, including type 2 diabetes mellitus, inflammation, and cardiovascular disease [1,2]. Obesity occurs when energy intake is greater than energy expenditure. Increasing energy expenditure is therefore a potential therapeutic strategy for the treatment of obesity [1,3].

Adipose tissue is involved in the regulation of whole-body energy metabolism, and is responsible for breaking down lipid droplets into free fatty acids (substrates for energy metabolism) as well as lipid storage through adipogenesis. This imbalance in energy metabolism regulation leads to obesity, where excess energy is stored in fat cells, causing hyperplasia (increase in cell number) and hypertrophy (increase in cell size) [4,5]. For that reason, it is considered important to develop anti-obesity drugs to properly understand and control the regulatory mechanisms of adipogenesis and lipogenesis [6].

Thermogenesis generally occurs in brown adipose tissue (BAT), but in adipocytes thermogenesis is also possible in brown-like white adipocytes (also known as beige adipocytes). The process by which adipocytes acquire the characteristics of BATs is referred to as browning, and mouse studies show a correlation between this process and improvements to metabolic disease [7]. Achieving a positive energy balance by inhibiting excessive white adipose tissue (WAT) deposition, while stimulating WAT browning and activating BAT thermogenesis are considered as potential therapeutic targets for the treatment of obesity.

Monoamine oxidases (MAOs) are widely distributed enzymes that catalyze oxidative deamination of biogenic amines involved adrenalin, dopamine, and serotonin to produce hydrogen peroxide. Previous studies of MAO enzymes showed they are also expressed in the adipocytes of humans [8,9] and rodents [10,11]. These enzymes have been shown to be increased in the differentiated 3T3-L1 and white adipocytes of obese animal models [11,12]. MAO also accelerates adipogenesis by generating reactive oxygen species (ROS) [13]. Furthermore, the MAO inhibitors not only stimulate glucose uptake [14] but also inhibit lipolysis [15] in the adipocytes of rats.

Selegiline, a selective MAO type B inhibitor, effectively reduced obesity induced by a high-fat and high-sugar (HFS) diet in rats. It also played a role in reducing adipose tissue metabolism and inflammation. However, it did not affect body weight gain, impaired glucose homeostasis, or behavior [16]. Previous research suggests that the combined administration of MAO and semicarbazide-sensitive amine oxidases (SSAOs) can help alleviate fat accumulation and reduce body weight in obese Zucker rats [17,18]. Pargyline, a monoamine oxidase inhibitor administered at a dosage of 30 mg/kg, promoted lipolysis and increased the levels of free fatty acids in rats [19]. A recent study reported that selegiline demonstrated a protective effect against HFD-induced dyslipidemia and hepatic steatosis [20]. Despite the established metabolic benefits of selegiline in obese rodents, the specific mechanisms behind MAOB inhibition and lipid metabolism remain unclear. Therefore, this study aims to investigate the effects of selegiline on obese mice fed an HFD and elucidate any potential underlying mechanisms.

In our research, we have demonstrated that selegiline influences lipid metabolism and induces the browning of white adipocytes by activating AMP-activated protein kinase (AMPK). This identified molecular signaling pathway in eWAT may explain the anti-obesity effects of selegiline in vivo.

2. Materials and Methods

2.1. Animal Experiments

In vivo animal experiments were performed consistent with the guidelines established by the Jeonbuk National University Institutional Animal Care and Use Committee (IACUC) (Approval number: JBNU 2022-026). C57BL/6 mice (male, 6 weeks old) were purchased from Nara Biotech (Kyunggi-do, Korea) and housed with a 12 h light/dark cycle (light on, 08:00). The animals were allowed to adapt to laboratory conditions for a minimum of 7 days prior to the experiment. After becoming acclimated, mice were randomly assigned to either cohort 1 or cohort 2 (Figure 1). All mice were fed either a normal chow diet (NCD; 18% kcal fat, 3.1 kcal/g) or a high-fat diet (HFD; 60% kcal fat, 5.24 kcal/g; Research Diets, NJ, USA) and provided with ad libitum access to water.

Cohort 1: Mice were randomly divided into four groups: NCD+Veh group ($n = 5$): administration with vehicle to NCD fed mice; NCD+Selegiline group ($n = 5$): administration with selegiline (30 mg/kg) to NCD fed mice; HFD+Veh group ($n = 5$): administration with vehicle to HFD-fed mice; HFD+Selegiline group ($n = 5$): administration with selegiline (30 mg/kg) to HFD-fed mice. After 3 weeks of treatment, eWAT was collected and Hematoxylin and Eosin (H&E) staining was performed.

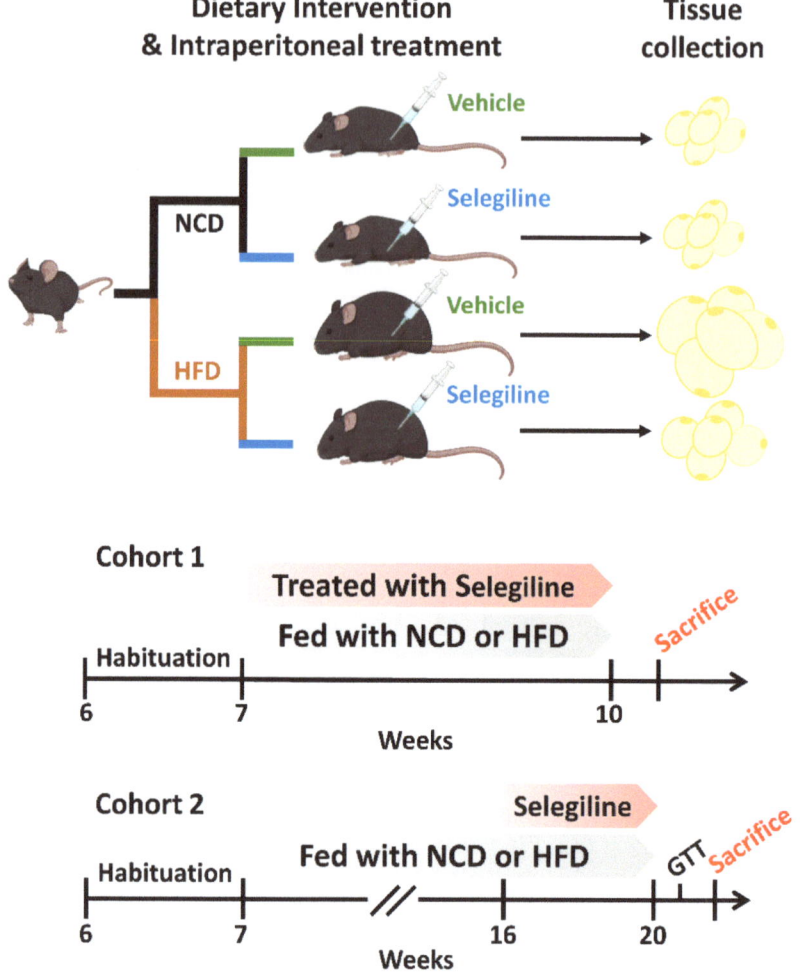

Figure 1. Schematic illustration of the experimental configuration.

Cohort 2: A total of 20 mice were randomly divided into two groups: those fed an NCD (18% kcal fat, 3.1 kcal/g) and those fed an HFD (60% kcal fat, 5.24 kcal/g, Research Diets, NJ, USA). Food was provided for 9 weeks to establish obese mice models. The 20 mice were then weight matched and divided further into four groups: (1) NCD+Veh group ($n = 5$): administration with vehicle to NCD fed mice, (2) NCD+Selegiline group ($n = 5$): administration with selegiline (30 mg/kg) to NCD fed mice, (3) HFD+Veh group ($n = 5$): administration with vehicle to HFD-fed mice, (4) HFD+Selegiline group ($n = 5$): administration with selegiline (30 mg/kg) to HFD-fed mice. The selegiline was administered intraperitoneally once per day over 4 weeks. During the animal experiments, body weight and food intake were measured every day. At the end of the experiments, adipose tissue [eWAT, inguinal white adipose tissue (iWAT), BAT] was collected and subjected to H&E staining, immunohistochemistry (IHC) and Western blot analyses.

2.2. Glucose Tolerance Test (GTT)

The GTT was performed by modifying a previously reported method [21]. At the end of administration vehicle or selegiline, mice were fasted for 15 h (18:00 p.m.–9:00 a.m.)

before GTT. The mice received an intraperitoneally injection of glucose (2 g/kg body weight, G8270, Sigma-Aldrich, St. Louis, MO, USA) and then, blood samples were collected from the tail at 0, 15, 30, 45, 60, 90, and 120 min to measure blood glucose concentration using a CareSensII Plus glucose meter (I-SENS Inc., Seoul, Korea). The area under the curve (AUC) was calculated using GraphPad Prism software, version 8.0.1 (GraphPad Software, San Diego, CA, USA).

2.3. Western Blotting Analysis

A Western blot was conducted as previously described [22]. Adipose tissues were homogenized in RIPA buffer with protease and a phosphatase inhibitor cocktail. Lysates were resolved on 8–10% sodium dodecyl sulfate-polyacrylamide gel and then transferred onto polyvinylidene fluoride membrane. The membranes were blocked with 5% skim milk in 0.1% Tween 20/Tris-buffered saline (TBST) and primary antibodies were incubated overnight at 4 °C using acetyl-CoA carboxylase (ACC: # (3662), phospho (p)ACC (#3661), AMPKα (#2532), p-AMPKα (#50081), CCAAT/enhancer-binding protein alpha (C/EBPα: #8178), fatty acid binding protein 4 (FABP4: #2120), peroxisome proliferator activated receptor gamma (PPARγ: #2435), Hormone-sensitive lipase (HSL: #4107), pHSL (#4137) (1:1000 dilution, Cell Signaling Technology, Beverly, MA, USA), Adipose triglyceride lipase (ATGL: sc-365278), PPARγ coactivator 1-alpha (PGC1α: sc-518025) (1:200 dilution, Santa Cruz Biotechnology Inc., Santa Cruz, CA, USA), PR/SET Domain 16 (PRDM16: Ab106410), Uncoupling Protein 1 (UCP1: ab155117) (1:1000 dilution, Abcam, Cambridge, UK), and Glyceralde-hyde-3-phosphate dehydrogenase (GAPDH: AP0066; 1:5000, Bioworld Technology, Bloomington, MN, USA). After washing with TBST, membranes were incubated with anti-rabbit (#7074) or mouse (#7076) HRP-conjugated secondary antibody (1:5000, Cell Signaling Technology) for 1 h at room temperature. The expression levels of target proteins were quantified by image density scanning using ImageJ software Version 1.54d (NIH, Bethesda, MD, USA) and adjusted for GAPDH expression.

2.4. Hematoxylin and Eosin (H&E)

The paraffin-embedded epididymal adipose tissue sections (10 μm) were stained with Hematoxylin (S3309, Dako, Copenhagen, Denmark) and Eosin (HT110216, Sigma-Aldrich, St. Louis, MO, USA). The slides were mounted with mounting medium (ab104139; Abcam, Waltham, MA, USA). Images were captured using LAS software, version V4.9 (Leica, Hessen, Germany) under a light microscope (ICC50E, Leica) and adipocyte areas in the H&E stained cross-sections were analyzed using pixel-based AdipoArea software. The size of adipocytes was expressed as μm^2.

2.5. Immunohistochemistry (IHC)

UCP1 immunofluorescence was performed using a method previously described in [23]. The tissue sections were placed for 10 min in a citrate buffer (pH of 6.0) at 60 °C for antigen retrieval and blocked with 5% normal goat serum/0.1 M PBS buffer. eWAT sections were incubated overnight in PBS at 4 °C with anti-UCP1 antibody (1:1000, Abcam) then further incubated in PBS for 2 h at room temperature with anti-rabbit IgG-Alexa 488 (ab150077, 1:1000, Abcam). After rinsing in PBS, the slides were mounted with Anti-Fade Fluorescence mounting medium (ab104135, Abcam). The images were acquired using a fluorescent microscope (CELENA S, Logos Biosystems, Anyang-si, Kyunggi-do, Korea).

2.6. Statistical Analysis

All data are presented as means ± SEM. Statistical analysis was performed using GraphPad Prism software version 8.0.1 (GraphPad Software, San Diego, CA, USA). The difference between groups was determined by one-way ANOVA followed by Dunnett's multiple comparison test. Time course comparison between groups was analyzed using a two-way repeated measures (RM) ANOVA with Dunnett's multiple comparisons. All p values < 0.05 were considered statistically significant.

3. Results

3.1. Selegiline Prevented Obesity in HFD-Fed Mice

We investigated if the processing of selegiline, a selective MAO-B inhibitor, is involved in body weight change in adipocytes from HFD-fed obese mice. Cohort 1, a group administered selegiline at the beginning of the trials, was established to elucidate the preventive effect of the MAO-B inhibitor on HFD-induced obesity. Selegiline (30 mg/kg, i.p.) was administered concurrently with feeding a normal chow or high-fat diet into mice (Figure 2A). We observed that the body weight and white fat pad weight (eWAT and iWAT) was significantly higher in the HFD+Veh group than in the NCD+Veh group (Figure 2B–D). Interestingly, simultaneous administration of selegiline over 3 weeks reduced body weight gain in HFD-fed mice. However, there was no change in body weight in the group fed regular food and the group administered selegiline in combination (Figure 2B,C). Additionally, simultaneous administration of HFD and selegiline decreased eWAT and iWAT weights compared to HFD mice, but there was no change in BAT (Figure 2D). We conducted H&E staining on eWAT and analyzed the impact of selegiline on adipocyte size change. Our experiment demonstrated that adipocytes in HFD mice were bigger than those in NCD mice. Co-administration of selegiline resulted in smaller adipocyte sizes in HFD mice compared to HFD alone (Figure 2E,F). Furthermore, based on a 3000 μm^2 size distribution analysis of fat cells, the combined HFD and selegiline group had a greater increase in fat cell size below 3000 μm^2 compared to just the HFD group, while the HFD group had a higher prevalence of fat cells larger than 3000 μm^2 than the selegiline group (Figure 2G). In sum, these findings suggest that a combination treatment of selegiline during the early stages of HFD could effectively reduce the accumulation of WAT and body weight.

3.2. Selegiline Reduced Body Weight and Fat Accumulation in HFD-Fed Obese Mice

Selegiline was administered to HFD-induced obese mice to confirm whether it was effective in treating the state of obesity. After being fed an NCD or HFD for 9 weeks, mice received intraperitoneal injections of selegiline (30 mg/kg) for 4 weeks (Figure 3A). Selegiline-treated mice exhibited significantly less body weight gain than mice in the HFD+Veh group (Figure 3B–D). We further examined whether selegiline could affect feeding behavior itself. As shown in Figure 3E, we observed that the daily food intake of mice fed an HFD was significantly higher than those fed an NCD. However, we observed no difference in daily food consumption amounts between selegiline-treated and untreated mice fed an HFD. This indicates that selegiline does not modulate food intake behavior. We next performed an intraperitoneal glucose tolerance test (GTT) to check for disturbances in glucose metabolism in all HFD mice. We found that selegiline treatment significantly improved the glucose tolerance of obese mice fed an HFD (Figure 3F). In sum, these results showed that the inhibition of MAO-B by the systemic administration of selegiline, while not changing the amount of food consumed by obese mice fed an HFD, nevertheless improved their glucose metabolism, thereby exerting a positive effect on the regulation of body weight and fat accumulation.

3.3. Selegiline Administration Reduced Epididymal Adipocyte Size

Comparing the size of adipocytes and the weight of adipose tissue is an important means of assessing the effectiveness of anti-obese agents. We examined whether selegiline treatment had any regulatory effect on the size of adipose cells or tissues by weighing eWATs and iWATs as well as BATs. As shown Figure 4A,B, selegiline treatment reduced fat mass in the eWATs and iWATs compared with the vehicle-treated HFD group, but the fat mass of the BAT did not change in either group. To investigate whether selegiline administration reduces adipocyte hypertrophy in HFD-induced obese mice, the size of eWATs, the primary component of WAT, was analyzed and compared between selegiline-treated and untreated groups. Tissue imaging analysis revealed that the eWATs were significantly smaller in the selegiline-treated groups than in the untreated groups (Figure 4C–F).

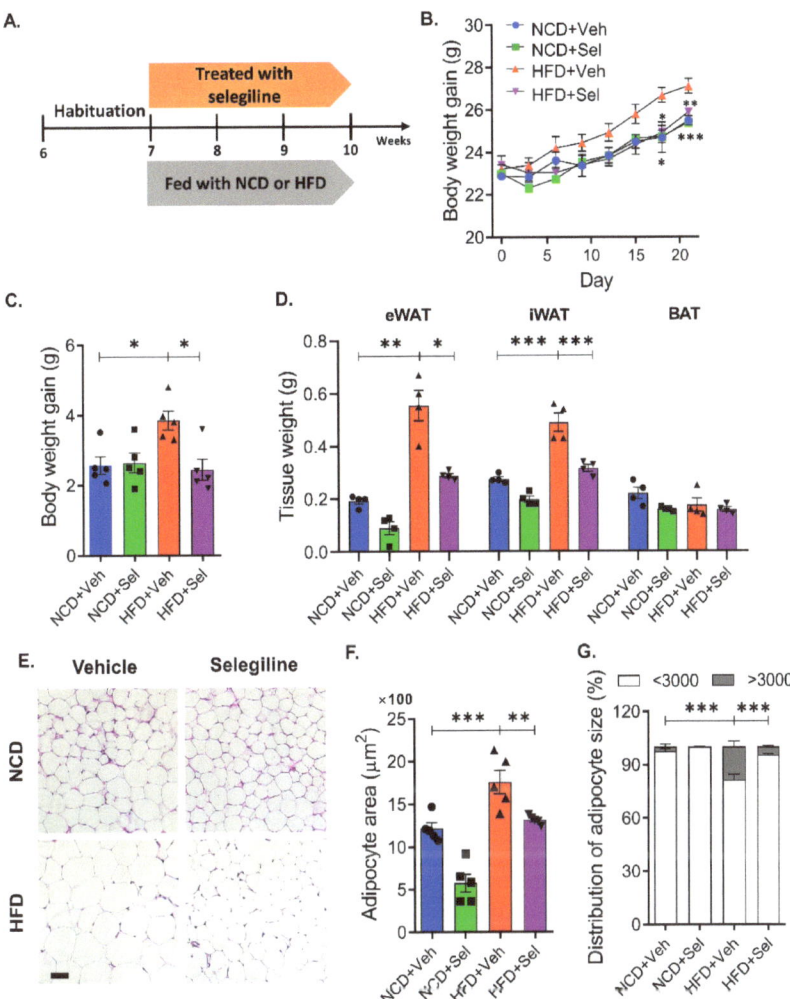

Figure 2. Selegiline prevented weight gain in HFD-fed mice. (**A**) Schematic diagram for this experiment. C57BL/6 mice were fed NCD or HFD and intraperitoneally treated with vehicle or selegiline (30 mg/kg) once a day for 3 weeks. (**B**) Body weight curves of vehicle- and selegiline-treated mice fed NCD or HFD (n = 5 per group). (**C**) Graph of body weight gain each groups. (**D**) Bar graph of weight of eWATs, iWATs, and BATs. (**E**) Representative of H&E staining of eWATs. Scale bar = 50 μm. (**F**) Summary plot of average of adipocyte areas. (**G**) Summary plot of frequency of large adipocytes, defined as having an adipocyte area greater than 3000 μm^2. Data are presented as the mean ± SEM and one-way ANOVA followed by Dunnett's multiple comparison test was employed for data analysis. Significance denoted by *: $p < 0.05$, **: $p < 0.01$, ***: $p < 0.001$ compared to HFD+Veh. NCD, normal chow diet; HFD, high-fat diet; Veh, vehicle; Sel, selegiline; eWAT, epididymal white adipose tissues; iWAT, inguinal white adipose tissue; BAT, brown adipose tissue.

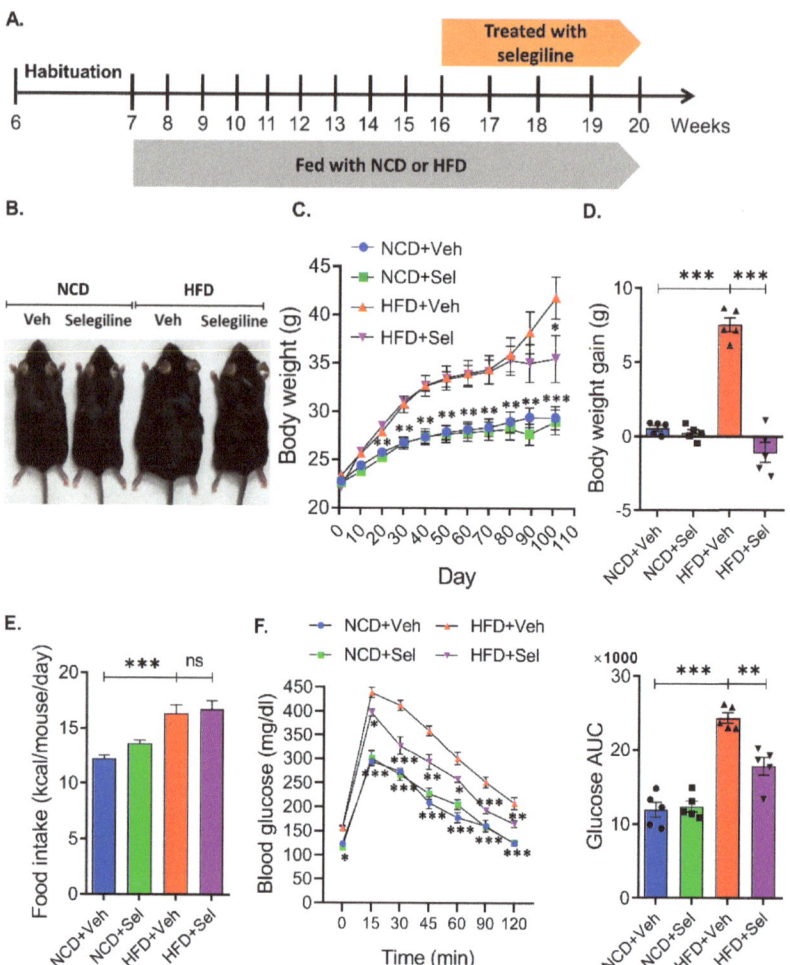

Figure 3. Selegiline markedly reduced body weight and fat accumulation in HFD-fed obese mice. (**A**) Schematic diagram for this experiment. C57BL/6 mice were fed an NCD or HFD for 9 weeks, and then intraperitoneal administrated 30 mg/kg of selegiline or saline once a day for 4 weeks. (**B**) Representative figure of body weight change in each group. (**C**) Polled data of body weight of each group. One-way ANOVA followed by Dunnett's multiple comparison test. (**D**) Graph of body weight gain by each group. One-way ANOVA followed by Dunnett's multiple comparison test. (**E**) Food intake of each group. (**F**) Left: Polled data of GTT of each group. Two-way RM ANOVA followed by Dunnett's multiple comparison test, interaction $F_{(6,108)} = 5.398$, $p < 0.0001$, time $F_{(6,108)} = 351.8$, $p < 0.0001$, between group $F_{(3,18)} = 71.06$, $p < 0.0001$. Right: Bar graphs showing area under the curve (AUC) values obtained from GTT experiments. Data are presented as the mean ± SEM. Significance was denoted by *: $p < 0.05$, **: $p < 0.01$, ***: $p < 0.001$ compared to HFD+Veh. NCD, normal chow diet; HFD, high-fat diet; Veh, vehicle; Sel, selegiline.

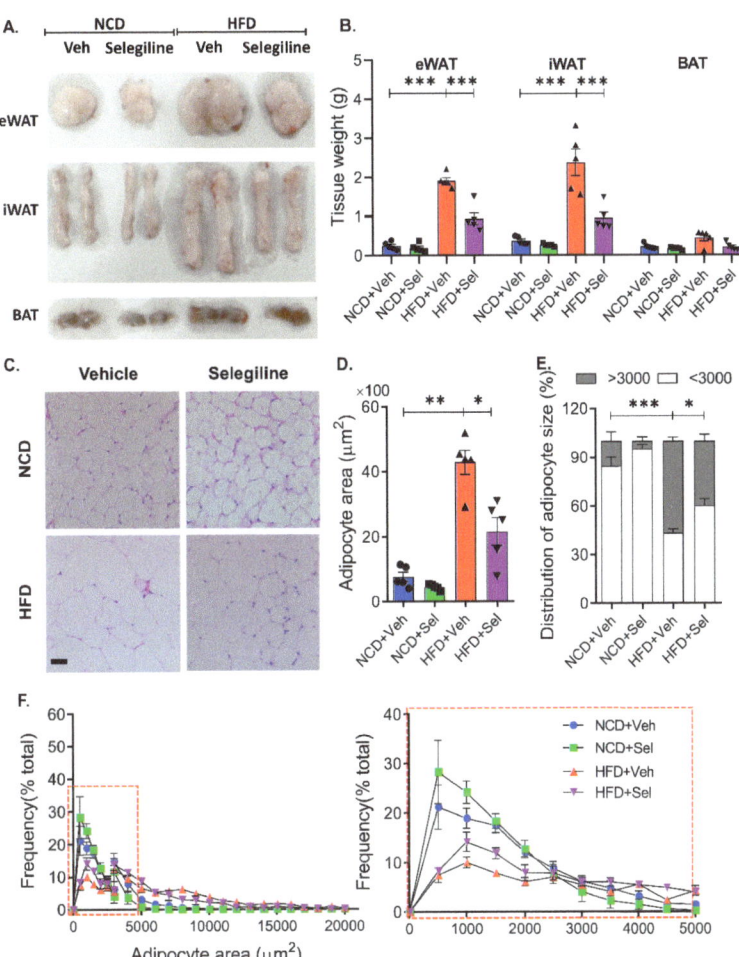

Figure 4. Selegiline administration reduced epididymal adipocyte size in HFD-fed obese mice. (**A**) Representative figure of eWATs, iWATs, and BATs. (**B**) Polled data of weight of eWATs, iWATs, and BATs. (**C**) Representative images of H&E staining of eWATs from each group. Scale bar = 50 μm. (**D**) Average of adipocyte size of WAT were measured from H&E images using AdipoArea software. n = 5 per group. (**E**) Frequency of large adipocytes, defined as having an adipocyte area greater than 3000 μm^2. (**F**) Summary plot of quantitative analysis of adipocyte area. Data are presented as the mean ± SEM and one-way ANOVA followed by Dunnett's multiple comparison test was employed for data analysis. Significance denoted by *: $p < 0.05$, **: $p < 0.01$, ***: $p < 0.001$ compared to HFD+Veh. NCD, normal chow diet; HFD, high fat diet; Veh (V), vehicle; Sel, selegiline; eWAT, epididymal white adipose tissues; iWAT, inguinal white adipose tissue; BAT, brown adipose tissue.

A more fine-grained analysis was performed to determine the mechanism by which the size of the adipocytes, such as eWAT, were reduced. Our experiments confirmed a change in the size distribution of adipocytes after treatment with selegiline; the number of small adipocytes (below 3000 μm^2) was higher than that of large adipocytes (above 3000 μm^2) post-treatment. This may be the cause of the overall decrease in body weight gain and fat mass that was observed to have followed selegiline treatment. Our results suggest that treatment of an obesity-induced mouse model with a MAO-B inhibitor can control the accumulation of adipocytes and exert an anti-obesity effect by regulating their distribution.

3.4. Selegiline Regulates Lipid Metabolism through an Activated AMPK Signaling Pathway in eWAT

To better understand the inhibitory effects of selegiline on fat accumulation in obese mice, we investigated the related molecular mechanisms for lipid metabolism. Protein levels of pAMPK, AMPK, PPARγ, C/EBPα, pACC, ACC, FABP4, ATGL, pHSL, and HSL were determined by Western blotting. Selegiline administration increased the ratio of p-AMPKα to AMPKα, indicating activation of the AMPKα signaling pathway (Figure 5A). In addition, selegiline significantly down-regulated the protein levels of adipogenic markers such as FABP4 and C/EBPα in the eWAT in obese mice, but slightly decreased PPARγ expression (though only to a degree that does not suggest statistical significance) (Figure 5A). Selegiline significantly increased phosphorylation of acetyl CoA carboxylase (pACC) by AMPK, indicating that the treatment inhibited the activity of ACC, a lipogenesis marker (Figure 5B). Phosphorylation of ATGL and hormone-sensitive lipase (HSL) was significantly higher in the selegiline-treated group than in the HFD-induced obese group, indicating that activated lipolysis occurred in the former. These results suggest that selegiline ameliorates HFD-induced obesity by inhibiting adipogenesis or lipogenesis and reducing fat pad storage through the activation of lipolysis.

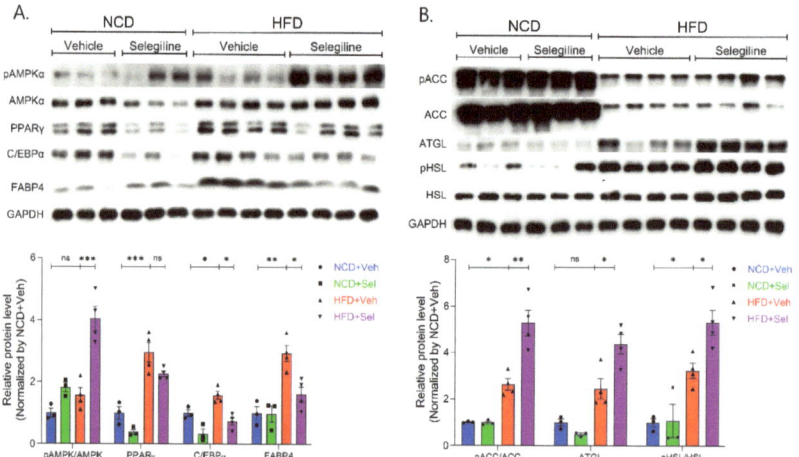

Figure 5. Selegiline-regulated lipid metabolism in epididymal WATs. (**A**) Upper panel: Images of Western blot of pAMPK, AMPK, PPARγ, C/EBPα, FABP4, and GAPDH in WATs from mice treated with selegiline or vehicle fed an NCD or HFD. Lower panel: Summary plot of expression of ratio of pAMPK/AMPK, PPARγ, C/EBPα, and FABP4. (**B**) Upper panel: Images of Western blot of pACC, ACC, ATGL, pHSL, HSL, and GAPDH in eWATs from mice treated with selegiline or vehicle fed an NCD or HFD. Lower panel: Summary plot of expression of ration of pACC/ACC, ATGL, ratio of pHSL/HSL. Data are presented as the mean ± SEM and one-way ANOVA followed by by Dunnett's multiple comparison test was employed for data analysis. Significance denoted by *: $p < 0.05$, **: $p < 0.01$, ***: $p < 0.001$ compared to HFD+Veh. p(Phospho)AMPKα, AMP-activated protein kinase α; PPARγ, Peroxisome proliferator activated receptor gamma; C/EBPα, CCAAT/enhancer-binding protein alpha; FABP4, fatty acid binding protein 4; GAPDH, Glyceraldehyde-3-phosphate dehydrogenase; pACC, Phospho-Acetyl-CoA Carboxylase; ATGL, Adipose triglyceride lipase; HSL, Hormone-sensitive lipase.

Phosphorylation of ATGL and hormone-sensitive lipase (HSL) was significantly higher in the selegiline-treated group than in the HFD-induced obese group, indicating that activated lipolysis occurred in the former. These results suggest that selegiline ameliorates

HFD-induced obesity by inhibiting adipogenesis or lipogenesis and reducing fat pad storage through the activation of lipolysis.

3.5. Selegiline Induced eWAT Browning of HFD-Fed Obese Mice

We further investigated whether eWAT browning was enhanced by selegiline treatment. We assessed this by quantifying PRDM16 and PGC1α protein levels, which are markers for brown-like adipocytes. As shown in Figure 6, PRDM16 and PGC1α protein expression was strongly induced by selegiline in eWATs from HFD mice, suggesting that the transition from white to brown-like adipocytes occurred. Treatment with selegiline was observed to have induced higher levels of UCP1 expression levels in the eWATs than in the untreated group (Figure 6A,B). This result was confirmed through fluorescence staining UCP1, which revealed more UCP1 positive staining in the HFD+Selegiline group than in the HFD-Veh group (Figure 6C). We did not have any significant difference in UCP1 expression levels in the BATs of the HFD-Veh and HFD+Selegiline groups (Figure 6D,E). Our results ultimately strongly suggest that the MAO-B inhibitor selegiline promotes the formation of brown or beige-like eWATs while simultaneously increasing thermogenesis in HFD-induced obese mice.

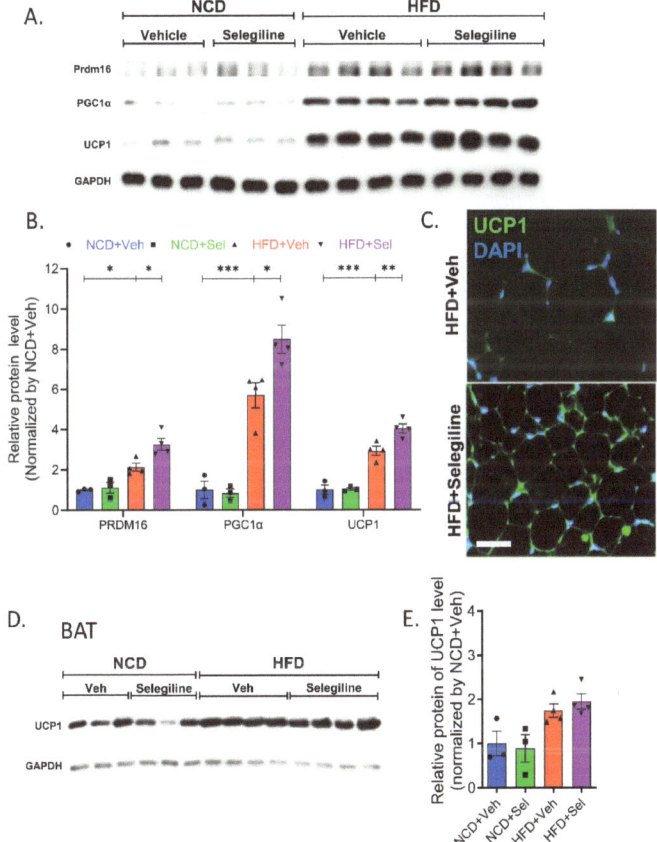

Figure 6. Selegiline promoted thermogenesis and epididymal WAT browning in HFD-fed obese mice. (**A**) Images of Western blot of PRDM16, PGC1α, UCP1, and GAPDH in eWAT from mice treated with

selegiline or vehicle fed an NCD or HFD. (**B**) Summary plot of expression of PRDM16, PGC1α, and UCP1 in eWATs from mice treated with selegiline or vehicle fed an NCD or HFD. (**C**) Representative of UCP1 immunostaining of eWAT. Scale bar = 50 μm. (**D**) Images of Western blot UCP1 and GAPDH in BATs from mice treated with selegiline or vehicle fed an NCD or HFD. (**E**) Summary plot of expression UCP1 in BATs from mice treated with selegiline or vehicle fed an NCD or HFD. Data are presented as the mean ± SEM and one-way ANOVA followed by Dunnett's multiple comparison test was employed for data analysis. Significance denoted by *: $p < 0.05$, **: $p < 0.01$, ***: $p < 0.001$ compared to HFD+Veh. Prdm16, PR/SET Domain 16; PGC1α, Peroxisome proliferator-activated receptor gamma coactivator 1-alpha; UCP1, Uncoupling Protein 1; GAPDH, Glyceraldehyde-3-phosphate dehydrogenase; NCD, normal chow diet; HFD, high-fat diet; Veh, vehicle; Sel, selegiline; BAT, brown adipose tissue.

4. Discussion

In this study, we investigated the anti-obesity impact of selegiline on eWAT lipid metabolism and the underlying molecular mechanism in an obese mouse model given HFD. Our findings indicate that co-administration of selegiline and HFD reduces body weight and fat accumulation in WAT and also decreases the size of eWAT. Selegiline treatment in an animal model, where obesity was induced by HFD, reduced the weight of obese mice, white fat accumulation, and eWAT size. Furthermore, our study showed that selegiline improved glucose homeostasis, lipid metabolism, and promoted browning of WAT.

MAO activity is found not only in the brain but also in peripheral organs such as adipocytes [24]. In adipose tissue, MAO is highly expressed in mature adipocytes and appears during adipocyte differentiation [9]. Previous studies have identified selegiline as responsible for improved energy metabolism and suppressed inflammation in the adipose tissues of high-fat and high-sugar diet obese rats, but observed no change to body weight [16]. Other studies concerning the effect of a selective/non-selective MAO-inhibitor have shown that MAO inhibitors repress adipogenesis in hBM-MSCs [18,25]. Also, selegiline improved lipid metabolism in the liver of HFD-fed mice due to regulating fatty acid oxidation [20]. Another MAO inhibitor, phenelzine, has been reported to improve obesity-related complications [26]. These research results showed the potential for anti-obesity effects by targeting adipocyte MAOs. Similar to previous findings, this study demonstrates that selegiline (30 mg/kg) has potential for anti-obesity prevention and treatment in a mouse model with obesity induced by HFD.

The HFD mouse model induces obesity and is commonly used to screen for anti-obesity compounds. The phenotype of mice changes due to the obesity induced by the HFD, leading to weight gain and altered expression of genes related to lipids. C/EBPα, PPARγ, and FABP4 are key regulators of adipocyte differentiation and have been reported to be highly expressed in HFD mice [27].

Activation of AMPK is essential in combatting obesity as it hinders lipid assimilation and suppresses adipocyte differentiation. AMPK phosphorylation inhibited adipogenesis and lipogenesis, and increased lipolysis and thermogenesis. AMPK is a cellular energy sensor and regulator of metabolic homeostasis, which controls lipid and glucose metabolisms [28–31]. The activation level of AMPK in HFD-induced obese mice is lower than that in normal mice. According to previous studies, AMPK activation in peripheral tissues (such as liver and adipose tissue) suppresses obesity, type 2 diabetes, and related metabolic disorders [32–35]. Thus, although limited to peripheral tissues, AMPK activators (such as metformin, which is provided as a treatment for diabetes), which directly regulate lipid metabolism and indirectly activate thermogenesis, are considered as potential therapeutic agents for obesity and metabolic diseases [28,34,36–38].

In mammals, ACC acts as a downstream signal of AMPK, which facilitates the conversion of acetyl-CoA to malonyl-CoA. AMPK inhibited ACC1 and ACC2 activity by phosphorylating ACC1 Ser79 and ACC2 Ser212 in mice [39]. In general, many anti-obesity compounds hinder lipid synthesis by phosphorylating AMPK or ACC, resulting in their effectiveness [40,41]. Changes in adipose tissue lipid metabolism significantly impact whole-body energy homeostasis [42,43].

We then tested the effect of selegiline on lipid metabolism in epididymal adipose tissue. Our data showed a significant reduction in the expression of adipogenic genes (C/EBPα, FABP4) and down-regulated lipogenesis by ACC to pACC in HFD-fed obese mice administered selegiline. Selegiline significantly increased ATGL expression and HSL phosphorylation in the epididymal adipose tissues of HFD obese mice, which in turn promoted lipolysis. WAT is known to contain HSL, and lipolysis is activated through the phosphorylation of this enzyme.

Lipolysis is the process of breaking down triglycerides (TGs) stored in adipose tissue into free fatty acids (FFAs) and glycerol. Lipolysis in the WAT of humans and rodents is regulated in a step-wise fashion by adipose triglyceride lipase (ATGL), hormone-sensitive lipase (HSL), and monoacylglycerol lipase (MAGL) [44]. During the development of obesity, adipose tissue expands tremendously and adipocyte size increases to neutralize and store nutritional overload. However, when the adipocytes are eventually unable to store excess lipids, two important pathological processes in adipose tissue are important for the development of metabolic diseases: adipose tissue inflammation and hypertrophy. Therefore, complete lipolysis in adipocytes seems to necessitate the coordinated activation of ATGL, HSL, and MAGL. The findings of this investigation indicate that selegiline inhibits the increased expression of lipid-related genes caused by a HFD and triggers the phosphorylation of AMPK, suggesting a possible link between AMPK phosphorylation and the anti-obesity effect of selegiline treatment.

UCP1 inhibits ATP production, and increased UCP1 in adipose tissue stimulates the breakdown of triglycerides stored as fat [45]. WAT plays an important role in maintaining systemic homeostasis [46]. Elevated UCP1 levels in WAT may be due to its conversion to BAT, which has thermogenic properties [45]. Several studies have shown that PRDM16 primarily regulates transcription factors such as PGC1α [47,48]. There is evidence that reducing the expression of PRDM16 reduces thermogenic properties in brown adipocytes [49,50]. Together, these proteins play an important role in regulating energy metabolism in adipocytes.

Our results revealed that selegiline stimulated the protein expression of UCP1 in the WAT of HFD-fed obese mice. Consistent with this upregulated expression, the expression of PGC1α and PRDM16 of the brown adipocyte marker was also upregulated by selegiline. In short, treatment with selegiline induced lipolysis and indirectly affected browning of white adipocyte and thermogenesis in the HFD-fed mice. Although we observed an increase in UCP1 expression in the eWATs, there was no change in UCP1 expression in the BATs, a major organ of thermogenesis. These outcomes implied that the activation of AMPKα, and the subsequent increased expression of brown adipocyte marker genes, might play a role in the selegiline-stimulated browning of eWAT in HFD obese mice.

Despite showing the anti-obesity effect of selegiline, our study has limitations. Selegiline is clinically administered orally to depression patients (5~10 mg/day) [51]. In previous studies, obese animals were subcutaneous administered dose of 0.25~0.6 mg/kg and 10 mg/kg daily dissolving the compound in drinking water [52], it is not known whether this dose is optimal for treatment of obese. Furthermore, our study is limited by using a single dose of 30 mg/kg (roughly 1 mg/day). And, using only an obese animal model, we were unable to conduct experiments on the anti-obesity effect of MAO-B inhibition by directly controlling the brain–adipose tissue axis, and by observing changes in dietary amount, there was no change in eating behavior.

Our study demonstrated the mechanism of action of selegiline, an MAO-B inhibitor, in HFD-induced obese mice. Selegiline inhibits adipogenesis through AMPK activation and exhibits preventive and therapeutic effects by inducing lipolysis in adipose tissue, reducing adipogenesis markers (C/EBPα and FABP4), an adipogenesis marker (pACC), and lipolysis markers (ATGL and pHSL) were increased resulting in a reduction in fat accumulation in adipose tissue. In addition, selegiline-activated AMPK induced WAT browning by increasing UCP1 levels, which triggers energy expenditure using fatty acids as substrates. Throughout this study, we have provided evidence to support the use of selegiline and its mechanisms as an anti-obesity agent.

Collectively, the present study demonstrated that selegiline prevents HFD-induced obesity in vivo, as well as inhibits the expression of adipogenesis- and lipogenesis-related proteins and stimulates the expression of lipolysis-related proteins in the eWAT of HFD-fed mice. Our results further show that selegiline induces the expression of thermogenesis-related proteins and promotes browning in the eWAT of obese mice. In conclusion, epididymal adipocyte browning was induced via phosphorylated AMPK, meaning that it may contribute to the anti-obesity effects of selegiline in HFD-induced obese mice.

Author Contributions: Conceptualization, H.-Y.J., J.-M.O. and S.C.; validation, H.-Y.J., J.-M.O. and S.C.; investigation, H.-Y.J. and J.-M.O.; writing—original draft preparation, H.-Y.J., J.-M.O., M.-S.S., Y.-B.K. and S.C.; writing—review and editing, J.-M.O., M.-S.S., Y.-B.K. and S.C.; supervision, S.C.; project administration, H.-Y.J., J.-M.O. and S.C.; funding acquisition, J.-M.O. and S.C. All authors have read and agreed to the published version of the manuscript.

Funding: This work was supported by the Medical Research Center Program (2017R1A5A2015061, S.C.), by the Brain Research Program (2019M3C7A1032551, S.C.), by the Basic Science Research Program (2022R1A2C1012142, S.C.), and by the Basic Science Research Program (2022R1I1A1A01070134, J.-M.O.) through the National Research Foundation funded by the Korean government.

Institutional Review Board Statement: The animal study protocol was approved by the Institutional Animal Care and Use Committee (IACUC) of Jeonbuk National University (Approval number: JBNU 2022-026).

Informed Consent Statement: Not applicable.

Data Availability Statement: All data is contained within this article. Further inquiries can be directed to the corresponding authors.

Acknowledgments: We thank the Writing Center at Jeonbuk National University for its skilled proofreading service.

Conflicts of Interest: The authors declare no conflict of interest.

References

1. Jung, D.Y.; Suh, N.; Jung, M.H. Tanshinone 1 prevents high fat diet-induced obesity through activation of brown adipocytes and induction of browning in white adipocytes. *Life Sci.* **2022**, *298*, 120488. [CrossRef]
2. Khafagy, R.; Dash, S. Obesity and Cardiovascular Disease: The Emerging Role of Inflammation. *Front. Cardiovasc. Med.* **2021**, *8*, 768119. [CrossRef]
3. Zhang, F.; Ai, W.; Hu, X.; Meng, Y.; Yuan, C.; Su, H.; Wang, L.; Zhu, X.; Gao, P.; Shu, G.; et al. Phytol stimulates the browning of white adipocytes through the activation of AMP-activated protein kinase (AMPK) alpha in mice fed high-fat diet. *Food Funct.* **2018**, *9*, 2043–2050. [CrossRef] [PubMed]
4. Shin, S.K.; Cho, H.W.; Song, S.E.; Im, S.S.; Bae, J.H.; Song, D.K. Oxidative stress resulting from the removal of endogenous catalase induces obesity by promoting hyperplasia and hypertrophy of white adipocytes. *Redox Biol.* **2020**, *37*, 101749. [CrossRef]
5. Ahmad, B.; Serpell, C.J.; Fong, I.L.; Wong, E.H. Molecular Mechanisms of Adipogenesis: The Anti-adipogenic Role of AMP-Activated Protein Kinase. *Front. Mol. Biosci.* **2020**, *7*, 76. [CrossRef]
6. Jakab, J.; Miskic, B.; Miksic, S.; Juranic, B.; Cosic, V.; Schwarz, D.; Vcev, A. Adipogenesis as a Potential Anti-Obesity Target: A Review of Pharmacological Treatment and Natural Products. *Diabetes Metab. Syndr. Obes.* **2021**, *14*, 67–83. [CrossRef]
7. Seale, P.; Conroe, H.M.; Estall, J.; Kajimura, S.; Frontini, A.; Ishibashi, J.; Cohen, P.; Cinti, S.; Spiegelman, B.M. Prdm16 determines the thermogenic program of subcutaneous white adipose tissue in mice. *J. Clin. Investig.* **2011**, *121*, 96–105. [CrossRef]
8. Pizzinat, N.; Marti, L.; Remaury, A.; Leger, F.; Langin, D.; Lafontan, M.; Carpene, C.; Parini, A. High expression of monoamine oxidases in human white adipose tissue: Evidence for their involvement in noradrenaline clearance. *Biochem. Pharmacol.* **1999**, *58*, 1735–1742. [CrossRef]
9. Bour, S.; Daviaud, D.; Gres, S.; Lefort, C.; Prevot, D.; Zorzano, A.; Wabitsch, M.; Saulnier-Blache, J.S.; Valet, P.; Carpene, C. Adipogenesis-related increase of semicarbazide-sensitive amine oxidase and monoamine oxidase in human adipocytes. *Biochimie* **2007**, *89*, 916–925. [CrossRef]
10. Barrand, M.A.; Callingham, B.A. Monoamine oxidase activities in brown adipose tissue of the rat: Some properties and subcellular distribution. *Biochem. Pharmacol.* **1982**, *31*, 2177–2184. [CrossRef]

11. Tong, J.H.; D'Iorio, A.; Kandaswami, C. On the characteristics of mitochondrial monoamine oxidase in pancreas and adipose tissues from genetically obese mice. *Can. J. Biochem.* **1979**, *57*, 197–200. [CrossRef] [PubMed]
12. Carpene, C.; Marti, L.; Morin, N. Increased monoamine oxidase activity and imidazoline binding sites in insulin-resistant adipocytes from obese Zucker rats. *World J. Biol. Chem.* **2022**, *13*, 15–34. [CrossRef]
13. Maggiorani, D.; Manzella, N.; Edmondson, D.E.; Mattevi, A.; Parini, A.; Binda, C.; Mialet-Perez, J. Monoamine Oxidases, Oxidative Stress, and Altered Mitochondrial Dynamics in Cardiac Ageing. *Oxid Med. Cell Longev.* **2017**, *2017*, 3017947. [CrossRef]
14. Marti, L.; Morin, N.; Enrique-Tarancon, G.; Prevot, D.; Lafontan, M.; Testar, X.; Zorzano, A.; Carpene, C. Tyramine and vanadate synergistically stimulate glucose transport in rat adipocytes by amine oxidase-dependent generation of hydrogen peroxide. *J. Pharmacol. Exp. Ther.* **1998**, *285*, 342–349. [PubMed]
15. Visentin, V.; Prevot, D.; Marti, L.; Carpene, C. Inhibition of rat fat cell lipolysis by monoamine oxidase and semicarbazide-sensitive amine oxidase substrates. *Eur. J. Pharmacol.* **2003**, *466*, 235–243. [CrossRef] [PubMed]
16. Nagy, C.T.; Koncsos, G.; Varga, Z.V.; Baranyai, T.; Tuza, S.; Kassai, F.; Ernyey, A.J.; Gyertyan, I.; Kiraly, K.; Olah, A.; et al. Selegiline reduces adiposity induced by high-fat, high-sucrose diet in male rats. *Br. J. Pharmacol.* **2018**, *175*, 3713–3726. [CrossRef]
17. Carpene, C.; Iffiu-Soltesz, Z.; Bour, S.; Prevot, D.; Valet, P. Reduction of fat deposition by combined inhibition of monoamine oxidases and semicarbazide-sensitive amine oxidases in obese Zucker rats. *Pharmacol. Res.* **2007**, *56*, 522–530. [CrossRef]
18. Carpene, C.; Abello, V.; Iffiu-Soltesz, Z.; Mercier, N.; Feve, B.; Valet, P. Limitation of adipose tissue enlargement in rats chronically treated with semicarbazide-sensitive amine oxidase and monoamine oxidase inhibitors. *Pharmacol. Res.* **2008**, *57*, 426–434. [CrossRef]
19. Mattila, M.; Torsti, P. Effect of monoamine oxidase inhibitors and some related compounds on lipid metabolism in rat. Plasma free fatty acids and lipoprotein lipase of the heart and adipose tissue. *Ann. Med. Exp. Biol. Fenn.* **1966**, *44*, 397–400.
20. Tian, Z.; Wang, X.; Han, T.; Sun, C. Selegiline ameliorated dyslipidemia and hepatic steatosis in high-fat diet mice. *Int. Immunopharmacol.* **2023**, *117*, 109901. [CrossRef]
21. Kwon, E.; Joung, H.Y.; Liu, S.M.; Chua, S.C., Jr.; Schwartz, G.J.; Jo, Y.H. Optogenetic stimulation of the liver-projecting melanocortinergic pathway promotes hepatic glucose production. *Nat. Commun.* **2020**, *11*, 6295. [CrossRef] [PubMed]
22. Oh, J.M.; Kim, E.; Chun, S. Ginsenoside Compound K Induces Ros-Mediated Apoptosis and Autophagic Inhibition in Human Neuroblastoma Cells In Vitro and In Vivo. *Int. J. Mol. Sci.* **2019**, *20*, 4279. [CrossRef]
23. Zaqout, S.; Becker, L.L.; Kaindl, A.M. Immunofluorescence Staining of Paraffin Sections Step by Step. *Front. Neuroanat.* **2020**, *14*, 582218. [CrossRef] [PubMed]
24. Les, F.; Prieto, J.M.; Arbones-Mainar, J.M.; Valero, M.S.; Lopez, V. Bioactive properties of commercialised pomegranate (*Punica granatum*) juice: Antioxidant, antiproliferative and enzyme inhibiting activities. *Food Funct.* **2015**, *6*, 2049–2057. [CrossRef] [PubMed]
25. Byun, Y.; Park, J.; Hong, S.H.; Han, M.H.; Park, S.; Jung, H.I.; Noh, M. The opposite effect of isotype-selective monoamine oxidase inhibitors on adipogenesis in human bone marrow mesenchymal stem cells. *Bioorg. Med. Chem. Lett.* **2013**, *23*, 3273–3276. [CrossRef]
26. Mercader, J.; Sabater, A.G.; Le Gonidec, S.; Decaunes, P.; Chaplin, A.; Gomez-Zorita, S.; Milagro, F.I.; Carpene, C. Oral Phenelzine Treatment Mitigates Metabolic Disturbances in Mice Fed a High-Fat Diet. *J. Pharmacol. Exp. Ther.* **2019**, *371*, 555–566. [CrossRef]
27. Garin-Shkolnik, T.; Rudich, A.; Hotamisligil, G.S.; Rubinstein, M. FABP4 attenuates PPARgamma and adipogenesis and is inversely correlated with PPARgamma in adipose tissues. *Diabetes* **2014**, *63*, 900–911. [CrossRef]
28. Herzig, S.; Shaw, R.J. AMPK: Guardian of metabolism and mitochondrial homeostasis. *Nat. Rev. Mol. Cell Biol.* **2018**, *19*, 121–135. [CrossRef]
29. Liu, H.; Liu, M.; Jin, Z.; Yaqoob, S.; Zheng, M.; Cai, D.; Liu, J.; Guo, S. Ginsenoside Rg2 inhibits adipogenesis in 3T3-L1 preadipocytes and suppresses obesity in high-fat-diet-induced obese mice through the AMPK pathway. *Food Funct.* **2019**, *10*, 3603–3614. [CrossRef]
30. Long, Y.C.; Zierath, J.R. AMP-activated protein kinase signaling in metabolic regulation. *J. Clin. Investig.* **2006**, *116*, 1776–1783. [CrossRef]
31. Garcia, D.; Shaw, R.J. AMPK: Mechanisms of Cellular Energy Sensing and Restoration of Metabolic Balance. *Mol. Cell* **2017**, *66*, 789–800. [CrossRef] [PubMed]
32. Hardie, D.G. Sensing of energy and nutrients by AMP-activated protein kinase. *Am. J. Clin. Nutr.* **2011**, *93*, 891S–896S. [CrossRef]
33. Zhou, G.; Sebhat, I.K.; Zhang, B.B. AMPK activators--potential therapeutics for metabolic and other diseases. *Acta Physiol.* **2009**, *196*, 175–190. [CrossRef]
34. Zhou, G.; Myers, R.; Li, Y.; Chen, Y.; Shen, X.; Fenyk-Melody, J.; Wu, M.; Ventre, J.; Doebber, T.; Fujii, N.; et al. Role of AMP-activated protein kinase in mechanism of metformin action. *J. Clin. Investig.* **2001**, *108*, 1167–1174. [CrossRef] [PubMed]
35. Jarzyna, R. [AMP-activated protein kinase—The key role in metabolic regulation]. *Postepy Biochem.* **2006**, *52*, 283–288. [PubMed]
36. Wu, L.; Zhang, L.; Li, B.; Jiang, H.; Duan, Y.; Xie, Z.; Shuai, L.; Li, J.; Li, J. AMP-Activated Protein Kinase (AMPK) Regulates Energy Metabolism through Modulating Thermogenesis in Adipose Tissue. *Front. Physiol.* **2018**, *9*, 122. [CrossRef]
37. Gauthier, M.S.; Miyoshi, H.; Souza, S.C.; Cacicedo, J.M.; Saha, A.K.; Greenberg, A.S.; Ruderman, N.B. AMP-activated protein kinase is activated as a consequence of lipolysis in the adipocyte: Potential mechanism and physiological relevance. *J. Biol. Chem.* **2008**, *283*, 16514–16524. [CrossRef]
38. Foretz, M.; Taleux, N.; Guigas, B.; Horman, S.; Beauloye, C.; Andreelli, F.; Bertrand, L.; Viollet, B. Regulation of energy metabolism by AMPK: A novel therapeutic approach for the treatment of metabolic and cardiovascular diseases. *Med. Sci.* **2006**, *22*, 381–388.
39. Galic, S.; Loh, K.; Murray-Segal, L.; Steinberg, G.R.; Andrews, Z.B.; Kemp, B.E. AMPK signaling to acetyl-CoA carboxylase is required for fasting- and cold-induced appetite but not thermogenesis. *eLife* **2018**, *7*, e32656. [CrossRef]

40. Jang, H.M.; Han, S.K.; Kim, J.K.; Oh, S.J.; Jang, H.B.; Kim, D.H. Lactobacillus sakei Alleviates High-Fat-Diet-Induced Obesity and Anxiety in Mice by Inducing AMPK Activation and SIRT1 Expression and Inhibiting Gut Microbiota-Mediated NF-kappaB Activation. *Mol. Nutr. Food Res.* **2019**, *63*, e1800978. [CrossRef]
41. Lee, Y.S.; Kim, W.S.; Kim, K.H.; Yoon, M.J.; Cho, H.J.; Shen, Y.; Ye, J.M.; Lee, C.H.; Oh, W.K.; Kim, C.T.; et al. Berberine, a natural plant product, activates AMP-activated protein kinase with beneficial metabolic effects in diabetic and insulin-resistant states. *Diabetes* **2006**, *55*, 2256–2264. [CrossRef] [PubMed]
42. Leiria, L.O.; Tseng, Y.H. Lipidomics of brown and white adipose tissue: Implications for energy metabolism. *Biochim. Biophys. Acta Mol. Cell Biol. Lipids* **2020**, *1865*, 158788. [CrossRef] [PubMed]
43. Ceddia, R.B. The role of AMP-activated protein kinase in regulating white adipose tissue metabolism. *Mol. Cell Endocrinol.* **2013**, *366*, 194–203. [CrossRef] [PubMed]
44. Roh, E.; Yoo, H.J. The Role of Adipose Tissue Lipolysis in Diet-Induced Obesity: Focus on Vimentin. *Diabetes Metab. J.* **2021**, *45*, 43–45. [CrossRef]
45. Machado, S.A.; Pasquarelli-do-Nascimento, G.; da Silva, D.S.; Farias, G.R.; de Oliveira Santos, I.; Baptista, L.B.; Magalhaes, K.G. Browning of the white adipose tissue regulation: New insights into nutritional and metabolic relevance in health and diseases. *Nutr. Metab.* **2022**, *19*, 61. [CrossRef]
46. de Pinho, L.; Andrade, J.M.; Paraiso, A.; Filho, A.B.; Feltenberger, J.D.; Guimaraes, A.L.; de Paula, A.M.; Caldeira, A.P.; de Carvalho Botelho, A.C.; Campagnole-Santos, M.J.; et al. Diet composition modulates expression of sirtuins and renin-angiotensin system components in adipose tissue. *Obesity* **2013**, *21*, 1830–1835. [CrossRef]
47. Kajimura, S.; Seale, P.; Kubota, K.; Lunsford, E.; Frangioni, J.V.; Gygi, S.P.; Spiegelman, B.M. Initiation of myoblast to brown fat switch by a PRDM16-C/EBP-beta transcriptional complex. *Nature* **2009**, *460*, 1154–1158. [CrossRef]
48. Hondares, E.; Rosell, M.; Diaz-Delfin, J.; Olmos, Y.; Monsalve, M.; Iglesias, R.; Villarroya, F.; Giralt, M. Peroxisome proliferator-activated receptor alpha (PPARalpha) induces PPARgamma coactivator 1alpha (PGC-1alpha) gene expression and contributes to thermogenic activation of brown fat: Involvement of PRDM16. *J. Biol. Chem.* **2011**, *286*, 43112–43122. [CrossRef]
49. Seale, P.; Bjork, B.; Yang, W.; Kajimura, S.; Chin, S.; Kuang, S.; Scime, A.; Devarakonda, S.; Conroe, H.M.; Erdjument-Bromage, H.; et al. PRDM16 controls a brown fat/skeletal muscle switch. *Nature* **2008**, *454*, 961–967. [CrossRef]
50. Seale, P.; Kajimura, S.; Yang, W.; Chin, S.; Rohas, L.M.; Uldry, M.; Tavernier, G.; Langin, D.; Spiegelman, B.M. Transcriptional control of brown fat determination by PRDM16. *Cell Metab.* **2007**, *6*, 38–54. [CrossRef]
51. Kitaichi, Y.; Inoue, T.; Mitsui, N.; Nakagawa, S.; Kameyama, R.; Hayashishita, Y.; Shiga, T.; Kusumi, I.; Koyama, T. Selegiline remarkably improved stage 5 treatment-resistant major depressive disorder: A case report. *Neuropsychiatr. Dis. Treat.* **2013**, *9*, 1591–1594. [CrossRef] [PubMed]
52. Sa, M.; Yoo, E.S.; Koh, W.; Park, M.G.; Jang, H.J.; Yang, Y.R.; Bhalla, M.; Lee, J.H.; Lim, J.; Won, W.; et al. Hypothalamic GABRA5-positive neurons control obesity via astrocytic GABA. *Nat. Metab.* **2023**, *5*, 1506–1525. [CrossRef] [PubMed]

Disclaimer/Publisher's Note: The statements, opinions and data contained in all publications are solely those of the individual author(s) and contributor(s) and not of MDPI and/or the editor(s). MDPI and/or the editor(s) disclaim responsibility for any injury to people or property resulting from any ideas, methods, instructions or products referred to in the content.

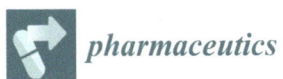

Review

DNA and RNA Molecules as a Foundation of Therapy Strategies for Treatment of Cardiovascular Diseases

Ljiljana Rakicevic

Institute of Molecular Genetics and Genetic Engineering, University of Belgrade, Vojvode Stepe 444a, 11042 Belgrade, Serbia; ljiljanarakicevic011@gmail.com or lili@imgge.ac.bg.rs; Tel.: +381-062-551-485; Fax: +381-11-3975-808

Abstract: There has always been a tendency of medicine to take an individualised approach to treating patients, but the most significant advances were achieved through the methods of molecular biology, where the nucleic acids are in the limelight. Decades of research of molecular biology resulted in setting medicine on a completely new platform. The most significant current research is related to the possibilities that DNA and RNA analyses can offer in terms of more precise diagnostics and more subtle stratification of patients in order to identify patients for specific therapy treatments. Additionally, principles of structure and functioning of nucleic acids have become a motive for creating entirely new therapy strategies and an innovative generation of drugs. All this also applies to cardiovascular diseases (CVDs) which are the leading cause of mortality in developed countries. This review considers the most up-to-date achievements related to the use of translatory potential of DNA and RNA in treatment of cardiovascular diseases, and considers the challenges and prospects in this field. The foundations which allow the use of translatory potential are also presented. The first part of this review focuses on the potential of the DNA variants which impact conventional therapies and on the DNA variants which are starting points for designing new pharmacotherapeutics. The second part of this review considers the translatory potential of non-coding RNA molecules which can be used to formulate new generations of therapeutics for CVDs.

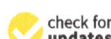

Citation: Rakicevic, L. DNA and RNA Molecules as a Foundation of Therapy Strategies for Treatment of Cardiovascular Diseases. *Pharmaceutics* **2023**, *15*, 2141. https://doi.org/10.3390/pharmaceutics15082141

Academic Editors: Cristina Manuela Drăgoi, Alicia Rodríguez-Gascón, Alina Crenguța Nicolae and Ion-Bogdan Dumitrescu

Received: 30 June 2023
Revised: 27 July 2023
Accepted: 11 August 2023
Published: 15 August 2023

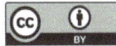

Copyright: © 2023 by the author. Licensee MDPI, Basel, Switzerland. This article is an open access article distributed under the terms and conditions of the Creative Commons Attribution (CC BY) license (https:// creativecommons.org/licenses/by/ 4.0/).

Keywords: personalized medicine; cardiovascular diseases; DNA markers; non-coding RNA; biomarkers

1. Introduction

There has always been a tendency of medicine to take an individualised approach to treating patients (adjusting drug doses according to patient's weight, selecting antibiotics according to antibiograms, etc.). However, the most significant advances in the field of personalised medicine are related to the development of methods of molecular biology. Methodological approaches of molecular biology have facilitated new and more precise insight into fundamental biological processes, the description of new diagnostic and prognostic markers, recognising new pharmacological targets, as well as setting a base for development of innovative treatment methods. DNA and RNA analyses have enabled more precise diagnostics and more subtle stratification of patients in order to identify patients for specific therapy treatments. All this leads us closer to the ideal of personalised medicine [1]. These research influence therapy strategies for certain diseases in a few ways. Firstly, we are provided with possibilities for more precise diagnostics, more precise prognostics and more precise stratification of patients which allow more successful therapeutic treatment [2,3]. Additionally, the founding and development of pharmacogenetics, which correlates genetics and the effects of certain drugs, have enabled us to reach explanations of interindividual differences in response to given therapy. This creates a basis for better prediction of reaction to certain drugs and more reliable algorithms for treatments [4]. Secondly, advanced research has allowed for the recognition of new pharmacological targets, as well as the formulation of innovative drugs based on the physical and chemical features and function of nucleic acids. What these new formulations promise will affect the essential biological processes as well as overcome the limitations of the currently existing generations of drugs [5]. Whether the protocols for use in already existing pharmacotherapeutics are being improved or entirely new innovative generations of drugs are being created, analyses of DNA and RNA force modern medicine to face both new possibilities and new challenges.

This review considers the most up-to-date achievements related to the use of translatory potential of DNA and RNA in treatment of cardiovascular diseases, and it considers the challenges and prospects in this field. The foundations that enable this translatory potential are also presented. The first part of this review focuses on the potential of the DNA variants which impact conventional therapies and on the DNA variants which are starting points for designing new pharmacotherapeutics. The second part of this review considers the translatory potential of non-coding RNA molecules which can be used to formulate new generations of therapeutics for CVDs.

2. Molecular Biology as a Promoter of Research and Treatment of Cardiovascular Diseases

Cardiovascular diseases (CVDs) are a class of illnesses which are a result of concurrence of genetic and acquired factors. They are the leading cause of mortality in developed countries and represent an important medical and social issue, considering their severity and frequency [6,7].

This class of diseases has various manifestations such as hypertension, arrhythmia, venous and arterial thrombosis, heart valve diseases, and myocardial and pericardial diseases etc, which can often be comorbid. Additionally, the presence of other diseases, such as metabolic disorder, hormonal disbalance, rheumatism, infectious diseases, etc., makes diagnostics and treatment even more demanding.

Issues regarding CVDs have spurred research into many directions, the results of which should be a part of the integral platform for treatment and prevention. The attempts of modern society to decrease the frequency of disease and mortality are made through fundamental research, the use of innovative technologies, and education of the population [6,7]. Just as molecular biology has sparked progress over many areas, it set cardiovascular research on an entirely new platform.

2.1. DNA Variants—Biomarkers in CVDs

The development of technologies, which has enabled the analysis and interpretation of genetic information, has led to new diagnostic and prognostic possibilities in medicine. The science has been able to describe the causes of monogenic heart diseases [8], as well as the risk factors for diseases such as hypertension [9,10], arrhythmia [11], atherosclerosis [12], and vein thrombosis [13].

Research in the field of pharmacogenetics is particularly important for the development of personalised drug therapy. It is through them that the genes which affect pharmacotherapeutics for cardiovascular system (CVS) have been identified. These genes control the synthesis of enzymes which are necessary for absorption, transport, and metabolism of drugs, as well as proteins which are the targets of pharmacologic substances [4]. In this context, the drugs used against venous and arterial thrombosis-coumarin derivatives and clopidogrel have been the most frequently considered. Both coumarins and clopidogrel are among the most commonly prescribed drugs in today's medicine. It is known that a division of the patients who take warfarin or clopidogrel can show hypersensitivity or resistance to these drugs, which puts them in life-threatening situations. The anticoagulation drug warfarin, the most prescribed among coumarins, is often referred to as the "poster child" of pharmacogenomics [14,15]. Although there is a large number of genes with an influence on the therapeutic effects of warfarin, it has been shown that of the genes encoding enzymes important for the pharmacodynamics and pharmacokinetics of this drug, these are the ones which are of greatest significance: VKORC1 (the vitamin K epoxide reductase complex subunit 1, pharmacological target of coumarin), P450 2C9 (the major metabolizing enzyme for S-warfarin) and P450 4F2 (acts in counterpart to VKORC1 and limits the accumulation of vitamin K). The variants of these genes with the greatest pharmacogenetic potential are the *VKORC1*2* (c.-1639G>A; rs9923231), the *CYP2C9*2* (c.430C>T; rs1799853), the *CYP2C9*3* (c.1075A>C; rs1057910), and the *CYP4F2*3* (c.1297G>A; *rs2108622*) [14]. In 2010, the American Food and Drug Administration (FDA) recommended pharmacogenetic testing in relation to warfarin. A recommendation for testing is also given by the Clinical Pharmacogenetics Implementation Consortium (CPIC) [16].

Clopidogrel (along with aspirin) is a cornerstone of antiplatelet therapy and requires enzymatic transformation into an active form of the drug. A number of cytochrome P450 enzymes is involved in the metabolism and activation of clopidogrel. Enzymes CYP1A2, CYP2B6, CYP3A4/5, CYP2C9, and CYP2C19, are involved in the activation, with CYP2C19 being the most engaged. It has been shown that the *CYP2C19* gene variants have the greatest pharmacogenetic potential, namely *CYP2C19*2* (681G>A; rs4244285), *CYP2C19*3* (636G>A; rs4986893), and *CYP2C19*17* (−806C>T; rs12248560) [17,18]. Recommendations for genotype-guided antiplatelet therapy are provided by the CPIC, as well as by the FDA and the DPWG (Dutch Pharmacogenetics Working Group) [19]. The subjects of pharmacogenetic studies were also other drugs relevant to cardiovascular diseases: acenocoumarol, β blockers, statins, hydralazine, flecainide, and propafenone [20], (listed in Table 1).

Table 1. The most relevant gene for pharmacogenetics in CVDs.

Farmacogenetics Factors	Drugs	Adverse Effects (Related to Genetic Factors)	Recommendations for Pharmacogenetics Testing
VKORC1, CYP2C9, CYP4F2	Coumarin derivatives warfarin acenocoumarol	Overdose (bleeding) Resistance (thrombosis)	CPIC*, FDA** DPWG***
CYP2C19	Clopidogrel	Overdose (bleeding) Resistance (thrombosis)	CPIC, FDA
SLCO1B1	Statins simvastatin atorvastatin	Myopathy	CPIC DPWG
ADRB1	β-Adrenergic receptor antagonists metoprolol	Bradycardia	DPWG
CYP2D6	Antiarrhythmics flecainide, propafenone	Drug accumulation	DPWG DPWG, FDA

CPIC*—Clinical Pharmacogenetics Implementation Consortium; FDA**—Food and Drug Administration; DPWG***—Dutch Pharmacogenetics Working Group.

Describing DNA markers has an impact on the effects and outcomes of therapy and allow and improvement of the existing therapy protocols. It is possible to design algorithms to predict the effects of a certain therapeutic by analysing pharmacogenetic markers, as well as non-genetic factors which may influence therapy. This enables us to select the safest therapy from drugs produced by the pharmaceutical industry. It has been shown that algorithms designed in this way allow for better predictions than previous interpretations of pharmacogenetic markers given in the form of the FDA-approved warfarin label table [21]. Also, it has been demonstrated that the use of algorithms based on pharmacogenetic analyses is more cost-effective for health systems [22]. Several consortia and working groups have recommended many gene–drug pairs in order to support medical professionals to tailor a unique therapy for an individual patient [16,19,20]. Nevertheless, despite the recommendations and the large amount of generated data, routine pharmacogenetic testing has not yet taken root in practice. Furthermore, it seems that response from the cardiology community is *lukewarm* [23]. Surprisingly, this is true even for clopidogrel which is one of the drugs highly recommended for pharmacogenetic testing. Routine acceptance of recommendations does meet obstacles, mainly due to lack of more precise data on patient adherence, variability in effect of therapy even within the same genotype, and the lack of data on the less frequent groups of patients [23]. The introduction of pharmacogenetic protocols into therapy is often challenged by economic strains, although financial investments which would offer transparent results are not the only issue to be addressed. Meeting these challenges demands innovation in pharmacogenetics and medicine, but also in other areas such as infrastructure, human resources, management, etc [24,25]. This was clearly shown in a study which analysed an attempt to implement pharmacogenetic testing in a large number of medical centres. The study concluded that identified issues were actually non-pharmacogenetic [26].

New challenges have emerged in the field of pharmacogenetics thanks to next-generation sequencing (NGS) [27–29]. This technology has enabled for the rapid acceleration in determining the sequence of DNA or RNA, including whole-genome sequencing (WGS), whole-exome sequencing (WES), and transcriptome analyses (RNA-Seq). Chronologically speaking, the first wave of significant results in pharmacogenetics was triggered by studies which focused on genes which were the logical candidates based on their roles in pharmacokinetics and pharmacodynamics of drugs. The studies explained the great deviation of effects that the explored drugs had. Later, with use of technology which allows WES and WGS, the abundance of DNA variants was detected and a large number of them are yet to be defined. The frequency of these variants is smaller [30], but it is expected that once they are interpreted, the distribution of drug responses could be presented as a continuum, rather than a polymodal distribution which corresponds to the pre-NGS era [4].

It is unquestionable that gathering data related to pharmacogenetic markers is a work in progress. The influx of a large amount of data requires tools for their faster analysis, as well as a larger number of studies that can validate potential genetic markers. Also, the integration of data from different fields is of particular importance, and in this sense, the development of bioinformatics and network medicine plays an important role [31].

DNA Variants and New Drugs Development

The results of research in the fields of genetics and genomics are also important for the development of new pharmacotherapeutics. It has been shown that proteins whose function is altered as a result of mutations in corresponding genes can be taken into consideration as models or targets for creating new pharmacotherapeutics. These strategies are also taken into consideration for the development of new drugs for several disorders which are closely related to the occurrence of cardiovascular diseases. Often, the focus of such research is on the genetic causes of lipid disorders, which is understandable considering the role lipids have in the development of CVDs [32]. For instance, the gene for PCSK9 (proprotein convertase subtilisin kexin 9), whose specific variants cause familial hypercholesterolemia (FH), as well as its variants lead to striking decreases in low-density lipoprotein cholesterol (LDL-C) and to atherosclerosis risk [33]. In the pharmacological battle against high level of LDL-C, variants of the NPC1L1 (Niemann–Pick C1-like 1) gene are being reconsidered as they have a deactivating effect on proteins, resulting in reduced plasma LDL-C levels and a reduced risk of coronary heart disease [34]. In terms of hyperlipidaemia, the gene of interest is ANGPTL4 (Angiopoietin Like 4) [35,36], while the variations of APOC3 (Apolipoprotein C3) are important for hypertriglyceridemia [37]. The variants of SLC30A8 (Solute Carrier Family 30 Member 8) are significant for the prevention of type 2 diabetes [38].

In general, the influence genomics has on the modern pharmaceutical industry is very strong. Genetic research is increasingly necessary when selecting pharmacological targets and in selecting indications for the process of development of specific pharmacotherapeutic. Certain studies indicate that the success of developing a drug is twofold higher if genetic research has been incorporated into its development [39–41].

2.2. Non-Coding RNAs (ncRNAs)

Messenger RNAs (mRNA), which code sequence of proteins, constitute less than 2% of the expressed genome. The majority of RNAs which are synthesised in the process of transcription are non-coding. Apart from transfer RNA (tRNA) and ribosomal RNA (rRNA) (which were defined first), a large number of non-coding RNAs have been described: long non-coding RNA (lncRNA), micro RNA (miRNA), short interfering RNA (siRNA), PIWI-interacting (piRNA), short nuclear RNA (snRNA), extracellular RNA (exRNA), and small Cajal body associated RNA (scaRNA) [42]. During the 1990s, extensive research on these molecules started and that is when the first mechanisms of expression regulation by non-coding RNA in *Caenorhabditis elegans* were described [43]. Non-coding RNAs were recognised as a special group of molecules essential for maintaining basic biological processes. At the same time, their extraordinary translatory potential in medicine was recognised too. First of all, it became apparent that many non-coding RNAs could be new types of biomarkers and new pharmaceutical targets. In addition, ncRNA research opened possibilities to use the structure and function of nucleic acids for formulating innovative therapeutic strategies and designing entirely novel kinds of therapeutics which could overcome the limitations of present drugs (small molecules, antibodies). In that respect, the principles of complementarity, hybridization, and interference are of the utmost importance [5]. One of the most studied processes in RNA interference is the mechanism for post-transcriptional silencing of gene expression in cells of eukaryotes [44]. Double-stranded RNAs (siRNAs and miRNAs), complementary to the target mRNA, take part in this process. Their presence leads to the activation of a specific RISC (RNA-induced silencing complex) enzyme complex, which results in sequence-specific suppression of gene expression (Figure 1).

NcRNAs were very actively studied in connection to cardiovascular diseases. The goal was to explain the molecular processes which lead to pathological conditions and/or to use principles of the way this class of molecules function in order to find new biomarkers and formulate new generation of drugs.

2.2.1. NcRNAs and Monitoring the Therapy

Some of the possibilities this group of molecules offer are potentially as diagnostically useful biomarkers, monitoring and treating CVDs.

It is known that most of miRNAs in human blood derive from thrombocytes and that they represent promising biomarker candidates [45]. There are data on both basic cellular processes involving thrombocyte miRNAs, as well as on potential significance of miRNAs in relation to analysis of thrombocytes' activity and the effects of anti-aggregation therapy. MiRNAs in circulation have been shown to indicate the status of thrombocytes in real time and that they can be used as biomarkers for the prediction of various aspects of their function, i.e., they can be used for monitoring and adjusting anti-aggregation therapy [46,47]. Additionally, it has been confirmed that miRNAs affect anticoagulation therapy with coumarin derivatives [48], therapy with direct anticoagulation drugs [49], and that they also affect therapy with statins, i.e., statin intolerance [50]. The predictive potential of long non-coding RNAs has also been recognised for the effects of anti-aggregation therapy [51]. Some databases that provide information regarding associations of ncRNA and drug effects already exist [52]. However, data related to ncRNAs and their association between drug effects are rapidly generated. The traditional biological experiments can recognize new ncRNA–drug-effects associations, but this approach faces challenges like time consumption and financial issues. Additionally, new efforts have been made on predicting the associations between ncRNAs and drugs' effects by computer methods which offer acceleration of this process and provide new possibilities for improving therapeutic treatments. So, in the near future, we can expect more precise and complete data on this matter [53–55].

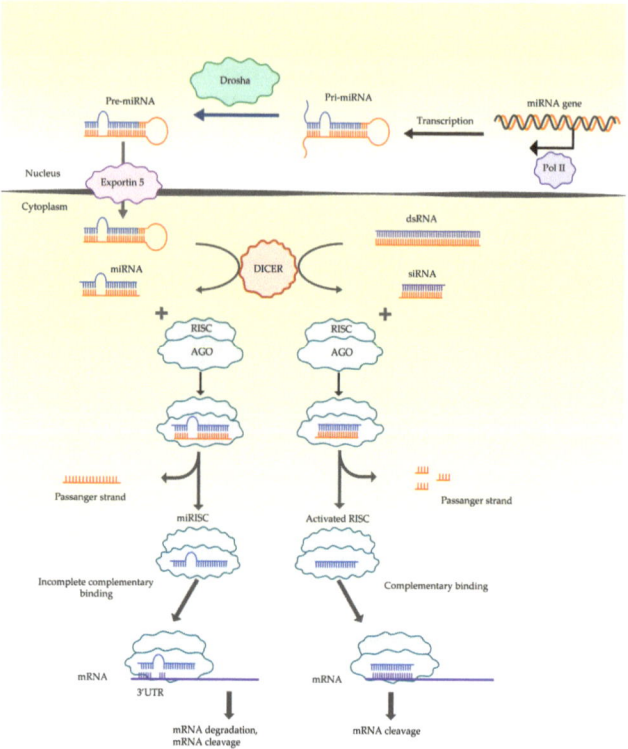

Figure 1. Mechanism of RNA interference. RNAi mechanism recognizes long dsRNA which is then cleaved by Dicer endonuclease into 21–25 nucleotide-long double-strand siRNAs. AGO2 (Argonaute 2) and RISC complexes recognize the new siRNA, it is followed by degradation of sense strand and complementary binding of antisense strand with targeted mRNA which leads to disintegration of mRNA. siRNAs are highly specific with only one mRNA target. MiRNAs biogenesis begins with the synthesis of long primary miRNAs (pri-miRNAs), which are processed into pre-miRNAs by nuclear ribonuclease. Pre-miRNAs are exported from the nucleus, followed by the cleavage by Dicer enzyme and then (as mature miRNA) they are joined to AGO2-RISK complex. The miRNAs bind to the target mRNAs through partial complementary base pairing, leading to translational repression, degradation, and cleavage of mRNAs. Endogenous miRNAs are able to target multiple mRNAs at once.

2.2.2. NcRNAs and New Generation of Therapeutics

RNA therapy is a strategy that involves use of RNA-based molecules for the treatment of diseases. This strategy is based on the use of structural and functional characteristics of RNA molecules, i.e., by mimicking or attenuating their function in the regulation of biological processes. Several types of technologies are used for these approaches: antisense oligonucleotides (ASOs), aptamers, siRNAs, miRNA mimics/attenuation (Table 2).

One of the biggest challenges related to the development of RNA therapy is achieving certain pharmacodynamic and pharmacokinetic properties of drugs. It is achieved by chemical modifications of nucleic acid molecules. The most often employed modifications are phosphate linkage modifications (phosphorothioate) and $2'$ ribose modifications such as $2'$-O-methyl ($2'$-OMe), $2'$-fluoro ($2'$-F), $2'$-O-methoxyethyl ($2'$-MOE), and locked nucleic. Also, a subject of great interest for development of the therapy is delivery platforms, i.e., technologies which allow the targeting of drugs to cell-specific ligands. The most considered technology is the binding of different structures to nucleic acid based agents, such as antibody fragments, an entire antibody, or the FDA approved N-Acetylgalactosamine (GalNAc), which binds to asialoglycoprotein receptor 1 (ASGR1), which is highly expressed in the liver [56,57]. The possibilities of RNA therapy use have been researched in a large number of severe diseases, where conventional treatments are not effective and one of the greatest expectations of this therapy is the possible treatment of molecules that have been "undruggable". Conventional pharmacotherapy mostly uses small molecules (and antibodies in part) and targets different proteins, such as enzymes, ion channels, nuclear receptors, G-protein coupled receptors, etc. A human organism contains about 20,000 proteins, but just a small number of these molecules can be targeted by small-molecule therapy ("druggable" proteins). It is estimated that only about 15% of human proteins are "druggable", including those already targeted by pharmacotherapeutics [58]. Using RNA-based therapy allows us to act on the upstream phase, i.e., at the level of mRNA, which can turn an "undruggable" protein "druggable". Additionally, recognising ncRNAs as pharmacological targets ensures a much higher capacity to act with therapeutics. This is due to the fact that more than 70% of the human genome is determined by ncRNAs, in contrast to just 2% determined by human protein [59]. In addition to the use of therapeutics that contain some type of nucleic acids as principle components, the possibility of acting on ncRNAs through small molecules is being considered [60].

Table 2. Technologies employed in RNA therapy development.

Formulatrion	Fundamental Basic
ASO	ASO are short, synthetic, single-stranded oligonucleotides that can be based on both DNA and RNA. ASOs bind their target RNAs in a sequence-specific manner modulating mRNA function and gene expression or inactivating miRNAs.
Aptamers	Aptamers are short, artificial single-stranded oligonucleotides, composed of DNA or RNA, that bind target molecules (proteins, peptides, carbohydrates, small molecules). The important quality of these molecules is conformation, which allows high affinity and high specificity towards ligands. That is precisely why aptamers are often referred to as chemical antibodies (aptemer derives from Latin "aptus" meaning "to fit").
siRNAs	SiRNAs are non-coding RNAs which are involved in RNA interference (RNAi). Synthetic siRNAs are 20–25 base pairs with 3′ overhangs long and they can avoid the action of Dicer enzyme directly engaging in RISC and control of gene expression.
MiRNA mimics/atenuation	MiRNAs are non-coding RNA involved in RNA interference. Endogenous miRNAs are able to target multiple mRNAs at once. The miRNA mimics is designed to have the same sequence as the endogenous miRNA and can target multiple mRNAs at once. Anti-miRNAs are ASOs designed to be (fully or partially) complementary to a selected endogenous miRNA to prevent interaction with its target genes.

The majority of approved RNA drugs for CVDs, as well as RNA drugs in various stages of clinical development, affect the metabolism of lipids. Such drugs are mipomersen, inclisiran, and volanesorsen (Table 3).

Mipomersen is an antisense oligonucleotide drug designed to target the apoB-100 mRNA and cause its degradation, thus inhibiting the synthesis of a particular protein. The use of this drug significantly reduces LDL-C and other lipoprotein levels. However, due to the probability of severe adverse effects, including hepatotoxicity, the use of mipomersen is highly limited. It is approved for the treatment of homozygous for familial hypercholesterolemia-autosomal dominant, a genetic disorder that leads to significantly elevated LDL-C levels and increased risk for cardiovascular diseases [61].

Table 3. RNA-based formulations for treatment of CVSs in humans.

Phase	Drug (Brend Name)	Chemical Specificity and Modification	Target
Approved for therapy (by FDA or/and EMA)	Mipomersen Kynamro®	ASO PS; 2'-MOE	*APOB* mRNA
	Inclisiran Leqvio®	siRNA 2'-F; 2'-MOE; 2'-O-Me; PS; GalNAc	*PCSK9* mRNA
	Volanesorsen Waylivra®	ASO 2'-MOE	*APOC3* mRNA
Various stages of clinical development	Olpasiran	siRNA PS; 2'-O-Me; 2'-F; GalNAc	*LPA* mRNA
	Pelacarsen	ASO 2'-O-MOE; GalNAc	*LPA* mRNA
	Vupanorsen	ASO GalNAc	*ANGPTL3* mRNA
	SLN360	siRNA 2'-O-Me; 2'-deoxy-2'-F; GalNAc	*LPA* mRNA;
	LY3819469	siRNA 2'-O-Me; 2'-F; GalNAc	*LPA* mRNA;
	MRG-110	Anti-mir	miRNA-92A
	CDR132L	Anti-mir	miRNA-132

2'-O-Me, 2'-methoxy; 2'-O-MOE, 2'-methoxyethyl; 2'-F, 2'-fluoro; PS, phosphorothioate; GalNAc, N–Acetylgalactosamine.

Inclisiran is a siRNA-based therapeutic that closely mirrors the function of natural, endogenous miRNA. This drug targets mRNA for PCSK9 which is a serine protease that regulates plasma LDL-C levels. Inclisiran is approved for the treatment of adults with primary (familial and non-familial) hypercholesterolemia or mixed dyslipidemia, and for patients with clinical atherosclerotic cardiovascular disease (ASCVD) who require additional lowering of LDL-C. It is intended for administration alone or in combination with other lipid-lowering drugs in patients who are statin-intolerant or patients for whom a statin therapy is contraindicated. During the conducted clinical trials there was no evidence of kidney, liver, muscle, or platelet toxicity [62,63].

Volanesorsen is an ASO designed to prevent the translation of apolipoprotein CIII (APOC3) by targeting APOC3 mRNA. Apolipoprotein CIII is a small protein, with a role in the inhibition of triglyceride metabolism and hepatic clearance of chylomicrons, so its overexpression is associated with the risk of atherosclerosis. A combined analysis of several conducted randomised controlled studies has shown that the administration of volanesorsen in patients with severe hypertriglyceridemia significantly reduces triglycerides, very low-density lipoprotein cholesterol (VLDL-C), Apo-B48, non- high-density lipoprotein cholesterol (HDL-C), and increases HDL-C in comparison to placebo. Additionally, volanesorsn, has shown an acceptable safety profile. Most of the registered adverse effects were mild and they were related to injection site reactions. Volanesorsen is approved by the EMA (European Medicines Agency) to treat familial chylomicronaemia syndrome (FCS), a genetic disorder characterised by high levels of triglycerides in the blood. Since FCF belongs to rare diseases, volanesorsen is designated as an orphan medicine (medicines used for the treatment of rare diseases) [64].

Apart from the formulations that have already been approved for therapy, there is a whole range of candidates for the treatment of cardiovascular diseases (Table 3).

Olpasiran is a siRNA molecule that prevents translation of apo(a) protein and consequently precludes assembly of the Lp(a) particles. The mechanism of olpasiran action occurs through targeting and degrading mRNA of the LPA gene that encodes apo(a). In the first phase of clinical trials in the first-in-human study, it was shown that the drug was potent in reducing plasma Lp(a) concentration [65,66]. Additionally, several clinical studies are being conducted to evaluate the efficacy, safety, tolerability and the impact of olpasiran on major cardiovascular events (NCT05489614, NCT05481411, NCT04987320, NCT04270760, NCT05581303).

Pelacarsen, another drug whose clinical development is still ongoing, is designed according to the principle of ASO action. It is directed against mRNA of the gene for apolipoprotein (a) which consequently inhibits synthesis of apolipoprotein (a) in the liver. This also leads to reduction in the level of Lp (a), which is recognized as an independent cause of CVDs. Interestingly, the use of pelacarsen also reduces LDL-C, apolipoprotein B (apo B), and oxidised phospholipids on apo B and apo(a) [67]. Future studies, as well as re-evaluating laboratory measurement procedures, could give answers to these phenomena. There are also ongoing clinical studies which are examining the effects and safety of this drug (NCT05900141, NCT05646381, NCT05305664, NCT04023552).

Vupanorsen is an antisense oligonucleotide that targets the mRNA for angiopoietin like 3 (ANGPTL3) in the liver and consequently inhibits ANGPTL3 protein synthesis. The published results of the first clinical studies show that administration of vupanorsen significantly reduced levels of serum ANGPTL3 protein and some lipid parameters including triglycerides and non–high-density lipoprotein cholesterol in comparison to placebo. Despite these findings, the Pfizer-led vupanorsen clinical development has been discontinued. The rationale behind this decision is that the evident decrease in lipid parameters was still not sufficiently effective to prevent CVDs [68,69].

An agent named *SLN360* is a siRNA that interferes with the biosynthesis of Lp(a). Inhibition of protein synthesis occurs through the formation of a complex between SLN360 and LPA mRNA, which leads to degradation of the targeted mRNA and inhibition of translation (NCT05537571, NCT04606602). According to the published results, SLN360 significantly reduced the plasma Lp(a) concentration, in dose-dependent manner and has a safety profile at a satisfactory level [70]. Another new siRNA agent, *LY3819469*, is still in the clinical development phase. It is designed to influence the level of Lp(a) in the plasma. The ongoing clinical trial aims to investigate the pharmacokinetics and pharmacodynamics of this agent, as well as its safety and tolerability (NCT04914546).

The synthetic agent *MRG-110* is designed to inhibit miRNA92a (NCT03603431). It was previously determined that miRNA92A in human cells performs inhibition of processes necessary for angiogenesis by silencing expression of proangiogenic factors (such as integrin alpha 5), blocking the build up vascular network, and slowing down migration of endothelial cells and their ability to connect to fibronectin. Preclinical studies on mammals have shown that the synthetic miRNA92a inhibitor increases expression of proangiogenic genes, which are targets for miRNA92a [71]. Also, it has been shown that inhibition of miRNK92a improved vascularization after myocardial infarction and blood circulation after hind limb ischemia, a model of peripheral occlusive disease [72]. In an ischemia/reperfusion model in pigs, anti-miR-92a significantly improved cardiac function and vascularization [73,74]. Additionally, it has been demonstrated that this miRNA can be an appropriate therapeutic target for treating cardiac microvascular dysfunction in diabetes [75]. The first results of testing the agent MRG-110 in humans were published in 2020 by Abplanalp and co-authors. In that study, the molecular effects of MRG-110 administration in healthy volunteers were investigated. It was shown that MRG-110 reduced miR-92a in whole blood, circulating CD31$^+$ cells, and in extracellular vesicles. Also, this agent has been shown to derepress miRNA92a target genes [76].

The use of synthetic *CDR132L* which inhibits miRNA132 (NCT04045405) has also been approved for testing in humans. MiRNA132 orchestrates the beginning of pathological remodelling of myocard by silencing a range of relevant genes such as *NOS3*

(Endothelial Nitric Oxide Synthase 3) and *SERCA2a* (Sarcoplasmic/Endoplasmic Reticulum Ca^{2+}ATPase 2a). During the preclinical studies, it was shown that CDR132L blocks adverse remodelling of myocard and restores coronary function, while, on a molecular level, it restores the expression of ATPase SERCA2a which is crucial for retaking in calcium during contractions of cardiomyocytes [77]. The results of the first application of CDR132L in humans were published in 2021 by Taubel and co-authors. They conducted a Phase 1b randomized, double-blind, placebo-controlled study in patients with heart failure and showed that CDR132L was safe and well tolerated; furthermore, the study showed that the use of CDR132L preparation leads to cardiac functional improvements-improvement in left ventricular ejection fraction (LVEF), significant QRS narrowing, reduction in the amino terminal fragment of pro-brain natriuretic peptide (NTproBNP) levels, and positive trends for relevant cardiac fibrosis biomarkers [78].

2.2.3. NcRNAs and Extracellular Vesicles

A particularly important aspect of the translation potential of non-coding RNAs is their natural presence in extracellular vesicles (EVs). EVs are released by all living cells. They are surrounded by a double membrane and contain numerous molecules, such as proteins, nucleic acids, bioactive lipids, etc. EVs are important mediators in intercellular and inter-organ communication which uses their contents to pass different signals to targeted cells and they participate in different processes within those cells [79]. Based on their biogenesis, size, and physicochemical properties, EVs can be classified into subcategories (exosomes, microvesicles, apoptotic bodies). The International Society of Extracellular Vesicles recommended defining all prepared vesicles (independent of their origin) as EVs [80].

There is a lot of available data related to the role of molecular mediators carried by exosomes originating from the heart as well as data on mediators carried by exosomes from other organs that affect the heart [81,82]. EVs are especially interesting for their potential regarding the regeneration of myocard [83,84]. The research on miRNA and lncRNA which originated from EVs is important because extracellular vesicles affect myocard with these two classes of non-coding RNAs [85].

EV-derived ncRNAs are a part of a wide range of cellular processes and many aspects of their functions may be considered for new therapeutic strategies. It has been shown that myocardial infarction is associated with increased levels of lncRNA, NEAT1, and miR-328-3p [86,87], as well as with decreased levels of lncRNA HCP5, miR-21, miR-24, miR-98-5p, miR-150p, miR-185, and miR-212-5p [88–94]. Additionally, there is enough convincing evidence related to heart damaged by infarction, which shows that restoring levels of decreased ncRNAs back to normal can be achieved by using ES-derived ncRNAs [88–91,94,95]. Experiments with models for myocardial infarction have also shown that ncRNAs derived from EVs are involved in processes which are essential for recovery of the heart, i.e., they increase cardiomyocyte survival and cardiac functional recovery [89,92,94–101]. Also, it has been confirmed that EV-derived ncRNAs influence other processes related to the cardiovascular system such as inflammatory response [90,95,102–104], as well as vascular protection and angiogenesis [105–111].

The results of this research indicate the great translatory potential of EVs. As natural delivery systems, EVs act as a safe vehicle because they allow for the stabilization and protection of ncRNAs (as well as other molecules they transfer) on the way to targeted cells. This, and their biocompatibility and targeting ability, makes them very attractive for innovative therapy technologies. On the other hand, there are a number of obstacles related to the biological production methods of EVs in large-scale production. The greatest challenges are related to isolation of undamaged EVs, purity and characterization, and high costs. However, a large number of ongoing studies promise to solve the mentioned problems in the near future [112].

The number of data related to non-coding RNAs is rapidly growing and it is obvious that various types of non-coding RNAs are joined into unique regulatory processes. This makes both setting the premises of research and the interpretation of results very complex. For that very reason, bioinformatic research is so important. It can facilitate extractions of clusters of molecules which are most important to the study of specific physiological and pathophysiological processes. At the same time, it would facilitate the selection of highly specific molecules related to specific diseases as the most relevant biomarkers or pharmacological targets [113].

3. Conclusions and Future Perspectives

It is usual to simultaneously use various kinds of therapies to target various pathogenic pathways when tackling problems which develop with CVDs. At the same time, it is still necessary to develop new treatments which can give better treatment results, and modern research into DNA and RNA molecules, and their role in new therapeutic approaches, makes a great contribution to this. The development of pharmacogenetics has led to the identification of DNA markers that allow more precise classification of patients to sub-phenotypes, which is important for more successful application of conventional therapy. Constant advancement in this field and the generation of new data forges a basis for designing multi-variant panels which can be used for prediction of a wide range of drug-induced adverse effects. We can also expect panels encompassing RNA pharmacogenetic markers. Additionally, studying the principals of RNA function led to formulations of innovative therapeutic strategies such as RNA therapies. Probably the most significant achievement of RNA based therapy so far is the possibility to influence molecules which have been "undruggable" until now. This field is rapidly advancing and it is followed by a huge data generation in fundamental and preclinical research. Investments in multi-omics research, as well as in non-biological disciplines such as computer science, should enable us to faster identify the most adequate molecule candidates for the further development of drugs.

Generally, modern medicine confronts a large quantity of data related to translatory potential of DNA and RNA molecules for treatment of cardiovascular diseases. However, new challenges have emerged simultaneously with it. For instance, the speed of generating data and new findings is not in proportion to their practical application. In a way, more subtle stratification on a molecular level makes cardiovascular diseases, which are already of complex nature, even more complex for consideration. A deluge of information related to DNA and RNA poses questions about the management and interpretation of results, about recognising specificities of potential biomarkers, and about the possibilities of formulating drugs which are safe for human use. Also, there are questions related to infrastructural and economic components of analysing a large number of potential biomarkers which may become an important element of comprehensive strategies for the diagnostics, monitoring, and treatment of diseases.

Overcoming these challenges demands social investments and the engagement of the scientific community on various levels (Figure 2). First of all, data processing and interpretation require employing within computer science and bioinformatics at proportional level. Also, it is necessary to continue studies in order to research and validate DNA and RNA biomarkers with high translatory potential in supervising treatment, as well as to research possible therapeutics for CDV. The cardiology community needs additional studies even for well defined DNA markers in pharmacogenetics in order to provide missing data (mentioned above)—precise medicine demands precise data and precise conclusions. At the same time, we are looking for efficient modes for the use of well-defined pharmacogenetic markers in routine practice. Finding these modes is a challenge even for developed economies and demands innovation in medicine and genetics, as well as innovation in the entire management of health systems.

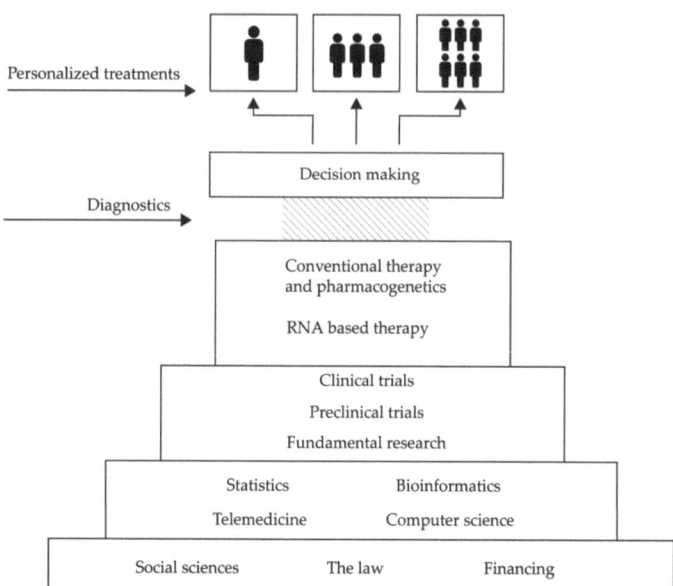

Figure 2. Different areas and activities involved in the development of personalized therapeutic approaches.

However, despite challenges, trends such as intensive development of bioinformatics tools and artificial intelligence, constant improvement of technological approaches to molecular biology analyses, as well as decreases in costs of analyses offer satisfactory answers. Finally, all present knowledge indicates that the foundation for developing the medicine of the future has already been laid, and DNA and RNA molecules play an important role in it.

Funding: This work was supported by the Ministry of Science, Technological Development and Innovation of the Republic of Serbia (Contract No. 451-03-47/2023-01/200042).

Institutional Review Board Statement: Not applicable.

Informed Consent Statement: Not applicable.

Data Availability Statement: Not applicable.

Conflicts of Interest: The author declares no conflict of interest.

References

1. Goetz, L.H.; Schork, N.J. Personalized medicine: Motivation, challenges, and progress. *Fertil. Steril.* **2018**, *109*, 952–963. [CrossRef] [PubMed]
2. Schulte, C.; Zeller, T. Biomarkers in primary prevention: Meaningful diagnosis based on biomarker scores? *Herz* **2020**, *45*, 10–16. [CrossRef] [PubMed]
3. Sethi, Y.; Patel, N.; Kaka, N.; Kaiwan, O.; Kar, J.; Moinuddin, A.; Goel, A.; Chopra, H.; Cavalu, S. Precision Medicine and the future of Cardiovascular Diseases: A Clinically Oriented Comprehensive Review. *J. Clin. Med.* **2023**, *12*, 1799. [CrossRef]
4. Roden, D.M.; McLeod, H.L.; Relling, M.V.; Williams, M.S.; Mensah, G.A.; Peterson, J.F.; Van Driest, S.L. Pharmacogenomics. *Lancet* **2019**, *394*, 521–532. [CrossRef]
5. Yu, A.M.; Tu, M.J. Deliver the promise: RNAs as a new class of molecular entities for therapy and vaccination. *Pharmacol. Ther.* **2022**, *230*, 107967. [CrossRef] [PubMed]
6. Tsao, C.W.; Aday, A.W.; Almarzooq, Z.I.; Anderson, C.A.M.; Arora, P.; Avery, C.L.; Baker-Smith, C.M.; Beaton, A.Z.; Boehme, A.K.; Buxton, A.E.; et al. Heart Disease and Stroke Statistics-2023 Update: A Report From the American Heart Ssociation. *Circulation* **2023**, *147*, e93–e621. [CrossRef] [PubMed]

7. Roth, G.A.; Mensah, G.A.; Johnson, C.O.; Addolorato, G.; Ammirati, E.; Baddour, L.M.; Barengo, N.C.; Beaton, A.Z.; Benjamin, E.J.; Benziger, C.P.; et al. Global Burden of Cardiovascular Diseases and Risk Factors, 1990–2019: Update from the GBD 2019 Study. *J. Am. Coll. Cardiol.* **2020**, *76*, 2982–3021. [CrossRef] [PubMed]
8. Richards, A.A.; Garg, V. Genetics of congenital heart disease. *Curr. Cardiol. Rev.* **2010**, *6*, 91–97. [CrossRef]
9. Padmanabhan, S.; Melander, O.; Johnson, T.; Di Blasio, A.M.; Lee, W.K.; Gentilini, D.; Hastie, C.E.; Menni, C.; Monti, M.C.; Delles, C.; et al. Genome-Wide Association Study of Blood Pressure Extremes Identifies Variant near UMOD Associated with Hypertension. *PLoS Genet.* **2010**, *6*, e1001177. [CrossRef]
10. Ehret, G.B.; Munroe, P.B.; Rice, K.M.; Bochud, M.; Johnson, A.D.; Chasman, D.I.; Smith, A.V.; Tobin, M.D.; Verwoert, G.C.; Hwang, S.J.; et al. Genetic variants in novel pathways influence blood pressure and cardiovascular disease risk. *Nature* **2011**, *478*, 103–109.
11. Gray, B.; Behr, E.R. New Insights Into the Genetic Basis of Inherited Arrhythmia Syndromes. *Circ. Cardiovasc. Genet.* **2016**, *9*, 569–577. [CrossRef] [PubMed]
12. Fava, C.; Montagnana, M. Atherosclerosis Is an Inflammatory Disease which Lacks a Common Antiinflammatory Therapy: How Human Genetics Can Help to This Issue. *Narrative Rev. Front. Pharmacol.* **2018**, *9*, 55. [CrossRef] [PubMed]
13. de Haan, H.G.; Bezemer, I.D.; Doggen, C.J.; Le Cessie, S.; Reitsma, P.H.; Arellano, A.R.; Tong, C.H.; Devlin, J.J.; Bare, L.A.; Rosendaal, F.R.; et al. Multiple SNP testing improves risk prediction of first venous thrombosis. *Blood* **2012**, *120*, 656–663. [CrossRef]
14. Drozda, K.; Pacanowski, M.A.; Grimstein, C.; Zineh, I. Pharmacogenetic Labeling of FDA-Approved Drugs: A Regulatory Retrospective. *JACC Basic Transl. Sci.* **2018**, *3*, 545–549. [CrossRef] [PubMed]
15. Pratt, V.M.; Cavallari, L.H.; Del Tredici, A.L.; Hachad, H.; Ji, Y.; Kalman, L.V.; Ly, R.C.; Moyer, A.M.; Scott, S.A.; Whirl-Carrillo, M.; et al. Recommendations for Clinical Warfarin Genotyping Allele Selection: A Report of the Association for Molecular Pathology and the College of American Pathologists. *J. Mol. Diagn.* **2020**, *22*, 847–859. [CrossRef]
16. Johnson, J.A.; Caudle, K.E.; Gong, L.; Whirl-Carrillo, M.; Stein, C.M.; Scott, S.A.; Lee, M.T.; Gage, B.F.; Kimmel, S.E.; Perera, M.A.; et al. Clinical Pharmacogenetics Implementation Consortium (CPIC) Guideline for Pharmacogenetics-Guided Warfarin Dosing: 2017 Update. *Clin. Pharmacol. Ther.* **2017**, *102*, 397–404. [CrossRef]
17. Curzen, N.; Sambu, N. Antiplatelet therapy in percutaneous coronary intervention: Is variability of response clinically relevant? *Heart* **2011**, *97*, 1433–1440. [CrossRef]
18. Kazui, M.; Nishiya, Y.; Ishizuka, T.; Hagihara, K.; Farid, N.A.; Okazaki, O.; Ikeda, T.; Kurihara, A. Identification of the human cytochrome P450 enzymes involved in the two oxidative steps in the bioactivation of clopidogrel to its pharmacologically active metabolite. *Drug Metab. Dispos.* **2010**, *38*, 92–99. [CrossRef]
19. Lee, C.R.; Luzum, J.A.; Sangkuhl, K.; Gammal, R.S.; Sabatine, M.S.; Stein, C.M.; Kisor, D.F.; Limdi, N.A.; Lee, Y.M.; Scott, S.A.; et al. Clinical Pharmacogenetics Implementation Consortium Guideline for CYP2C19 Genotype and Clopidogrel Therapy: 2022 Update. *Clin. Pharmacol. Ther.* **2022**, *112*, 959–967. [CrossRef]
20. Duarte, J.D.; Cavallari, L.H. Pharmacogenetics to guide cardiovascular drug therapy. *Nat. Rev. Cardiol.* **2021**, *18*, 649–665. [CrossRef]
21. Finkelman, B.; Gage, B.F.; Johnson, J.A.; Brensinger, C.M.; Kimmel, S.E. Genetic warfarin dosing: Tables versus algorithms. *J. Am. Coll. Cardiol.* **2011**, *57*, 612–618. [CrossRef] [PubMed]
22. Mitropoulou, C.; Fragoulakis, V.; Rakicevic, L.B.; Novkovic, M.M.; Vozikis, A.; Matic, D.M.; Antonijevic, N.M.; Radojkovic, D.P.; van Schaik, R.H.; Patrinos, G.P.; et al. Economic analysis of pharmacogenomicguided clopidogrel treatment in Serbian patients with myocardial infarction undergoing primary percutaneous coronary intervention. *Pharmacogenomics* **2016**, *17*, 1775–1784. [CrossRef] [PubMed]
23. Roden, D.M. Clopidogrel Pharmacogenetics—Why the Wait? *N. Engl. J. Med.* **2019**, *381*, 1677–1678. [CrossRef] [PubMed]
24. Blagec, K.; Swen, J.J.; Koopmann, R.; Cheung, K.C.; Crommentuijn-van Rhenen, M.; Holsappel, I.; Konta, L.; Ott, S.; Steinberger, D.; Xu, H.; et al. Pharmacogenomics decision support in the U-PGx project: Results and advice from clinical implementation across seven European countries. *PLoS ONE* **2022**, *17*, e0268534. [CrossRef]
25. Wake, D.T.; Smith, D.M.; Kazi, S.; Dunnenberger, H.M. Pharmacogenomic clinical decision support: A review, how-to guide, and future vision. *Clin. Pharmacol. Ther.* **2022**, *112*, 44–57. [CrossRef]
26. Herr, T.M.; Bielinski, S.J.; Bottinger, E.; Brautbar, A.; Brilliant, M.; Chute, C.G.; Cobb, B.L.; Denny, J.C.; Hakonarson, H.; Hartzler, A.L.; et al. Practical considerations in genomic decision support: The eMERGE experience. *J. Pathol. Inform.* **2015**, *6*, 50. [CrossRef]
27. Genomes Project Consortium; Abecasis, G.R.; Auton, A.; Brooks, L.D.; DePristo, M.A.; Durbin, R.M.; Handsaker, R.E.; Kang, H.M.; Marth, G.T.; McVean, G.A. An integrated map of genetic variation from 1,092 human genomes. *Nature* **2012**, *491*, 56–65.
28. Dewey, F.E.; Murray, M.F.; Overton, J.D.; Habegger, L.; Leader, J.B.; Fetterolf, S.N.; O'dushlaine, C.; Van Hout, C.V.; Staples, J.; Gonzaga-Jauregui, C.; et al. Distribution and clinical impact of functional variants in 50,726 whole-exome sequences from the DiscovEHR study. *Science* **2016**, *354*, aaf6814. [CrossRef]
29. Schwarz, U.I.; Gulilat, M.; Kim, R.B. The Role of Next-Generation Sequencing in Pharmacogenetics and Pharmacogenomics. *Cold Spring Harb. Perspect. Med.* **2019**, *9*, a033027. [CrossRef]
30. Nelson, M.R.; Wegmann, D.; Ehm, M.G.; Kessner, D.; St Jean, P.; Verzilli, C.; Shen, J.; Tang, Z.; Bacanu, S.-A.; Fraser, D.; et al. An Abundance of Rare Functional Variants in 202 Drug Target Genes Sequenced in 14,002 People. *Science* **2012**, *337*, 100–104. [CrossRef]

31. Lee, L.Y.; Pandey, A.K.; Maron, B.A.; Loscalzo, J. Network medicine in Cardiovascular Research. *Cardiovasc. Res.* **2021**, *117*, 2186–2202. [CrossRef]
32. Hamilton, M.C.; Fife, J.D.; Akinci, E.; Yu, T.; Khowpinitchai, B.; Cha, M.; Barkal, S.; Thi, T.T.; Yeo, G.H.T.; Ramos Barroso, J.P.; et al. Systematic elucidation of genetic mechanisms anderlying cholesterol uptake. *Cell Genom.* **2023**, *3*, 100304. [CrossRef] [PubMed]
33. Cohen, J.C.; Boerwinkle, E.; Mosley, T.H., Jr.; Hobbs, H.H. Sequence variations in PCSK9, low LDL, and protection against coronary heart disease. *N. Engl. J. Med.* **2006**, *354*, 1264–1272. [CrossRef]
34. Stitziel, N.O.; Won, H.H.; Morrison, A.C.; Peloso, G.M.; Do, R.; Lange, L.A.; Fontanillas, P.; Gupta, N.; Duga, S.; Goel, A.; et al. Inactivating mutations in NPC1L1 and protection from coronary heart disease. *N. Engl. J. Med.* **2014**, *371*, 2072–2082.
35. Stitziel, N.O.; Stirrups, K.E.; Masca, N.G.; Erdmann, J.; Ferrario, P.G.; König, I.R.; Weeke, P.E.; Webb, T.R.; Auer, P.L.; Schick, U.M.; et al. Coding Variation in ANGPTL4, LPL, and SVEP1 and the Risk of Coronary Disease. *N. Engl. J. Med.* **2016**, *374*, 1134–1144.
36. Dewey, F.E.; Gusarova, V.; O'Dushlaine, C.; Gottesman, O.; Trejos, J.; Hunt, C.; Van Hout, C.V.; Habegger, L.; Buckler, D.; Lai, K.-M.; et al. Inactivating Variants in ANGPTL4 and Risk of Coronary Artery Disease. *N. Engl. J. Med.* **2016**, *374*, 1123–1133. [CrossRef]
37. Crosby, J.; Peloso, G.M.; Auer, P.L.; Crosslin, D.R.; Stitziel, N.O.; Lange, L.A.; Lu, Y.; Tang, Z.Z.; Zhang, H.; Hindy, G.; et al. Loss-of-function mutations in APOC3, triglycerides, and coronary disease. *N. Engl. J. Med.* **2014**, *371*, 22–31.
38. Flannick, J.; Thorleifsson, G.; Beer, N.L.; Jacobs, S.B.; Grarup, N.; Burtt, N.P.; Mahajan, A.; Fuchsberger, C.; Atzmon, G.; Benediktsson, R.; et al. Loss-of-function mutations in SLC30A8 protect against type 2 diabetes. *Nat. Genet.* **2014**, *46*, 357–363. [CrossRef]
39. Nelson, M.R.; Tipney, H.; Painter, J.L.; Shen, J.; Nicoletti, P.; Shen, Y.; Floratos, A.; Sham, P.C.; Li, M.J.; Wang, J.; et al. The support of human genetic evidence for approved drug indications. *Nat. Genet.* **2015**, *47*, 856–860. [CrossRef]
40. King, E.A.; Davis, J.W.; Degner, J.F. Are drug targets with genetic support twice as likely to be approved? Revised estimates of the impact of genetic support for drug mechanisms on the probability of drug approval. *PLoS Genet.* **2019**, *15*, e1008489. [CrossRef]
41. Narganes-Carlón, D.; Crowther, D.J.; Pearson, E.R. A publication-wide association study (PWAS), historical language models to prioritise novel therapeutic drug targets. *Sci. Rep.* **2023**, *13*, 8366. [CrossRef]
42. Hombach, S.; Kretz, M. Non-coding RNAs: Classification, Biology and Functioning. *Adv. Exp. Med. Biol.* **2016**, *937*, 3–17. [CrossRef]
43. Fire, A.; Xu, S.; Montgomery, M.K.; Kostas, S.A.; Driver, S.E.; Mello, C.C. Potent and specific genetic interference by double-stranded RNA in Caenorhabditis elegans. *Nature* **1998**, *391*, 806–811. [CrossRef]
44. Elbashir, S.M.; Harborth, J.; Lendeckel, W.; Yalcin, A.; Weber, K.; Tuschl, T. Duplexes of 21-nucleotide RNAs mediate RNA interference in cultured mammalian cells. *Nature* **2001**, *411*, 494–498. [CrossRef]
45. Krammer, T.L.; Mayr, M.; Hackl, M. microRNAs as Promising Biomarkers of Platelet Activity in Antiplatelet Therapy Monitoring. *Int. J. Mol. Sci.* **2020**, *21*, 3477. [CrossRef]
46. Zapilko, V.; Fish, R.J.; Garcia, A.; Reny, J.-L.; Dunoyer-Geindre, S.; Lecompte, T.; Neerman-Arbez, M.; Fontana, P. MicroRNA-126 is a regulator of platelet-supported thrombin generation. *Platelets* **2020**, *31*, 746–755. [CrossRef]
47. Garcia, A.; Dunoyer-Geindre, S.; Nolli, S.; Reny, J.-L.; Fontana, P. An Ex Vivo and In Silico Study Providing Insights into the Interplay of Circulating miRNAs Level, Platelet Reactivity and Thrombin Generation: Looking beyond Traditional Pharmacogenetics. *J. Pers. Med.* **2021**, *11*, 323. [CrossRef]
48. Benincasa, G.; Costa, D.; Infante, T.; Lucchese, R.; Donatelli, F.; Napoli, C. Interplay between genetics and epigenetics in modulating the risk of venous thromboembolism: A new challenge for personalized therapy. *Thromb. Res.* **2019**, *177*, 145–153. [CrossRef] [PubMed]
49. Zhang, H.; Zhang, Z.; Liu, Z.; Mu, G.; Xie, Q.; Zhou, S.; Wang, Z.; Cao, Y.; Tan, Y.; Wei, X.; et al. Circulating miR-320a-3p and miR-483-5p level associated with pharmacokinetic-pharmacodynamic profiles of riva-roxaban. *Hum. Genom.* **2022**, *16*, 72.
50. Mangas, A.; Pérez-Serra, A.; Bonet, F.; Muñiz, O.; Fuentes, F.; Gonzalez-Estrada, A.; Campuzano, O.; Rodriguez Roca, J.S.; Alonso-Villa, E.; Toro, R. A microRNA Signature for the Diagnosis of Statins Intolerance. *Int. J. Mol. Sci.* **2022**, *23*, 8146. [CrossRef] [PubMed]
51. Liu, Y.L.; Hu, X.L.; Song, P.Y.; Li, H.; Li, M.P.; Du, Y.X.; Li, M.Y.; Ma, Q.L.; Peng, L.M.; Song, M.Y.; et al. Influence of GAS5/MicroRNA-223-3p/P2Y12 Axis on Clopidogrel Response in Coronary Artery Disease. *J. Am. Heart Assoc.* **2021**, *10*, e021129. [CrossRef] [PubMed]
52. Dai, E.; Yang, F.; Wang, J.; Zhou, X.; Song, Q.; An, W.; Wang, L.; Jiang, W. ncDR: A comprehensive resource of non-coding RNAs involved in drug resistance. *Bioinformatics* **2017**, *33*, 4010–4011. [CrossRef]
53. Gao, M.; Shang, X. Identification of associations between lncRNA and drug resistance based on deep learning and attention mechanism. *Front. Microbiol.* **2023**, *14*, 1147778. [CrossRef]
54. Li, Y.; Wang, R.; Zhang, S.; Xu, H.; Deng, L. LRGCPND: Predicting Associations between ncRNA and Drug Resistance via Linear Residual Graph Convolution. *Int. J. Mol. Sci.* **2021**, *22*, 10508. [CrossRef]
55. Niu, Y.; Song, C.; Gong, Y.; Zhang, W. MiRNA-drug resistance association prediction through the attentive multimodal graph convolutional network. *Front. Pharmacol.* **2022**, *12*, 799108. [CrossRef] [PubMed]
56. Kulkarni, J.A.; Witzigmann, D.; Thomson, S.B.; Chen, S.; Leavitt, B.R.; Cullis, P.R.; van der Meel, R. The current landscape of nucleic acid therapeutics. *Nat. Nanotechnol.* **2021**, *16*, 630–643. [CrossRef] [PubMed]

57. Crooke, S.T.; Liang, X.-H.; Crooke, R.M.; Baker, B.F.; Geary, R.S. Antisense drug discovery and development technology considered in a pharmacological context. *Biochem. Pharmacol.* **2020**, *189*, 114196. [CrossRef]
58. Makley, L.N.; Gestwicki, J.E. Expanding the number of "druggable" targets: Non-enzymes and protein-protein interactions. *Chem. Biol. Drug Des.* **2013**, *81*, 22–32. [CrossRef]
59. Djebali, S.; Davis, C.A.; Merkel, A.; Dobin, A.; Lassmann, T.; Mortazavi, A.; Tanzer, A.; Lagarde, J.; Lin, W.; Schlesinger, F.; et al. Landscape of transcription in human cells. *Nature* **2012**, *489*, 101–108. [CrossRef]
60. Costales, M.G.; Childs-Disney, J.L.; Haniff, H.S.; Disney, M.D. How We Think about Targeting RNA with Small Molecules. *J. Med. Chem.* **2020**, *63*, 8880–8900. [CrossRef]
61. Chambergo-Michilot, D.; Alur, A.; Kulkarni, S.; Agarwala, A. Mipomersen in Familial Hypercholesterolemia: An Update on Health-Related Quality of Life and Patient-Reported Outcomes. *Vasc. Health Risk Manag.* **2022**, *18*, 73–80. [CrossRef]
62. Lamb, Y.N. Inclisiran: First Approval. *Drugs* **2021**, *81*, 389–395, Erratum in **2021**, *81*, 1129. [CrossRef] [PubMed]
63. Winkle, M.; El-Daly, S.M.; Fabbri, M.; Calin, G.A. Noncoding RNA therapeutics—Challenges and potential solutions. *Nat. Rev. Drug Discov.* **2021**, *20*, 629–651. [CrossRef] [PubMed]
64. Calcaterra, I.; Lupoli, R.; Di Minno, A.; Di Minno, M.N.D. Volanesorsen to treat severe hypertriglyceridaemia: A pooled analysis of randomized controlled trials. *Eur. J. Clin. Investig.* **2022**, *52*, e13841. [CrossRef]
65. Koren, M.J.; Moriarty, P.M.; Baum, S.J.; Neutel, J.; Hernandez-Illas, M.; Weintraub, H.S.; Florio, M.; Kassahun, H.; Melquist, S.; Varrieur, T.; et al. Preclinical development and phase 1 trial of a novel siRNA targeting lipoprotein(a). *Nat. Med.* **2022**, *28*, 96–103. [CrossRef] [PubMed]
66. O'donoghue, M.L.; Rosenson, R.S.; Gencer, B.; López, J.A.G.; Lepor, N.E.; Baum, S.J.; Stout, E.; Gaudet, D.; Knusel, B.; Kuder, J.F.; et al. Small Interfering RNA to Reduce Lipoprotein(a) in Cardiovascular Disease. *N. Engl. J. Med.* **2022**, *387*, 1855–1864. [CrossRef]
67. Yeang, C.; Karwatowska-Prokopczuk, E.; Su, F.; Dinh, B.; Xia, S.; Witztum, J.L.; Tsimikas, S.J. Effect of pelacarsen on lipoprotein(a) cholesterol and corrected low-density lipoprotein Cholesterol. *Am. Coll. Cardiol.* **2022**, *79*, 1035–1046. [CrossRef]
68. Bergmark, B.A.; Marston, N.A.; Bramson, C.R.; Curto, M.; Ramos, V.; Jevne, A.; Kuder, J.F.; Park, J.-G.; Murphy, S.A.; Verma, S.; et al. Effect of Vupanorsen on Non–High-Density Lipoprotein Cholesterol Levels in Statin-Treated Patients with Elevated Cholesterol: TRANSLATE-TIMI. *Circulation* **2022**, *145*, 1377–1386. [CrossRef]
69. Fukuhara, K.; Furihata, K.; Matsuoka, N.; Itamura, R.; Ramos, V.; Hagi, T.; Kalluru, H.; Bramson, C.; Terra, S.G.; Liu, J. A multipurpose Japanese phase I study in the global development of vupanorsen: Randomized, placebocontrolled, single-ascending dose study in adults. *Clin. Transl. Sci.* **2023**, *16*, 886–897. [CrossRef]
70. Nissen, S.E.; Wolski, K.; Balog, C.; Swerdlow, D.I.; Scrimgeour, A.C.; Rambaran, C.; Wilson, R.J.; Boyce, M.; Ray, K.K.; Cho, L.; et al. Single Ascending Dose Study of a Short Interfering RNA Targeting Lipoprotein(a) Production in Individuals With Elevated Plasma Lipoprotein(a) Levels. *JAMA* **2022**, *327*, 1679–1687. [CrossRef]
71. Gallant-Behm, C.L.; Piper, J.; Dickinson, B.A.; Dalby, C.M.; Pestano, L.A.; Jackson, A.L. A synthetic mi-croRNA-92a inhibitor (MRG-110) accelerates angiogenesis and wound healing in diabetic and nondiabetic wounds. *Wound Repair. Regen.* **2018**, *26*, 311–323.
72. Bonauer, A.; Carmona, G.; Iwasaki, M.; Mione, M.; Koyanagi, M.; Fischer, A.; Burchfield, J.; Fox, H.; Doebele, C.; Ohtani, K.; et al. MicroRNA-92a Controls Angiogenesis and Functional Recovery of Ischemic Tissues in Mice. *Science* **2009**, *324*, 1710–1713. [CrossRef] [PubMed]
73. Hinkel, R.; Penzkofer, D.; Zühlke, S.; Fischer, A.; Husada, W.; Xu, Q.F.; Baloch, E.; van Rooij, E.; Zeiher, A.M.; Kupatt, C.; et al. Inhibition of microRNA-92a protects against ischemia/reperfusion injury in a large animal model. *Circulation* **2013**, *128*, 1066–1075. [PubMed]
74. Bellera, N.; Barba, I.; Rodriguez-Sinovas, A.; Ferret, E.; Asín, M.A.; Gonzalez-Alujas, M.T.; Pérez-Rodon, J.; Esteves, M.; Fonseca, C.; Toran, N.; et al. Single Intracoronary Injection of Encapsulated Antagomir-92a Promotes Angiogenesis and Prevents Adverse Infarct Remodeling. *J. Am. Heart Assoc.* **2014**, *3*, e000946. [CrossRef]
75. Samak, M.; Kaltenborn, D.; Kues, A.; Le Noble, F.; Hinkel, R.; Germena, G. Micro-RNA 92a as a Therapeutic Target for Cardiac Microvascular Dysfunction in Diabetes. *Biomedicines* **2021**, *10*, 58. [CrossRef] [PubMed]
76. Abplanalp, W.; Fischer, A.; John, D.; Zeiher, A.M.; Gosgnach, W.; Darville, H.; Montgomery, R.; Pestano, L.; Allée, G.; Paty, I.; et al. Efficiency and Target Derepression of Anti-miR-92a: Results of a First in Human Study. *Nucleic Acid. Ther.* **2020**, *30*, 335. [CrossRef]
77. Foinquinos, A.; Batkai, S.; Genschel, C.; Viereck, J.; Rump, S.; Gyöngyösi, M.; Traxler, D.; Riesenhuber, M.; Spannbauer, A.; Lukovic, D.; et al. Preclinical development of a miR-132 inhibitor for heart failure treat-ment. *Nat. Commun.* **2020**, *11*, 633. [CrossRef]
78. Täubel, J.; Hauke, W.; Rump, S.; Viereck, J.; Batkai, S.; Poetzsch, J.; Rode, L.; Weigt, H.; Genschel, C.; Lorch, U.; et al. Novel antisense therapy targeting microRNA-132 in patients with heart failure: Results of a first-in-human Phase 1b randomized, double-blind, placebo-controlled study. *Eur. Heart J.* **2021**, *42*, 178–188. [CrossRef]
79. Veziroglu, E.M.; Mias, G.I. Characterizing Extracellular Vesicles and Their Diverse RNA Contents. *Front. Genet.* **2020**, *11*, 700. [CrossRef]
80. Thery, C.; Witwer, K.W.; Aikawa, E.; Alcaraz, M.J.; Anderson, J.D.; Andriantsitohaina, R. Minimal information for studies of extracellular vesicles 2018 (MISEV2018): A position statement of the International Society for Extracellular Vesicles and update of the MISEV2014 guidelines. *J. Extracell. Vesicles* **2018**, *7*, 1535750. [CrossRef]

81. Gabisonia, K.; Khan, M.; Recchia, F.A. Extracellular vesicle-mediated bidirectional communication between heart and other organs. *Am. J. Physiol. Circ. Physiol.* **2022**, *322*, H769–H784. [CrossRef]
82. Hermann, D.M.; Xin, W.; Bähr, M.; Giebel, B.; Doeppner, T.R. Emerging roles of extracellular vesicle-associated non-coding RNAs in hypoxia: Insights from cancer, myocardial infarction and ischemic stroke. *Theranostics* **2022**, *12*, 5776–5802. [CrossRef]
83. Sahoo, S.; Losordo, D.W. Exosomes and Cardiac Repair After Myocardial Infarction. *Circ. Res.* **2014**, *114*, 333–344. [CrossRef]
84. Kervadec, A.; Bellamy, V.; El Harane, N.; Arakélian, L.; Vanneaux, V.; Cacciapuoti, I.; Nemetalla, H.; Périer, M.-C.; Toeg, H.D.; Richart, A.; et al. Cardiovascular progenitor–derived extracellular vesicles recapitulate the beneficial effects of their parent cells in the treatment of chronic heart failure. *J. Heart Lung Transplant.* **2016**, *35*, 795–807. [CrossRef]
85. Wu, Q.; Wang, J.; Tan, W.L.W.; Jiang, Y.; Wang, S.; Li, Q.; Yu, X.; Tan, J.; Liu, S.; Zhang, P.; et al. Extracellular vesicles from human embryonic stem cell-derived cardiovascular progenitor cells promote cardiac infarct healing through reducing cardiomyocyte death and promoting angiogenesis. *Cell Death Dis.* **2020**, *11*, 354. [CrossRef] [PubMed]
86. Huang, J.; Wang, F.; Sun, X.; Chu, X.; Jiang, R.; Wang, Y. Myocardial infarction cardiomyocytes-derived exosomal miR-328-3p promote apoptosis via Caspase signaling. *Am. J. Transl. Res.* **2021**, *13*, 2365–2378.
87. Kenneweg, F.; Bang, C.; Xiao, K.; Boulanger, C.M.; Loyer, X.; Mazlan, S.; Schroen, B.; Hermans-Beijnsberger, S.; Foinquinos, A.; Hirt, M.N.; et al. Long Noncoding RNA-Enriched Vesicles Secreted by Hypoxic Cardiomyocytes Drive Cardiac Fibrosis. *Mol. Ther.—Nucleic Acids* **2019**, *18*, 363–374. [CrossRef] [PubMed]
88. Li, K.; Bai, Y.; Li, J.; Li, S.; Pan, J.; Cheng, Y.; Li, K.; Wang, Z.G.; Ji, W.J.; Zhou, Q.; et al. LncRNA HCP5 in hBMSC-derived exosomes alleviates myocardial ischemia reperfusion injury by sponging miR-497 to activate IGF1/PI3K/AKT pathway. *Int. J. Cardiol.* **2021**, *342*, 72–81. [CrossRef] [PubMed]
89. Gu, H.; Liu, Z.; Li, Y.; Xie, Y.; Yao, J.; Zhu, Y.; Xu, J.; Dai, Q.; Zhong, C.; Zhu, H.; et al. Serum-Derived Extracellular Vesicles Protect Against Acute Myocardial Infarction by Regulating miR-21/PDCD4 Signaling Pathway. *Front. Physiol.* **2018**, *9*, 348. [CrossRef]
90. Zhang, L.; Wei, Q.; Liu, X.; Zhang, T.; Wang, S.; Zhou, L.; Zou, L.; Fan, F.; Chi, H.; Sun, J.; et al. Exosomal microRNA-98-5p from hypoxic bone marrow mesenchymal stem cells inhibits myocardial ischemia-reperfusion injury by reducing TLR4 and activating the PI3K/Akt signaling pathway. *Int. Immunopharmacol.* **2021**, *101*, 107592. [CrossRef]
91. Wu, Z.; Cheng, S.; Wang, S.; Li, W.; Liu, J. BMSCs-derived exosomal microRNA-150-5p attenuates myocardial infarction in mice. *Int. Immunopharmacol.* **2021**, *93*, 107389. [CrossRef]
92. Li, Y.; Zhou, J.; Zhang, O.; Wu, X.; Guan, X.; Xue, Y.; Li, S.; Zhuang, X.; Zhou, B.; Miao, G.; et al. Bone marrow mesenchymal stem cells-derived exosomal microRNA-185 represses ventricular remolding of mice with myocardial infarction by inhibiting SOCS. *Int. Immunopharmacol.* **2020**, *80*, 106156. [CrossRef]
93. Wu, Y.; Peng, W.; Fang, M.; Wu, M.; Wu, M. MSCs-Derived Extracellular Vesicles Carrying miR-212-5p Alleviate Myocardial Infarction-Induced Cardiac Fibrosis via NLRC5/VEGF/TGF-β1/SMAD Axis. *J. Cardiovasc. Transl. Res.* **2022**, *5*, 302–316. [CrossRef]
94. Zhang, C.-S.; Shao, K.; Liu, C.-W.; Li, C.-J.; Yu, B.-T. Hypoxic preconditioning BMSCs-exosomes inhibit cardiomyocyte apoptosis after acute myocardial infarction by upregulating microRNA-24. *Eur. Rev. Med. Pharmacol. Sci.* **2019**, *23*, 6691–6699.
95. Wang, X.; Zhu, Y.; Wu, C.; Liu, W.; He, Y.; Yang, Q. Adipose-Derived Mesenchymal Stem Cells-Derived Exosomes Carry MicroRNA-671 to Alleviate Myocardial Infarction Through Inactivating the TGFBR2/Smad2 Axis. *Inflammation* **2021**, *44*, 1815–1830. [CrossRef]
96. Zhu, L.P.; Tian, T.; Wang, J.Y.; He, J.N.; Chen, T.; Pan, M.; Xu, L.; Zhang, H.X.; Qiu, X.T.; Li, C.C.; et al. Hypoxia-elicited mesenchymal stem cell-derived exosomes facilitates cardiac repair through miR-125b-mediated prevention of cell death in myocardial infarction. *Theranostics* **2018**, *8*, 6163–6177. [CrossRef]
97. Zhu, W.; Sun, L.; Zhao, P.; Liu, Y.; Zhang, J.; Zhang, Y.; Hong, Y.; Zhu, Y.; Lu, Y.; Zhao, W.; et al. Macrophage migration inhibitory factor facilitates the therapeutic efficacy of mesenchymal stem cells derived ex-osomes in acute myocardial infarction through upregulating miR-133a-3p. *J. Nanobiotechnol.* **2021**, *19*, 61. [CrossRef]
98. Ke, X.; Yang, R.; Wu, F.; Wang, X.; Liang, J.; Hu, X.; Hu, C. Exosomal miR-218-5p/miR-363-3p from Endothelial Progenitor Cells Ameliorate Myocardial Infarction by Targeting the p53/JMY Signaling Pathway. *Oxid. Med. Cell Longev.* **2021**, *2021*, 5529430. [CrossRef]
99. Chen, J.; Cui, C.; Yang, X.; Xu, J.; Venkat, P.; Zacharek, A.; Yu, P.; Chopp, M. MiR-126 Affects Brain-Heart Interaction after Cerebral Ischemic Stroke. *Transl. Stroke Res.* **2017**, *8*, 374–385. [CrossRef]
100. Cheng, H.; Chang, S.; Xu, R.; Chen, L.; Song, X.; Wu, J.; Qian, J.; Zou, Y.; Ma, J. Hypoxia-challenged MSC-derived exosomes deliver miR-210 to attenuate post-infarction cardiac apoptosis. *Stem Cell Res. Ther.* **2020**, *11*, 224. [CrossRef]
101. Peng, Y.; Zhao, J.L.; Peng, Z.Y.; Xu, W.F.; Yu, G.L. Exosomal miR-25-3p from mesenchymal stem cells alleviates myocardial infarction by targeting pro-apoptotic proteins and EZH2. *Cell Death Dis.* **2020**, *11*, 317. [CrossRef]
102. Zheng, S.; Wang, L.; Ma, H.; Sun, F.; Wen, F. microRNA-129 overexpression in endothelial cell-derived extracellular vesicle influences inflammatory response caused by myocardial ischemia/reperfusion injury. *Cell Biol. Int.* **2021**, *45*, 1743–1756. [CrossRef]
103. Pan, J.; Alimujiang, M.; Chen, Q.; Shi, H.; Luo, X. Exosomes derived from miR-146a-modified adipose-derived stem cells attenuate acute myocardial infarction−induced myocardial damage via downregulation of early growth response factor 1. *J. Cell. Bichem.* **2019**, *120*, 4433–4443. [CrossRef]

104. Lin, B.; Chen, X.; Lu, C.; Xu, J.; Qiu, Y.; Liu, X.; Song, H.; Chen, A.; Xiong, J.; Wang, K.; et al. Loss of exosomal LncRNA HCG15 prevents acute myocardial ischemic injury through the NF-κB/p65 and p38 pathways. *Cell Death Dis.* **2021**, *12*, 1007. [CrossRef]
105. Sánchez-Sánchez, R.; Gómez-Ferrer, M.; Reinal, I.; Buigues, M.; Villanueva-Bádenas, E.; Ontoria-Oviedo, I.; Hernándiz, A.; González-King, H.; Peiró-Molina, E.; Dorronsoro, A.; et al. miR-4732-3p in Extracellular Vesicles From Mesenchymal Stromal Cells Is Cardioprotective During Myocardial Ischemia. *Front. Cell Dev. Biol.* **2021**, *9*, 734143. [CrossRef]
106. Ning, W.; Li, S.; Yang, W.; Yang, B.; Xin, C.; Ping, X.; Huang, C.; Gu, Y.; Guo, L. Blocking exosomal miRNA-153-3p derived from bone marrow mesenchymal stem cells ameliorates hypoxia-induced myocardial and microvascular damage by targeting the ANGPT1-mediated VEGF/PI3k/Akt/eNOS pathway. *Cell. Signal.* **2021**, *77*, 109812. [CrossRef]
107. He, Q.; Ye, A.; Ye, W.; Liao, X.; Qin, G.; Xu, Y.; Yin, Y.; Luo, H.; Yi, M.; Xian, L.; et al. Cancer-secreted exosomal miR-21-5p induces angiogenesis and vascular permeability by targeting KRIT1. *Cell Death Dis.* **2021**, *12*, 576. [CrossRef]
108. Li, Q.; Xu, Y.; Lv, K.; Wang, Y.; Zhong, Z.; Xiao, C.; Zhu, K.; Ni, C.; Wang, K.; Kong, M.; et al. Small extracellular vesicles containing miR-486-5p promote angiogenesis after myocardial infarction in mice and nonhuman primates. *Sci. Transl. Med.* **2021**, *13*, eabb0202. [CrossRef]
109. Liu, H.; Zhang, Y.; Yuan, J.; Gao, W.; Zhong, X.; Yao, K.; Lin, L.; Ge, J. Dendritic cell derived exosomal miR 494 3p promotes angiogenesis following myocardial infarction. *Int. J. Mol. Med.* **2021**, *47*, 315–325. [CrossRef] [PubMed]
110. Yang, M.; Liao, M.; Liu, R.; Zhang, Q.; Zhang, S.; He, Y.; Jin, J.; Zhang, P.; Zhou, L. Human umbilical cord mesenchymal stem cell-derived extracellular vesicles loaded with miR-223 ameliorate myocardial infarction through P53/S100A9 axis. *Genomics* **2022**, *114*, 110319. [CrossRef]
111. Zhu, D.; Wang, Y.; Thomas, M.; McLaughlin, K.; Oguljahan, B.; Henderson, J.; Yang, Q.; Chen, Y.E.; Liu, D. Exosomes from adipose-derived stem cells alleviate myocardial infarction via microRNA-31/FIH1/HIF-1α pathway. *J. Mol. Cell Cardiol.* **2022**, *162*, 10–19. [CrossRef]
112. Oshchepkova, A.; Zenkova, M.; Vlassov, V. Extracellular Vesicles for Therapeutic Nucleic Acid Delivery: Loading Strategies and Challenges. *Int. J. Mol. Sci.* **2023**, *24*, 7287. [CrossRef]
113. Tao, L.; Shi, J.; Huang, X.; Hua, F.; Yang, L. Identification of a lncRNA-miRNA-mRNA network based on competitive endogenous RNA theory reveals functional lncRNAs in hypertrophic cardiomyopathy. *Exp. Ther. Med.* **2020**, *20*, 1176–1190. [CrossRef]

Disclaimer/Publisher's Note: The statements, opinions and data contained in all publications are solely those of the individual author(s) and contributor(s) and not of MDPI and/or the editor(s). MDPI and/or the editor(s) disclaim responsibility for any injury to people or property resulting from any ideas, methods, instructions or products referred to in the content.

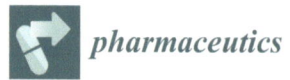

Article

Toward Stability Enhancement of NTS$_1$R-Targeted Radioligands: Structural Interventions on [^{99m}Tc]Tc-DT1

Panagiotis Kanellopoulos [1], Berthold A. Nock [1], Eric P. Krenning [2] and Theodosia Maina [1,*]

[1] Molecular Radiopharmacy, INRaSTES, NCSR "Demokritos", 15341 Athens, Greece; kanelospan@gmail.com (P.K.); nock_berthold.a@hotmail.com (B.A.N.)
[2] Cyclotron Rotterdam BV, Erasmus MC, 3015 CE Rotterdam, The Netherlands; erickrenning@gmail.com
* Correspondence: maina_thea@hotmail.com; Tel.: +30-210-650-3891

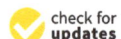

Citation: Kanellopoulos, P.; Nock, B.A.; Krenning, E.P.; Maina, T. Toward Stability Enhancement of NTS$_1$R-Targeted Radioligands: Structural Interventions on [^{99m}Tc]Tc-DT1. *Pharmaceutics* 2023, 15, 2092. https://doi.org/10.3390/pharmaceutics15082092

Academic Editors: Cristina Manuela Drăgoi, Alina Crenguţa Nicolae and Ion-Bogdan Dumitrescu

Received: 25 July 2023
Revised: 4 August 2023
Accepted: 5 August 2023
Published: 7 August 2023

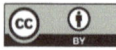

Copyright: © 2023 by the authors. Licensee MDPI, Basel, Switzerland. This article is an open access article distributed under the terms and conditions of the Creative Commons Attribution (CC BY) license (https://creativecommons.org/licenses/by/4.0/).

Abstract: The neurotensin subtype 1 receptor (NTS$_1$R) is overexpressed in a number of human tumors, thereby representing a valid target for cancer theranostics with radiolabeled neurotensin (NT) analogs like [^{99m}Tc]Tc-DT1 (DT1, N$_4$-Gly^7-NT(8-13)). Thus far, the fast degradation of intravenously injected NT–radioligands by neprilysin (NEP) and angiotensin-converting enzyme (ACE) has compromised their clinical applicability. Aiming at metabolic stability enhancements, we herein introduce (i) DT7 ([DAsn^{14}]DT1) and (ii) DT8 ([β-Homoleucine^{13}]DT1), modified at the C-terminus, along with (iii) DT9 ([(palmitoyl)Lys^7]DT1), carrying an albumin-binding domain (ABD) at Lys^7. The biological profiles of the new [^{99m}Tc]Tc–radioligands were compared with [^{99m}Tc]Tc-DT1, using NTS$_1$R-expressing AsPC-1 cells and mice models without or during NEP/ACE inhibition. The radioligands showed enhanced in vivo stability vs. [^{99m}Tc]Tc-DT1, with [^{99m}Tc]Tc-DT9 displaying full resistance to both peptidases. Furthermore, [^{99m}Tc]Tc-DT9 achieved the highest cell internalization and tumor uptake even without NEP/ACE-inhibition but with unfavorably high background radioactivity levels. Hence, unlike C-terminal modification, the introduction of a pendant ABD group in the linker turned out to be the most promising strategy toward metabolic stability, cell uptake, and tumor accumulation of [^{99m}Tc]Tc-DT1 mimics. To improve the observed suboptimal pharmacokinetics of [^{99m}Tc]Tc-DT9, the replacement of palmitoyl on Lys^7 by other ABD groups is currently being pursued.

Keywords: neurotensin subtype 1 receptor; radiolabeled neurotensin; targeted tumor imaging; Tc-99m; metabolic stability; neprilysin; angiotensin-converting enzyme; peptidase-inhibition

1. Introduction

The overexpression of neurotensin subtype 1 receptor (NTS$_1$R) has been documented in a number of human cancers, mainly in exocrine pancreatic ductal carcinoma (PDAC) [1–4], Ewing's sarcoma [5], and colon [6], prostate [7], and breast cancer [8], and is therefore regarded as a valid biomolecular target for cancer theranostics [9]. Several analogs of the C-terminal hexapeptide fragment of native neurotensin (NT, pyroGlu-Leu-Tyr-Glu-Asn-Lys-Pro-Arg-Arg-Pro-Tyr-Ile-Leu-OH) have been coupled to suitable chelators for stable binding of diagnostic (e.g., Tc-99m, In-111: SPECT imaging; Ga-68: PET imaging) or particle emitters (e.g., Lu-177) for use in the management of NTS$_1$R-expressing tumors [10–12]. However, results in patients have been suboptimal thus far, a fact attributed to the fast degradation of NT-derived radioligands following their entry in the circulation. Hence, supply to tumor sites and, consequently, tumor-targeting efficacy is compromised [13–17]. Previous studies have revealed the predominant role of two peptidases in the catabolism of NT and its analogs, neprilysin (NEP) and angiotensin-converting enzyme (ACE) [18–21]. Based on these findings, we recently achieved in situ stabilization of fast biodegradable [^{99m}Tc]Tc-DT1 (DT1, N$_4$-Gly^7-NT(8-13); N$_4$, 6-(carboxy)-1,4,8,11-tetraazaundecane) and its analogs [22,23] in peripheral mice blood by means of NEP/ACE inhibitors. As expected, tumor uptake in mice was markedly improved, highlighting NEP/ACE-resistance as a crucial feature in the performance of NT–radioligands [24,25].

Translation of the NEP/ACE-inhibition approach in the clinic has to circumvent a number of regulatory challenges related to the administration of two distinct peptidase inhibitors to patients, even though registered drugs for ACE or NEP inhibition are currently available. Thus, lisinopril is a widely used antihypertensive drug with high ACE-inhibition potency [26]. On the other hand, the potent and selective NEP inhibitors thiorphan (released from racecadotril in the anti-diarrhea drug hidrasec [27,28]) or sacubitrilat (released from sacubitril in the anti-hypertensive drug Entresto® [29–31]) can be applied following oral administration of hidrasec or Entresto® pills, respectively. It should be noted that hidrasec has been safely and successfully applied in medullary thyroid cancer patients to in situ stabilize a biodegradable gastrin radioligand, thereby indeed improving diagnostic accuracy [32]. Yet, the implementation of double NEP and ACE inhibition in patients, required in the case of NT analogs, undeniably remains a challenging goal. Therefore, we have next directed our efforts in search of [^{99m}Tc]Tc-DT1 mimics, which are resistant to at least one of the two peptidases, namely ACE.

ACE, also known as peptidyl dipeptidase A, primarily cleaves a C-terminal dipeptide from substrates including NT and its analogs [20,21]. For obtaining ACE-resistant [^{99m}Tc]Tc-DT1 mimics, we first pursued the Ile^{12} to Tle^{12}-replacement route. However, Tle^{12}-modified [^{99m}Tc]Tc-DT6 (DT6, [N$_4$-βAla^7,Dab^9,Tle^{12}]NT(8-13)) displayed low internalization efficacy and only slightly improved tumor uptake compared to both [^{99m}Tc]Tc-DT5 (DT5, [N$_4$-βAla^7,Dab^9]NT(8-13)) and the [^{99m}Tc]Tc-DT1 reference [24]. Most importantly, during ACE/NEP inhibition in mice models, tumor uptake of these analogs remained significantly inferior vs. [^{99m}Tc]Tc-DT1 [22–25]. Our next step toward ACE-robust [^{99m}Tc]Tc-DT1 mimics was prompted by reports on the resistance of peptide analogs containing D-amino acids at the C-terminus to the hydrolytic action of ACE [33]. Luckily, high-affinity binding of NT(8-13) analogs elongated by a D-amino acid residue at the C-terminus, such as NT(8-13)-DAsn (Ki = 2.2 ± 0.71 nM), was reported [34]. Thus, [^{99m}Tc]Tc-DT7 ([DAsn^{14}]DT1; Figure 1a) was considered as the first new analog in our study. Another route proposed to stabilize NT–radioligands in human plasma/serum is "homologation" [35–37]. Interestingly, replacement of C-terminal Leu^{13} by β-Homoleucine did not impair the binding affinity of [β-Homoleucine^{13}]NT(8-13) for the human NTS$_1$R (Ki = 3.2 ± 0.75 nM) [37]. Therefore, [^{99m}Tc]Tc-DT8 ([β-Homoleucine^{13}]DT8; Figure 1b) was selected as the second analog in our study.

As a third analog, we chose [^{99m}Tc]Tc-DT9 ([(palmitoyl)Lys^7]DT1; Figure 1c) based on a different stabilization strategy, namely the introduction of a lipid acid albumin-binding domain (ABD) on the linker. Lipidation of peptides has been often proposed as a useful means to increase metabolic stability and bioavailability [38–41]. The position of introducing the lipid acid should be carefully selected to avoid interference with receptor binding. In this context, we were intrigued by contulakin-G, a 16-amino-acid peptide (pGlu-Ser-Glu-Glu-Gly-Gly-Ser-Asn-Ala-Thr(R)-Lys-Lys-Pro-Tyr-Ile-Leu-OH; R, the disaccharide beta-D-Galp-(1-->3)-alpha-D-GalpNAc-(1-->); Galp, Galactopyranosyl and GalpNAc, N-acetylgalactosaminepyranosyl) isolated from the venom of the predatory sea snail *Conus geographus*, which displayed binding affinity to the human NTS$_1$R [42]. Replacement of the Thr^{10}-attached disaccharide by a variety of functional groups, including palmitoyl, led to analogs of improved bioavailability and high resistance to enzymatic degradation [43,44]. Notably, similarly modified NT analogs with improved characteristics were soon developed with pendant groups introduced at the corresponding position 7 in NT [43,44]. These reports provided the rationale for designing [^{99m}Tc]Tc-DT9.

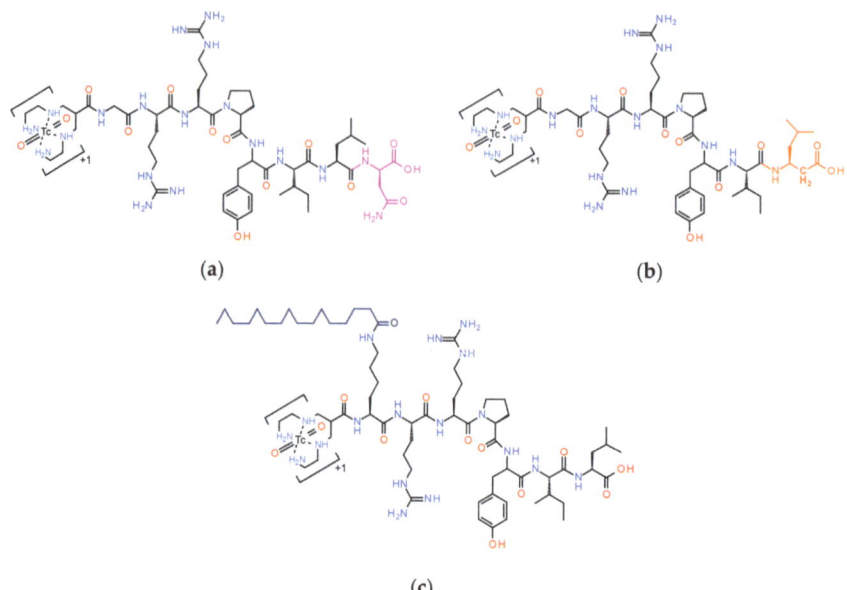

Figure 1. Chemical structures of C-terminal-modified [^{99m}Tc]Tc-DT1 mimics (DT1, N$_4$-Gly^7-Arg-Arg-Pro-Tyr-Ile-Leu-OH; N$_4$, 6-(carboxy)-1,4,8,11-tetraazaundecane): (**a**) [^{99m}Tc]Tc-DT7 (DT7, [DAsn^{14}]DT1); (**b**) [^{99m}Tc]Tc-DT8 (DT8, ([β-Homoleucine^{13}]DT1); and (**c**) [^{99m}Tc]Tc-DT9 (DT9, [(palmitoyl)Lys^7]DT1), carrying a pendant ABD palmitoyl-group at the Lys^7-linker.

In the present work, we compared the biological performance of the newly introduced peptide analogs DT7/8/9 and their [^{99m}Tc]Tc–radioligands in NTS$_1$R-positive cells and mice models vs. the [^{99m}Tc]Tc-DT1 reference, focusing on particular features like metabolic stability, receptor affinity, and internalization capacity. The effects of ACE/NEP inhibition were investigated as well to reveal the best candidates for subsequent evaluation in tumor-bearing mice. Conclusions on the suitability of the two structural intervention approaches on [^{99m}Tc]Tc-DT1 were drawn, and further steps to follow are herein discussed.

2. Materials and Methods
2.1. Chemicals and Radioligands
2.1.1. Peptides and Protease Inhibitors

Except for the solvents used in high-performance liquid chromatography (HPLC), which were HPLC grade, all other chemicals used were reagent grade. Neurotensin (NT) was obtained from Bachem (Bubendorf, Switzerland). Entresto® pills (200 mg corresponding to 24 mg/26 mg sacubitril/valsartan per pill; Novartis AG, Basel, Switzerland) were obtained from a local pharmacy. Individual doses were prepared by grinding pills in a mortar to a fine powder, dividing, and suspending in tap water forming a slurry for oral gavage to mice (12 mg/200 µL per animal) [24,25]. The ACE inhibitor lisinopril (Lis, lisinopril dehydrate, ((S)1–1-[N2-(1-carboxy-3-phenylpropyl)-lysyl-proline dehydrate, MK 521) was provided by Sigma-Aldrich (St. Louis, MO, USA).

The peptide conjugates DT1 (N$_4$-Gly-Arg-Arg-Pro-Tyr-Ile-Leu-OH, N$_4$ = 6-(carboxy)-1,4,8,11-tetraazaundecane; reference), DT7 (N$_4$-Gly-Arg-Arg-Pro-Tyr-Ile-Leu-DAsn-OH), DT8 (N$_4$-Gly-Arg-Arg-Pro-Tyr-Ile-β-Homoleucine-OH; β-Homoleucine = 3-amino-5-methylhexanoic acid), and DT9 (N$_4$-(palmitoyl)Lys-Arg-Arg-Pro-Tyr-Ile-Leu-OH; palmitoyl = hexadecanoyl) were purchased from PiChem Forschungs- und Entwicklungs GmbH (Raaba-Grambach, Austria); chemical structures are presented in Figure 1. Analytical data, including purity determined by HPLC analysis and matrix-assisted laser desorption/

ionization–time of flight (MALDI-TOF) mass spectrometry (MS) findings, is summarized in Table S1.

Technetium-99m, used for labeling, was eluted as [^{99m}Tc]NaTcO$_4$ in normal saline from a [^{99}Mo]Mo/[^{99m}Tc]Tc generator (Ultra-Technekow V4 Generator, Curium Pharma, Petten, The Netherlands). For preparation of [^{125}I]I-Tyr^3-NT, [^{125}I]NaI in dilute sodium hydroxide solution (pH 8–11) was obtained from Perkin Elmer (Waltham, MA, USA).

2.1.2. Radiolabeling

The peptide conjugates were dissolved at 2 mg/mL in doubly distilled H$_2$O and were stored in 50 µL aliquots in Eppendorf Protein LoBind tubes at −20 °C. Labelling was performed in a LoBind Eppendorf tube containing phosphate buffer (0.5 M, pH 11.5, 50 µL) to which [^{99m}Tc]NaTcO$_4$ (420 µL generator eluate) was added, followed by sodium citrate (0.1 M, 5 µL), the peptide stock solution (15 µL, 15 nmol), and SnCl$_2$ freshly dissolved in EtOH (10 µL, 10 µg). The mixture was incubated for 30 min at room temperature (RT), and the pH was adjusted to 7.4 using 0.1 M HCl.

For the quality control, HPLC and instant thin-layer chromatography (iTLC) were applied. HPLC analyses were conducted on a Waters Chromatograph coupled to a 2998-photodiode array UV detector (Waters, Vienna, Austria) and a Gabi gamma detector (Raytest RSM Analytische Instrumente GmbH, Straubenhardt, Germany). Data acquisition and processing were achieved by the Empower Software 3.0 (Waters, Milford, MA, USA). A Symmetry Shield RP-18 (5 µm, 3.9 mm × 20 mm) cartridge column (Waters, Eschborn, Germany) was eluted with a flow rate of 1 mL/min with a linear gradient (system 1): from 100% A/0% B to 60% A/40% B in 20 min (A: 0.1% aqueous TFA and B: MeCN). For [^{99m}Tc]Tc-DT9, analyses were performed on an XTerra RP-8 (5 µm, 3.9 mm × 20 mm) cartridge column (Waters, Vienna, Austria) eluted with a with a flow rate of 1 mL/min linear gradient (system 1b): from 60% A/40% B to 20% A/80% B in 20 min (A: 0.1% aqueous TFA supplemented with 10 mM 1-Heptanesulfonic acid sodium salt; B: MeCN/0.1% TFA 8/2, supplemented with 10 mM 1-Heptanesulfonic acid sodium salt). For iTLC, Whatman 3 mm chromatography paper strips (GE Healthcare, Chicago, IL, USA) were developed up to 10 cm from the point of origin with 5 M NH$_4$AcO/MeOH 1:1 (v/v) as mobile phase for the detection of reduced, hydrolyzed technetium (R_f = 0 cm) or acetone for the detection of free unreduced [^{99m}Tc]TcO$_4^-$ (R_f = 10 cm). Sample radioactivity was measured in a γ-counter (automated multi-sample, well-type instrument with a NaI(Tl) 3″ crystal, Canberra Packard Cobra^{TM} Quantum U5003/1, Auto-Gamma® counting system; Canberra Packard, Ramsey, MN, USA). Radioligand samples used in all biological experiments were prepared in a phosphate-buffered saline (PBS, pH 7.4)/EtOH v/v 9/1 solution and tested before and after completion of all experiments. In the case of [^{99m}Tc]Tc-DT9, this solution additionally contained 0.1% Tween-80 (Sigma-Aldrich Inc., St. Louis, MO, USA) to combat sticking to plastic and glass containers.

For I-125 labeling of NT, the chloramine T method was applied based on a published protocol [45]. Separation of [^{125}I]I-Tyr^3-NT from the reaction mixture was achieved by RP-HPLC on a Symmetry Shield RP-18 (5 µm, 3.9 mm × 150 mm) cartridge column (Waters, Eschborn, Germany) eluted with a flow rate of 1 mL/min with the following gradient: from 100% A/0% B to 80% A/20% B in 5 min and then to 70% A/30% B in 40 min (A: 0.1% TFA/0.05% Et$_3$N (pH 2–2.5); B: 0.1% TFA/0.05% Et$_3$N in MeCN). Elution time (t_R) [^{125}I]I-Tyr^3-NT: 28 min ([^{125}I]I-Tyr^{11}-NT: 29 min, NT: 20.5 min). A stock solution of purified [^{125}I]I-Tyr^3-NT in 0.1% BSA-PBS buffer was kept in aliquots at −20 °C for use in competition binding assays (molar activity of 74 GBq/µmol).

All procedures involving radioactive materials were performed by trained and authorized personnel using suitable shielding in licensed laboratories complying with European radiation-safety guidelines and supervised by the Greek Atomic Energy Commission (license # A/435/17092/2019).

2.2. Cell Studies

2.2.1. Cell Culture

The two human NTS_1R-expressing cell lines, the colorectal adenocarcinoma WiDr (LGC Promochem; Teddington, UK) and the pancreatic adenocarcinoma AsPC-1 cell lines (LGC Standards GmbH; Wesel, Germany), were used in this study. The WiDr cells were grown in McCoy's GLUTAMAX-I medium and the AsPC-1 cells in Roswell Park Memorial Institute-1640 (RPMI), both supplemented with 10% (v/v) fetal bovine serum (FBS), 100 U/mL penicillin, and 100 µg/mL streptomycin. Cells were cultured in 75 cm^2 flasks at 37 °C (95% humidity, 5% CO_2) in a Heal Force SMART CELL HF-90 incubator (Shanghai, China) and split at 80–90% confluency applying a Trypsin/EDTA (0.05%/0.02% w/v) solution. Culture media were obtained from Gibco BRL, Life Technologies (Grand Island, NY, USA) and supplements as well as the Trypsin/EDTA solution from Biochrom KG Seromed (Berlin, Germany).

2.2.2. Competition Binding Experiments

Cell membrane homogenates from WiDr cells were collected and stored in Tris/EDTA (10 mM Tris, 0.1 mM EDTA, pH 7.4) solution at −80 °C, as previously described. On the day of the experiment, the aliquots thereof were thawed, combined, and diluted in cold binding buffer (BB: 50 mM HEPES, 5.5 mM $MgCl_2$, 0.1 mg/mL bacitracin, 1% w/v BSA, pH 7.4). A dilution series of each test peptide (10^{-12}–10^{-5} M) and a fresh solution of [^{125}I]I-Tyr^3-NT (~40,000 cpm/70 µL, 214 pM) were prepared and kept on ice. In each RIA tube per placed on ice (in triplicate for each concentration point), the following ice-cold solutions were added: test peptide solution (30 µL), the [^{125}I]I-Tyr^3-NT radioligand (70 µL), and membrane homogenate (200 µL). Tubes were incubated under constant stirring for 1 h at 22 °C in an Incubator-Orbital Shaker (MPM Instr. Srl; Bernareggio, Italy). The incubation was terminated by placing the tubes on ice and adding ice-cold washing buffer (10 mM HEPES, 150 mM NaCl, pH 7.4). Samples were rapidly passed through Whatman GF/B filters (presoaked for 1 h in BB) on a 48-sample Brandel Cell Harvester (Adi Hassel Ingenieur Büro, Munich, Germany). Separate filters were measured for radioactivity on the γ-counter, and the half maximal inhibition concentration (IC_{50}) was calculated applying a non-linear one-site model (GraphPad Prism Software 6.0, San Diego, CA, USA). Results represent average IC_{50} values ± standard deviation (sd), n = 3.

2.2.3. Internalization in AsPC-1 Cells

The NTS_1R-specific internalization of [^{99m}Tc]Tc-DT1/7/8/9 radioligands was compared in AsPC-1 cells. The cells were seeded in 6-well plates (1×10^6 cells per well) and left to grow overnight. The following day, the medium was aspirated, and the cells were washed twice with internalization medium (2 mL IM: RPMI supplemented with 1% v/v FBS) on ice. They were placed on the bench, and warm IM (1200 µL 37 °C) was added per well, followed by radioligand solution (150 µL, 250 fmol) and either IM (150 µL total: T; upper wells) or NT (10^{-5} M in IM, non-specific: NS; lower wells). The plates were placed in the Incubator-Orbital Shaker at 37 °C for 1 h, and the incubation was interrupted by placing the plates on ice. The supernatant was collected in RIA tubes, and the cells were washed with 1 mL phosphate-buffered saline (PBS, pH 7.4, 4 °C) containing 0.5% w/v BSA, and the washing was also collected in the same RIA tube. Cells were treated twice for 5 min with glycine buffer (600 µL, 50 mM glycine, 0.1 M NaCl, pH 2.8), and supernatants were collected (membrane bound fraction, MB). The cells were washed again with 1 mL ice-cold PBS-BSA buffer, which was discarded. Finally, cells were lysed (2×600 µL 1 M NaOH), and the lysates were collected (internalized fraction, IF). Sample radioactivity was measured on the γ-counter. Specific values for MB and IF were acquired by subtracting NS values from T ones. Results are expressed as mean percentage of added radioactivity ± sd, n = 3. In addition, time-dependent internalization in AsPC-1 cells was directly compared for [^{99m}Tc]Tc-DT1/9 by incubation at 37 °C for 15 min, 30 min, 1 h, and 2 h, following the above-described protocol for each time point.

2.3. Animal Studies

2.3.1. Stability Studies

For the assessment of in vivo stability of [^{99m}Tc]Tc-DT7/8/9, healthy Swiss Albino mice (33 animals, >8 weeks of age, body weight: 30 ± 5 g) were obtained from NCSR "Demokritos" Animal House (Athens, Greece). Animals were injected through the tail vein with the radioligand (100 µL, 2 nmol in vehicle: PBS/EtOH 9/1 v/v, with the addition of 0.1% Tween-80 in the case of [^{99m}Tc]Tc-DT9) plus vehicle (100 µL; controls) or plus Lis (100 µg in 100 µL vehicle; Lis). Additional mice groups received per os a suspension of Entresto® (200 µL, 12 mg, 30 min prior to the i.v. injection of the radioligand plus vehicle—Entresto® group; or the i.v. injection of the radioligand plus Lis—Entresto®+Lis group). Animals were euthanized 5 min post injection (pi), and blood samples were drawn from the heart via a prechilled insulin syringe and transferred rapidly into pre-cooled 1.5 mL LoBind Eppendorf tubes containing EDTA (20 µL, 0.1 mM EDTA), and the collected radioactivity was measured in a dose calibrator (CURIEMENTOR 4, PTW Freiburg-GmbH; Freiburg, Germany). The tubes were centrifuged for 10 min at 2000× g at 4 °C in a Hettich Universal 320 R centrifuge (Tuttlingen, Germany). The plasma was collected, diluted in a 1:1 v/v ratio with MeCN, and thoroughly mixed; sample tubes were again centrifuged for 10 min at 15000× g at 4 °C. The supernatant was collected and the volume reduced to 50–100 µL under a gentle flux of N$_2$ and mild heating at 60 °C. Samples were diluted in physiological saline to a final volume of 450–500 µL and filtered through Millex GV filters (0.22 µm, 13 mm diameter, Millipore; Milford, CT, USA). Sample activity was measured in the dose calibrator, and aliquots were analyzed by radio-HPLC on a Symmetry Shield RP18 cartridge column (5 µm, 3.9 mm × 20 mm; Waters, Eschborn, Germany) eluted at a flow rate of 1 mL/min with the linear gradient (system 2): from 100% A/0% B to 60% A/40% B in 40 min (A: 0.1% aqueous TFA; B: MeCN). For [^{99m}Tc]Tc-DT9, analyses were performed on an XTerra RP-8 (5 µm, 3.9 mm × 20 mm) cartridge column (Waters, Vienna, Austria) eluted with a with a flow rate of 1 mL/min linear gradient (system 2b): from 90% A/10% B to 0% A/100% B in 45 min (A: 0.1% aqueous TFA supplemented with 10 mM 1-Heptanesulfonic acid sodium salt; B: MeCN/0.1% TFA 8/2, supplemented with 10 mM 1-Heptanesulfonic acid sodium salt). The t_R of intact [^{99m}Tc]Tc-DT7, [^{99m}Tc]Tc-DT8, or [^{99m}Tc]Tc-DT9 was determined by co-injection of blood samples processed as above with an aliquot of the labeling solution. Results were obtained from three mice per analog per treatment and are presented as average percentage of intact radiopeptide ± sd.

2.3.2. Biodistribution of [^{99m}Tc]Tc-DT9 in SCID Mice Bearing AsPC-1 Xenografts

Twenty male severe combined immunodeficiency (SCID) mice (23.1 ± 1.6 g body weight, six weeks of age on arrival day; NCSR "Demokritos" Animal House, Athens, Greece) were used in the biodistribution experiments. Animals were subcutaneously inoculated in their right flanks with a sterile suspension of freshly harvested AsPC-1 cells (150 µL, 5 × 10^6 cells/animal), and 3–4 weeks later, they developed well-palpable tumors at the implantation sites. During this period, mice were housed in suitable facilities under sterile conditions with 12 h day/night cycles and were provided with sterilized chow food and drinking water ad libitum. At the date of the experiment, animals were randomly divided in groups of four and received through the tail vein a bolus of [^{99m}Tc]Tc-DT9 (100 µL, 3 pmol in vehicle: PBS/EtOH 9/1 v/v with the addition of 0.1% Tween-80) plus vehicle (100 µL; controls at 4 and 24 h pi) or plus Lis (100 µg in 100 µL vehicle); the latter groups had additionally received per os 30 min in advance Entresto® (200 µL, 12 mg; Entresto®+Lis groups at 4 and 24 h pi). A further 4 h group of animals was treated with Entresto®, and 30 min later, mice were co-injected with excess NT and Lis (100 µg NT and 100 µg Lis in 100 µL vehicle—NTS$_1$R block). At the predetermined time intervals, mice were euthanized and weighted, and their blood, organs, and tissue samples of choice as well as the implanted tumors were collected and weighted. Sample radioactivity was measured on the γ-counter together with proper standards of the injected dose. Results were calculated as percentage of injected activity per gram tissue (%IA/g) and provided as mean %IA/g

and [^{99m}Tc]Tc-DT9, while cumulative results are presented in Table 1, including findings previously reported for [^{99m}Tc]Tc-DT1 for easy comparison purposes [24,25].

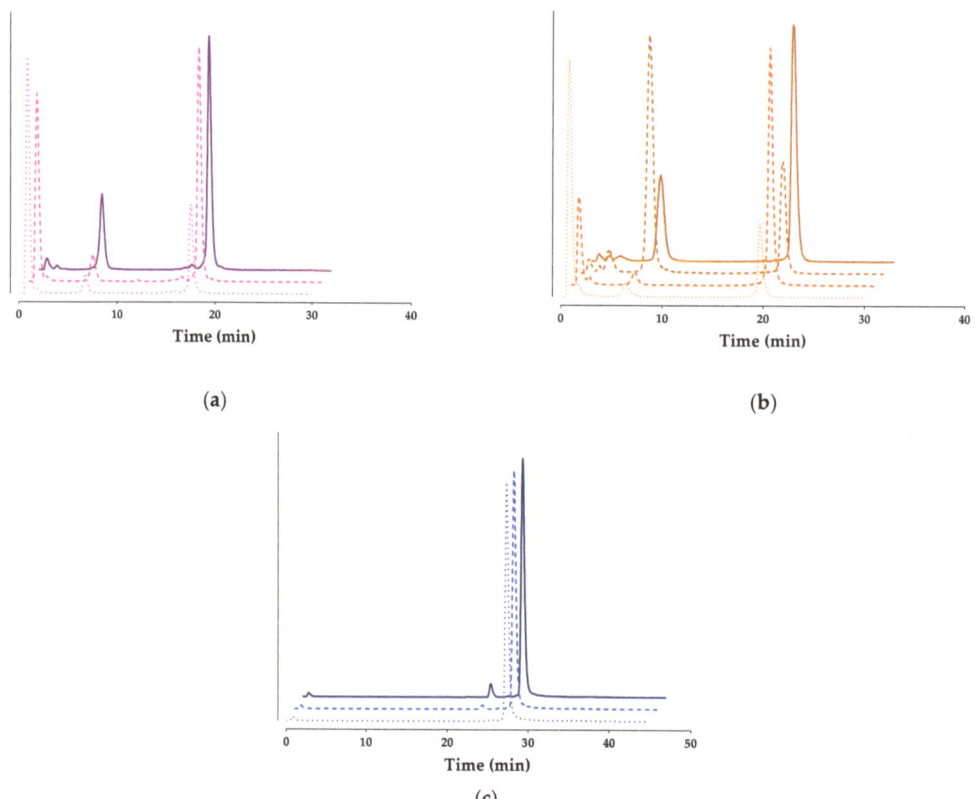

Figure 4. Representative radiochromatograms of HPLC analysis of mouse blood samples collected 5 min pi of (**a**) [^{99m}Tc]Tc-DT7 (pink lines), (**b**) [^{99m}Tc]Tc-DT8 (orange lines), or (**c**) [^{99m}Tc]Tc-DT9 (blue lines) administered without treatment (controls ......) or treated with Entresto® (– – –) or with Lis (darker – – –) or with the Entresto®+Lis combination (darker solid lines ———; HPLC system 2); percentages of intact radioligand are summarized in Table 1.

Table 1. Stabilities of [^{99m}Tc]Tc-DT1, [^{99m}Tc]Tc-DT7, [^{99m}Tc]Tc-DT8, and [^{99m}Tc]Tc-DT9 in peripheral mouse blood 5 min pi without treatment with NEP/ACE inhibitor(s) (controls) or treated with Entresto® or Lis or their combination (Entresto®+Lis).

	[^{99m}Tc]Tc-DT1 [1]	[^{99m}Tc]Tc-DT7	[^{99m}Tc]Tc-DT8	[^{99m}Tc]Tc-DT9
Control	1.81 ± 0.77 (n = 4)	26.91 ± 1.91 (n = 3)	20.68 ± 3.10 (n = 3)	98.06 ± 1.18 (n = 3)
Entresto®	5.46 ± 3.86 (n = 5)	56.61 ± 7.92 (n = 6)	60.72 ± 8.35 (n = 3)	97.33 ± 1.7 (n = 3)
Lis	18.77 ± 2.54 (n = 3)	-	28.82 ± 4.59 (n = 3)	-
Entresto®+Lis	63.80 ± 7.51 (n = 3)	60.27 ± 11.82 (n = 3)	64.06 ± 4.07 (n = 3)	93.72 ± 3.7 (n = 3)

[1] Metabolic stability results for [^{99m}Tc]Tc-DT1 have been adapted from [24,25]; data represents the mean percentage of intact radioligand ± sd; number of experiments are shown in parentheses.

It is interesting to observe that the structural interventions on the [^{99m}Tc]Tc-DT1 motif significantly increased the metabolic stability of all new analogs albeit to a different extent. Thus, the C-terminal modifications in [^{99m}Tc]Tc-DT7 and [^{99m}Tc]Tc-DT8 increased the stability by more than 200-fold, but only [^{99m}Tc]Tc-DT9 achieved clear resistance to both NEP and ACE. As a result, treatment of mice with Entresto® or Entresto®+Lis had no effect on the stability of [^{99m}Tc]Tc-DT9 in peripheral mice blood at 5 min pi ($p > 0.05$ amongst these animal groups). In the case of [^{99m}Tc]Tc-DT7 and [^{99m}Tc]Tc-DT8 though, treatment of mice with Entresto® alone resulted in pronounced increases in metabolic stability (56.61 ± 7.92 vs. 26.91 ± 1.91 in controls, $p < 0.0001$; 60.72 ± 8.35 vs. 20.68 ± 3.10 in controls, $p < 0.0001$, respectively). Interestingly, treatment of mice with the Entresto®+Lis combination further increased these values but not significantly ($p > 0.05$), a finding consistent with a predominant role of NEP in the catabolism of these particular analogs. In contrast, [^{99m}Tc]Tc-DT1 was exposed to the combined action of NEP and ACE (1.81 ± 0.77 in controls vs. 5.46 ± 3.86 in the Entresto® group, $p < 0.0001$; vs. 18.77 ± 2.54 in the Lis group, $p < 0.0001$; vs. 63.80 ± 7.51 in the Entresto®+Lis combination group; $p < 0.0001$).

3.3.2. Biodistribution of [^{99m}Tc]Tc-DT9 in Mice Bearing AsPC-1 Xenografts

The biodistribution results of [^{99m}Tc]Tc-DT9 in SCID mice bearing subcutaneous AsPC-1 tumors are summarized for 4 and 24 h pi in Table 2. Animals include subgroups without or after treatment with the Entresto®+Lis combination for both time points; for the 4 h pi interval, a further group additionally received excess i.v. NT for in vivo NTS$_1$R blockade. Results are expressed as mean %IA/g ± sd (n = 4). Selected biodistribution data for AsPC-1 tumors, kidneys, liver, and intestines, including both untreated and Entresto®+Lis treated subgroups, of [^{99m}Tc]Tc-DT9 are compared vs. [^{99m}Tc]Tc-DT1 at 4 and 24 h pi and their statistically significant differences indicated in Figure 5.

Table 2. Comparative biodistribution data of [^{99m}Tc]Tc-DT9 in SCID mice bearing AsPC-1 xenografts at 4 h (block, controls, and Entresto®+Lis treated) and 24 h pi (controls and Entresto®+Lis treated); data are expressed as %IA/g and represent average values ± sd, n = 4.

Organs/Tissues	[^{99m}Tc]Tc-DT9				
	4 h			24 h	
	Block	Controls	Entresto®+Lis	Controls	Entresto®+Lis
Blood	4.25 ± 0.37	4.63 ± 0.55	4.32 ± 0.42	0.68 ± 0.18	0.70 ± 0.06
Liver	30.93 ± 4.25	29.56 ± 3.77	28.42 ± 2.48	12.93 ± 1.66	16.96 ± 0.94
Heart	2.79 ± 0.47	3.12 ± 0.43	2.85 ± 2.48	0.64 ± 0.11	0.71 ± 0.06
Kidneys	8.56 ± 0.87	9.53 ± 1.18	9.15 ± 0.62	3.81 ± 0.54	4.63 ± 0.15
Stomach	2.06 ± 0.47	3.09 ± 1.06	2.27 ± 0.38	1.73 ± 0.50	1.56 ± 0.31
Intestines	6.27 ± 0.72	13.02 ± 4.60	7.90 ± 0.88	4.26 ± 0.61	5.37 ± 1.61
Spleen	6.18 ± 1.37	6.82 ± 1.11	5.47 ± 0.47	3.42 ± 0.54	4.47 ± 0.83
Muscle	0.82 ± 0.11	0.93 ± 0.13	0.81 ± 0.04	0.22 ± 0.02	0.24 ± 0.01
Lungs	8.46 ± 1.26	8.80 ± 1.42	7.61 ± 0.64	3.42 ± 0.67	3.62 ± 0.94
Pancreas	1.84 ± 0.41	2.10 ± 0.30	1.85 ± 0.18	0.75 ± 0.17	0.80 ± 0.07
AsPC-1 Tumor	3.68 ± 0.92	6.15 ± 0.92	5.24 ± 0.27	3.32 ± 0.35	2.84 ± 0.43

It is interesting to note that the uptake of [^{99m}Tc]Tc-DT9 in the AsPC-1 tumors in controls is significantly higher than that of [^{99m}Tc]Tc-DT1 (6.15 ± 0.92%IA/g vs. 1.25 ± 0.14%IA/g; $p < 0.0001$) at 4 h pi, most probably a result of its higher in vivo stability. This hypothesis is further supported by the lack of significant change in the tumor uptake of [^{99m}Tc]Tc-DT9 between controls and the Entresto®+Lis group of animals (6.15 ± 0.92%IA/g vs. 5.24 ± 0.27%IA/g; $p > 0.05$) at 4 h pi. Co-injection of excess NT to in vivo block the NTS$_1$R sites on the tumor caused a drop of uptake (6.15 ± 0.92%IA/g vs. 3.68 ± 0.92%IA/g; $p < 0.01$), which is in line with a receptor-mediated process. However, the observed reduction was far below the 90% previously reported for other NT-based radioligands [24,25], a finding assigned to the exceptionally high radioactivity levels found in the blood of all animal groups at 4 h pi (>4%IA/g vs. 0.07 ± 0.01%IA/g of [^{99m}Tc]Tc-DT1 in controls; $p < 0.0001$ and 0.08 ± 0.02%IA/g in the Entresto®+Lis group; $p < 0.0001$). Notably, the tumor uptake of [^{99m}Tc]Tc-DT9 at 24 h pi remained significantly higher than [^{99m}Tc]Tc-DT1 in controls (3.32 ± 0.35%IA/g vs. 0.71 ± 0.10%IA/g, respectively; $p < 0.01$), emphasizing the impact of metabolic stability at early time points on tumor uptake at much later time intervals. Interestingly, a statistically significant difference was not observed in the treated groups of animals at 24 h pi ($p > 0.05$).

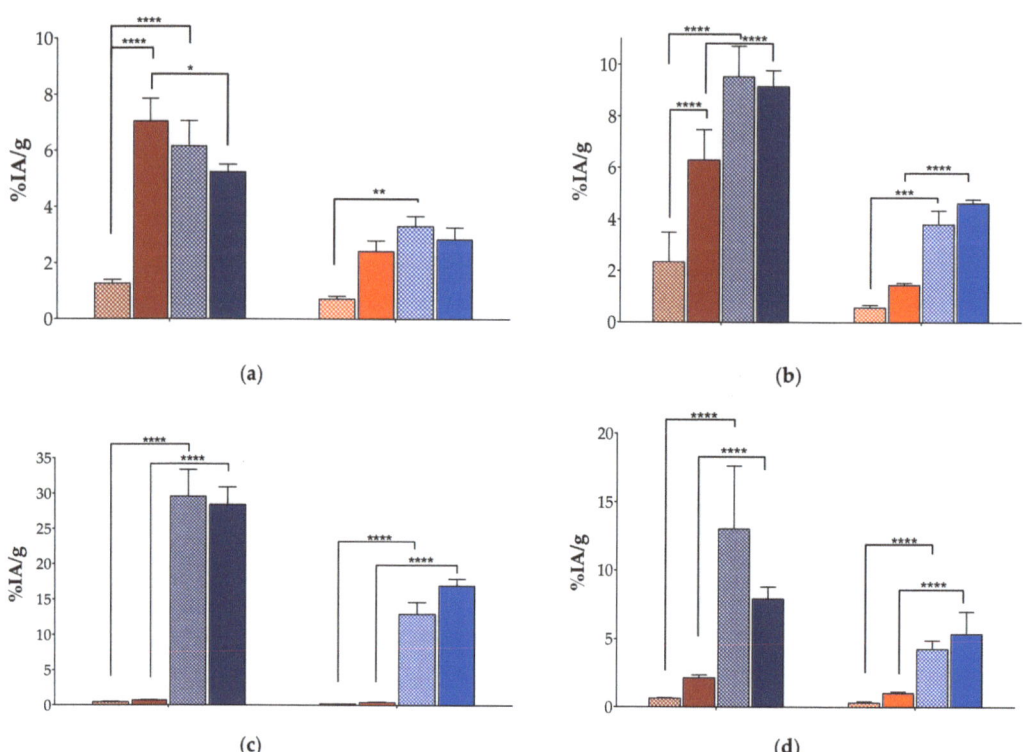

Figure 5. Comparative biodistribution data of [^{99m}Tc]Tc-DT9 (blue bars) and [^{99m}Tc]Tc-DT1 (reference; red bars) in SCID mice bearing AsPC-1 xenografts at 4 h (controls—dark checkered bars; Entresto®+Lis treated—dark solid bars) and 24 h pi (controls—light checkered bars; Entresto®+Lis treated—light solid bars) for (**a**) AsPC-1 tumors and (**b**) kidneys, (**c**) liver, and (**d**) intestines; data are expressed as %IA/g and represent average values ± sd, n = 4; statistically significant differences between treatments and radioligands at 4 and 24 h pi: ****: $p < 0.0001$, ***: $p < 0.001$, **: $p < 0.01$, and *: $p < 0.05$.

High uptake and retention was observed for [^{99m}Tc]Tc-DT9 in most tissues of the body and especially in the kidneys, the liver, and intestines, which surpassed by far that of [^{99m}Tc]Tc-DT1 (Figure 5). For example, the uptake of [^{99m}Tc]Tc-DT9 at 4 h pi was markedly increased compared with the unmodified reference in the liver (29.56 ± 3.77%IA/g vs. 0.44 ± 0.05%IA/g in controls; $p < 0.0001$) and intestines (13.02 ± 4.60%IA/g vs. 0.65 ± 0.04%IA/g in controls; $p < 0.0001$). This pronounced and persisting uptake could be partially attributed to the high blood levels of the ABD-modified radioligand combined with the high lipophilicity of the pendant palmitoyl group, resulting in an overall unfavorable in vivo profile for further clinical translation.

4. Discussion

The performance of radioligands based on the NT(8-13) motif has been largely compromised by suboptimal metabolic stability following their entry into circulation. In this respect, they are exposed to the rapid hydrolytic action of two major peptidases, ACE and NEP, with which they come into contact on their way to the NTS_1R target, while evading degradation by peptidases compartmentalized within cells, such as EC 3.4.24.15 (TOP, thimet-oligopeptidase, cleaving the Arg^8–Arg^9 bond) or EC 3.4.24.16 (neurolysin, hydrolyzing the Pro^{10}–Tyr^{11} bond) [18,20,21,24,46–48]. The peptidyl dipeptidase ACE hydrolyzes NT and its analogs at the Tyr^{11}–Ile^{12} bond, whereas the endopeptidase NEP cleaves both the Pro^{10}–Tyr^{11} and the Tyr^{11}–Ile^{12} bonds [18–21]. In the field of nuclear medicine, most metabolic stability assessments are typically performed by analysis of radioligand incubates in plasma or serum. While ACE is present in considerable levels in these biological fluids [17,33,49], NEP is scarcely present, and thus, its degrading role was inadvertently overlooked till recently [24,25,28,50]. Thus, efforts were initially directed at the stabilization of the ACE-hydrolyzed Tyr^{11}–Ile^{12} bond, predominantly via Ile^{12} substitution by Tle^{12} [17,23].

Following this route, we have indeed observed metabolic stability enhancement in mice plasma incubates and NTS_1R-mediated tumor uptake in mice in the case of [^{99m}Tc]Tc-DT6, a Tle^{12} [^{99m}Tc]Tc-DT1 mimic, compared with [^{99m}Tc]Tc-DT5 [23]. On these grounds, [^{99m}Tc]Tc-DT6 was selected for diagnostic imaging of NTS_1R-expressing tumors in human but proved unsuccessful in this respect [14]. We were able to recently demonstrate that [^{99m}Tc]Tc-DT6, albeit less degraded in peripheral mice blood than [^{99m}Tc]Tc-DT1 ($55.1 \pm 3.9\%$ vs. $1.8 \pm 0.8\%$ intact at 5 min pi; $p < 0.0001$), reached full metabolic stability only during in situ inhibition of NEP (to $89.3 \pm 6.7\%$ intact; $p < 0.0001$), revealing NEP as the major catabolizing peptidase [24]. Furthermore, the Tle^{12} substitution impaired cell internalization and final tumor uptake of [^{99m}Tc]Tc-DT6 during NEP inhibition when compared with the [^{99m}Tc]Tc-DT1 reference during double ACE/NEP inhibition [25]. In search of ACE-resistant [^{99m}Tc]Tc-DT1 mimics retaining high affinity to the human NTS_1R as well as favorable internalization capabilities, we developed the $DAsn^{14}$-elongated [^{99m}Tc]Tc-DT7 and the β-Homoleucine^{13}-substituted [^{99m}Tc]Tc-DT8 (Figure 1a,b). Although high receptor affinities were reported for the respective motifs [$DAsn^{14}$-]NT(8-13) [34] and [β-Homoleucine^{13}]NT(8-13) [35], in our study, only DT8 retained high NTS_1R affinity, while DT7 showed considerable affinity loss (Figure 2). On the other hand, both [^{99m}Tc]Tc-DT7 and [^{99m}Tc]Tc-DT8 achieved increased stability in peripheral mice blood compared with [^{99m}Tc]Tc-DT1, which increased by single NEP inhibition (Figure 3, Table 1). Further stabilization could not be achieved by combined NEP/ACE inhibition, a finding implying their becoming resistant to ACE. This assumption is further supported in the case of [^{99m}Tc]Tc-DT8 showing no significant improvement of stability during ACE inhibition vs. control. However, receptor specific internalization and uptake in AsPC-1 cells proved to be disappointingly poor for both radioligands, and consequently, they were not considered for further evaluation in tumor-bearing mice.

We subsequently directed our forces to derivatizing [^{99m}Tc]Tc-DT1 via the introduction of a pendant ABD handle to enhance metabolic stability. The type and position of this group was carefully selected based on existing reports on lipidation strategies proposed to prolong the bioavailability of peptide ligands [38–41]. In particular, conjugation of palmitoyl acid at positions Trp^{10} in contulakin-G and Pro^7 in NT led to improved analogs, thus attracting our attention [42–44]. To insert a second functionality in [^{99m}Tc]Tc-DT1, the Gly^7 linker was replaced by Lys^7, thus offering the ε-primary amine for attachment of the palmitoyl group. This modification led to DT9, which, as expected, preserved high affinity binding for the human NTS_1R (Figure 2). Furthermore, the respective [^{99m}Tc]Tc-DT9 radioligand, unlike the C-terminus-modified [^{99m}Tc]Tc-DT7 and [^{99m}Tc]Tc-DT8, displayed very high internalization capacity in AsPC-1 cells. Notably, internalization values surpassed even that of the [^{99m}Tc]Tc-DT1 reference at incubation times longer than 1 h (Figure 3). This finding is in agreement with previous studies showing that lipidation boosts the internalization of peptide analogs [38].

Of particular interest are the results of the in vivo stability study of palmitoylated [^{99m}Tc]Tc-DT9, confirming its full resistance to both ACE and NEP (Table 1, Figure 3). This positive outcome was further supported by the fact that treatment of animals with Entresto® (releasing in vivo the potent and selective NEP-inhibitor sacubitrilat [29–31]) or the Entresto® plus Lis combination (Lis a potent and selective inhibitor of ACE [26]) had no effect on stability results. It should be emphasized that [^{99m}Tc]Tc-DT9 is the first [^{99m}Tc]Tc-DT1 mimic that is stable in peripheral mice blood while preserving a high NTS$_1$R affinity and high internalization rates in NTS$_1$R-expressing cells. These qualities clearly show that the attachment of ABD groups at the linker of NT(8-13) analogs is a promising new strategy.

Next, we evaluated the biodistribution profile of [^{99m}Tc]Tc-DT9 in immunosuppressed mice bearing human NTS$_1$R-expressing pancreatic cancer xenografts (Table 2, Figure 5). As expected from the stability and internalization results, the tumor uptake of [^{99m}Tc]Tc-DT9 was significantly higher than that of unmodified [^{99m}Tc]Tc-DT1 at both 4 and 24 h pi. During treatment of mice with the Entresto® plus Lis combination, tumor uptake was improved only for the biodegradable [^{99m}Tc]Tc-DT1 reference but not for [^{99m}Tc]Tc-DT9, once again confirming the successful in vivo targeting of the palmitoylated mimic. However, the overall pharmacokinetic profile of [^{99m}Tc]Tc-DT9 turned out to be suboptimal, mainly due to high radioactivity levels found in the blood. High radioactivity levels in the blood resulted in elevated background radioactivity, especially in the liver and intestines, as previously reported for other albumin-binding lipophilic compounds [51]. It is evident that palmitoyl does not represent the ABD group of choice for Lys^7 attachment, but [^{99m}Tc]Tc-DT1 mimics derivatized from different groups may prove to be appropriate candidates for clinical translation.

5. Conclusions

Aiming at [^{99m}Tc]Tc-DT1 mimics for combined resistance to ACE and/or NEP with high NTS$_1$R affinity and high internalization rates, we followed two major strategies. Firstly, we developed the C-terminus-modified DT7 ([DAsn^{14}]DT1) and DT8 ([β-Homoleucine^{13}]DT1) and, secondly, the palmitoyl-decorated DT9 ([(palmitoyl)Lys^7]DT1). During head-to-head comparisons in NTS$_1$R-expressing cells, only [^{99m}Tc]Tc-DT9 achieved high internalization rates. It also proved to be the only radioligand stable in peripheral mice blood, displaying resistance to both ACE and NEP. In mice bearing NTS$_1$R-expressing pancreatic cancer xenografts, [^{99m}Tc]Tc-DT9 showed significantly higher tumor uptake compared with the [^{99m}Tc]Tc-DT1 reference, while during twin ACE/NEP inhibition, uptake was comparable between these analogs. The high background activity levels of [^{99m}Tc]Tc-DT9 in mice, however, led to an unfavorable pharmacokinetic profile. In conclusion, coupling of an ABD group on Lys^7 in [^{99m}Tc]Tc-DT1 mimics showed to be the preferred approach toward metabolic stability, cell internalization, and tumor targeting compared with the hitherto less successful C-terminal modification. Replacement of palmitoyl by other ABD groups to improve pharmacokinetics is warranted and is currently being pursued.

Supplementary Materials: The following supporting information can be downloaded at: https://www.mdpi.com/article/10.3390/pharmaceutics15082092/s1, Table S1: Analytical data for DT7, DT8, and DT9.

Author Contributions: Conceptualization, B.A.N. and T.M.; methodology, P.K., B.A.N. and T.M.; validation, B.A.N., P.K. and T.M.; formal analysis, P.K.; investigation, P.K., B.A.N. and T.M.; resources, T.M. and E.P.K.; writing—original draft preparation, P.K. and T.M.; writing—review and editing, all authors; visualization, P.K., B.A.N. and T.M.; supervision, T.M. and E.P.K.; project administration, T.M. and E.P.K.; funding acquisition, E.P.K. All authors have read and agreed to the published version of the manuscript.

Funding: This research received no external funding.

Institutional Review Board Statement: Mice experiments were conducted in licensed facilities (EL 25 BIO exp021) in accordance with the Declaration of Helsinki and complied with European and national regulations. The study protocols were approved by the Department of Agriculture and Veterinary Service of the Prefecture of Athens (#1609, 24-04-2019 for the stability studies and #1610, 24-04-2019 for the biodistribution studies).

Informed Consent Statement: Not applicable.

Data Availability Statement: Data is contained within the article or Supplementary Material.

Conflicts of Interest: The authors declare no conflict of interest.

References

1. Reubi, J.C.; Waser, B.; Friess, H.; Buchler, M.; Laissue, J. Neurotensin receptors: A new marker for human ductal pancreatic adenocarcinoma. *Gut* **1998**, *42*, 546–550. [CrossRef]
2. Körner, M.; Waser, B.; Ströbel, O.; Büchler, M.; Reubi, J.C. Neurotensin receptors in pancreatic ductal carcinomas. *EJNMMI Res.* **2015**, *5*, 17. [CrossRef] [PubMed]
3. Ishizuka, J.; Townsend, C.M., Jr.; Thompson, J.C. Neurotensin regulates growth of human pancreatic cancer. *Ann. Surg.* **1993**, *217*, 439–445; discussion 446. [CrossRef]
4. Fendler, W.P.; Baum, R.P. NTR is the new SSTR? Perspective for neurotensin receptor 1 (NTR)-directed theranostics. *J. Nucl. Med.* **2017**, *58*, 934–935. [CrossRef]
5. Reubi, J.C.; Waser, B.; Schaer, J.C.; Laissue, J.A. Neurotensin receptors in human neoplasms: High incidence in Ewing's sarcomas. *Int. J. Cancer* **1999**, *82*, 213–218. [CrossRef]
6. Gui, X.; Guzman, G.; Dobner, P.R.; Kadkol, S.S. Increased neurotensin receptor-1 expression during progression of colonic adenocarcinoma. *Peptides* **2008**, *29*, 1609–1615. [CrossRef] [PubMed]
7. Morgat, C.; Chastel, A.; Molinie, V.; Schollhammer, R.; Macgrogan, G.; Vélasco, V.; Malavaud, B.; Fernandez, P.; Hindié, E. Neurotensin Receptor-1 Expression in Human Prostate Cancer: A Pilot Study on Primary Tumors and Lymph Node Metastases. *Int. J. Mol. Sci.* **2019**, *20*, 1721. [CrossRef]
8. Souaze, F.; Dupouy, S.; Viardot-Foucault, V.; Bruyneel, E.; Attoub, S.; Gespach, C.; Gompel, A.; Forgez, P. Expression of neurotensin and NT1 receptor in human breast cancer: A potential role in tumor progression. *Cancer Res.* **2006**, *66*, 6243–6249. [CrossRef] [PubMed]
9. Kitabgi, P. Targeting neurotensin receptors with agonists and antagonists for therapeutic purposes. *Curr. Opin. Drug Discov. Devel.* **2002**, *5*, 764–776. [PubMed]
10. Achilefu, S.; Srinivasan, A.; Schmidt, M.A.; Jimenez, H.N.; Bugaj, J.E.; Erion, J.L. Novel bioactive and stable neurotensin peptide analogues capable of delivering radiopharmaceuticals and molecular beacons to tumors. *J. Med. Chem.* **2003**, *46*, 3403–3411. [CrossRef]
11. Mascarin, A.; Valverde, I.E.; Mindt, T.L. Structure-activity relationship studies of amino acid substitutions in radiolabeled neurotensin conjugates. *ChemMedChem* **2016**, *11*, 102–107. [CrossRef]
12. Maschauer, S.; Prante, O. Radiopharmaceuticals for imaging and endoradiotherapy of neurotensin receptor-positive tumors. *J. Label. Comp. Radiopharm.* **2018**, *61*, 309–325. [CrossRef]
13. Buchegger, F.; Bonvin, F.; Kosinski, M.; Schaffland, A.O.; Prior, J.; Reubi, J.C.; Blauenstein, P.; Tourwé, D.; Garcia Garayoa, E.; Bischof Delaloye, A. Radiolabeled neurotensin analog, ^{99m}Tc-NT-XI, evaluated in ductal pancreatic adenocarcinoma patients. *J. Nucl. Med.* **2003**, *44*, 1649–1654.
14. Gabriel, M.; Decristoforo, C.; Woll, E.; Eisterer, W.; Nock, B.; Maina, T.; Moncayo, R.; Virgolini, I. [^{99m}Tc]Demotensin VI: Biodistribution and initial clinical results in tumor patients of a pilot/phase I study. *Cancer Biother. Radiopharm.* **2011**, *26*, 557–563. [CrossRef]
15. De Visser, M.; Janssen, P.J.J.M.; Srinivasan, A.; Reubi, J.C.; Waser, B.; Erion, J.L.; Schmidt, M.A.; Krenning, E.P.; de Jong, M. Stabilised In-111-labelled DTPA- and DOTA-conjugated neurotensin analogues for imaging and therapy of exocrine pancreatic cancer. *Eur. J. Nucl. Med. Mol. Imaging* **2003**, *30*, 1134–1139. [CrossRef]
16. Fröberg, A.C.; van Eijck, C.; Verdijsseldonck, M.C.; Melis, M.; Bakker, H.; Krenning, E.P. Use of neurotensin analogue In-111-DTPA-neurotensin (In-111-MP2530) in diagnosis of pancreatic adenocarcinoma. *Eur. J. Nucl. Med. Mol. Imaging* **2004**, *31* (Suppl. S2), S392.
17. Schubiger, P.A.; Allemann-Tannahill, L.; Egli, A.; Schibli, R.; Alberto, R.; Carrel-Remy, N.; Willmann, M.; Blauenstein, P.; Tourwé, D. Catabolism of neurotensins. Implications for the design of radiolabeling strategies of peptides. *Q. J. Nucl. Med.* **1999**, *43*, 155–158.
18. Kitabgi, P.; De Nadai, F.; Rovere, C.; Bidard, J.N. Biosynthesis, maturation, release, and degradation of neurotensin and neuromedin n. *Ann. N. Y. Acad. Sci.* **1992**, *668*, 30–42. [CrossRef] [PubMed]
19. Kitabgi, P.; Dubuc, I.; Nouel, D.; Costentin, J.; Cuber, J.C.; Fulcrand, H.; Doulut, S.; Rodriguez, M.; Martinez, J. Effects of thiorphan, bestatin and a novel metallopeptidase inhibitor JMV 390-1 on the recovery of neurotensin and neuromedin N released from mouse hypothalamus. *Neurosci. Lett.* **1992**, *142*, 200–204. [CrossRef] [PubMed]

20. Checler, F.; Vincent, J.P.; Kitabgi, P. Degradation of neurotensin by rat brain synaptic membranes: Involvement of a thermolysin-like metalloendopeptidase (enkephalinase), angiotensin-converting enzyme, and other unidentified peptidases. *J. Neurochem.* **1983**, *41*, 375–384. [CrossRef] [PubMed]
21. Skidgel, R.A.; Engelbrecht, S.; Johnson, A.R.; Erdös, E.G. Hydrolysis of substance P and neurotensin by converting enzyme and neutral endopeptidase. *Peptides* **1984**, *5*, 769–776. [CrossRef] [PubMed]
22. Nock, B.A.; Nikolopoulou, A.; Reubi, J.C.; Maes, V.; Conrath, P.; Tourwé, D.; Maina, T. Toward stable N4-modified neurotensins for NTS1-receptor-targeted tumor imaging with ^{99m}Tc. *J. Med. Chem.* **2006**, *49*, 4767–4776. [CrossRef]
23. Maina, T.; Nikolopoulou, A.; Stathopoulou, E.; Galanis, A.S.; Cordopatis, P.; Nock, B.A. [^{99m}Tc]Demotensin 5 and 6 in the NTS1-R-targeted imaging of tumours: Synthesis and preclinical results. *Eur. J. Nucl. Med. Mol. Imaging* **2007**, *34*, 1804–1814. [CrossRef] [PubMed]
24. Kanellopoulos, P.; Kaloudi, A.; de Jong, M.; Krenning, E.P.; Nock, B.A.; Maina, T. Key-Protease Inhibition Regimens Promote Tumor Targeting of Neurotensin Radioligands. *Pharmaceutics* **2020**, *12*, 528. [CrossRef]
25. Kanellopoulos, P.; Nock, B.A.; Krenning, E.P.; Maina, T. Optimizing the profile of [^{99m}Tc]Tc-NT(7-13) tracers in pancreatic cancer models by means of protease inhibitors. *Int. J. Mol. Sci.* **2020**, *21*, 7926. [CrossRef]
26. Armayor, G.M.; Lopez, L.M. Lisinopril: A new angiotensin-converting enzyme inhibitor. *Drug Intell. Clin. Pharm.* **1988**, *22*, 365–372. [CrossRef]
27. Salazar-Lindo, E.; Santisteban-Ponce, J.; Chea-Woo, E.; Gutierrez, M. Racecadotril in the treatment of acute watery diarrhea in children. *N. Engl. J. Med.* **2000**, *343*, 463–467. [CrossRef] [PubMed]
28. Roques, B.P.; Noble, F.; Dauge, V.; Fournie-Zaluski, M.C.; Beaumont, A. Neutral endopeptidase 24.11: Structure, inhibition, and experimental and clinical pharmacology. *Pharmacol. Rev.* **1993**, *45*, 87–146.
29. Schiering, N.; D'Arcy, A.; Villard, F.; Ramage, P.; Logel, C.; Cumin, F.; Ksander, G.M.; Wiesmann, C.; Karki, R.G.; Mogi, M. Structure of neprilysin in complex with the active metabolite of sacubitril. *Sci. Rep.* **2016**, *6*, 27909. [CrossRef]
30. Ayalasomayajula, S.; Langenickel, T.; Pal, P.; Boggarapu, S.; Sunkara, G. Clinical pharmacokinetics of sacubitril/valsartan (LCZ696): A novel angiotensin receptor-neprilysin inhibitor. *Clin. Pharmacokinet.* **2017**, *56*, 1461–1478. [CrossRef]
31. Han, Y.; Ayalasomayajula, S.; Pan, W.; Yang, F.; Yuan, Y.; Langenickel, T.; Hinder, M.; Kalluri, S.; Pal, P.; Sunkara, G. Pharmacokinetics, safety and tolerability of sacubitril/valsartan (LCZ696) after single-dose administration in healthy chinese subjects. *Eur. J. Drug Metab. Pharmacokinet.* **2017**, *42*, 109–116. [CrossRef]
32. Valkema, R.; Schonebaum, L.E.; Fröberg, A.C.; Maina, T.; Nock, B.A.; de Blois, E.; Konijnenberg, M.W.; Koolen, S.L.W.; Peeters, R.P.; Visser, W.E.; et al. PepProtect: Improved detection of cancer and metastases by peptide scanning under the protection of enzyme inhibitors. *Eur. J. Nucl. Med. Mol. Imaging* **2022**, *49* (Suppl. S1), S81. [CrossRef]
33. Rohrbach, M.S.; Williams, E.B., Jr.; Rolstad, R.A. Purification and substrate specificity of bovine angiotensin-converting enzyme. *J. Biol. Chem.* **1981**, *256*, 225–230. [CrossRef]
34. Kling, R.C.; Burchardt, C.; Einsiedel, J.; Hubner, H.; Gmeiner, P. Structure-based exploration of an allosteric binding pocket in the NTS1 receptor using bitopic NT(8-13) derivatives and molecular dynamics simulations. *J. Mol. Model.* **2019**, *25*, 193. [CrossRef]
35. Einsiedel, J.; Hubner, H.; Hervet, M.; Harterich, S.; Koschatzky, S.; Gmeiner, P. Peptide backbone modifications on the C-terminal hexapeptide of neurotensin. *Bioorg. Med. Chem. Lett.* **2008**, *18*, 2013–2018. [CrossRef] [PubMed]
36. Seebach, D.; Lukaszuk, A.; Patora-Komisarska, K.; Podwysocka, D.; Gardiner, J.; Ebert, M.O.; Reubi, J.C.; Cescato, R.; Waser, B.; Gmeiner, P.; et al. On the terminal homologation of physiologically active peptides as a means of increasing stability in human serum--neurotensin, opiorphin, B27-KK10 epitope, NPY. *Chem. Biodivers.* **2011**, *8*, 711–739. [CrossRef]
37. Sparr, C.; Purkayastha, N.; Yoshinari, T.; Seebach, D.; Maschauer, S.; Prante, O.; Hubner, H.; Gmeiner, P.; Kolesinska, B.; Cescato, R.; et al. Syntheses, receptor bindings, in vitro and in vivo stabilities and biodistributions of DOTA-neurotensin(8-13) derivatives containing beta-amino acid residues—A lesson about the importance of animal experiments. *Chem. Biodivers.* **2013**, *10*, 2101–2121. [CrossRef] [PubMed]
38. Erak, M.; Bellmann-Sickert, K.; Els-Heindl, S.; Beck-Sickinger, A.G. Peptide chemistry toolbox—Transforming natural peptides into peptide therapeutics. *Bioorg. Med. Chem.* **2018**, *26*, 2759–2765. [CrossRef] [PubMed]
39. Kostelnik, K.B.; Els-Heindl, S.; Kloting, N.; Baumann, S.; von Bergen, M.; Beck-Sickinger, A.G. High metabolic in vivo stability and bioavailability of a palmitoylated ghrelin receptor ligand assessed by mass spectrometry. *Bioorg. Med. Chem.* **2015**, *23*, 3925–3932. [CrossRef]
40. Zhang, L.; Bulaj, G. Converting peptides into drug leads by lipidation. *Curr. Med. Chem.* **2012**, *19*, 1602–1618. [CrossRef]
41. Bellmann-Sickert, K.; Elling, C.E.; Madsen, A.N.; Little, P.B.; Lundgren, K.; Gerlach, L.O.; Bergmann, R.; Holst, B.; Schwartz, T.W.; Beck-Sickinger, A.G. Long-acting lipidated analogue of human pancreatic polypeptide is slowly released into circulation. *J. Med. Chem.* **2011**, *54*, 2658–2667. [CrossRef] [PubMed]
42. Craig, A.G.; Norberg, T.; Griffin, D.; Hoeger, C.; Akhtar, M.; Schmidt, K.; Low, W.; Dykert, J.; Richelson, E.; Navarro, V.; et al. Contulakin-G, an O-glycosylated invertebrate neurotensin. *J. Biol. Chem.* **1999**, *274*, 13752–13759. [CrossRef]
43. Green, B.R.; White, K.L.; McDougle, D.R.; Zhang, L.; Klein, B.; Scholl, E.A.; Pruess, T.H.; White, H.S.; Bulaj, G. Introduction of lipidization-cationization motifs affords systemically bioavailable neuropeptide Y and neurotensin analogs with anticonvulsant activities. *J. Pept. Sci.* **2010**, *16*, 486–495. [CrossRef]

44. Lee, H.K.; Zhang, L.; Smith, M.D.; Walewska, A.; Vellore, N.A.; Baron, R.; McIntosh, J.M.; White, H.S.; Olivera, B.M.; Bulaj, G. A marine analgesic peptide, contulakin-G, and neurotensin are distinct agonists for neurotensin receptors: Uncovering structural determinants of desensitization properties. *Front. Pharmacol.* **2015**, *6*, 11. [CrossRef]
45. Bidard, J.N.; de Nadai, F.; Rovere, C.; Moinier, D.; Laur, J.; Martinez, J.; Cuber, J.C.; Kitabgi, P. Immunological and biochemical characterization of processing products from the neurotensin/neuromedin N precursor in the rat medullary thyroid carcinoma 6-23 cell line. *Biochem. J.* **1993**, *291 Pt 1*, 225–233. [CrossRef]
46. Schindler, L.; Bernhardt, G.; Keller, M. Modifications at Arg and Ile give neurotensin(8-13) derivatives with high stability and retained NTS1 receptor affinity. *ACS Med. Chem. Lett.* **2019**, *10*, 960–965. [CrossRef]
47. Paschoalin, T.; Carmona, A.K.; Rodrigues, E.G.; Oliveira, V.; Monteiro, H.P.; Juliano, M.A.; Juliano, L.; Travassos, L.R. Characterization of thimet oligopeptidase and neurolysin activities in B16F10-NEX2 tumor cells and their involvement in angiogenesis and tumor growth. *Mol. Cancer* **2007**, *6*, 44. [CrossRef]
48. Berti, D.A.; Morano, C.; Russo, L.C.; Castro, L.M.; Cunha, F.M.; Zhang, X.; Sironi, J.; Klitzke, C.F.; Ferro, E.S.; Fricker, L.D. Analysis of intracellular substrates and products of thimet oligopeptidase in human embryonic kidney 293 cells. *J. Biol. Chem.* **2009**, *284*, 14105–14116. [CrossRef]
49. Lieberman, J. Elevation of serum angiotensin-converting-enzyme (ACE) level in sarcoidosis. *Am. J. Med.* **1975**, *59*, 365–372. [CrossRef] [PubMed]
50. Nortier, J.; Pauwels, S.; De Prez, E.; Deschodt-Lanckman, M. Human neutrophil and plasma endopeptidase 24.11: Quantification and respective roles in atrial natriuretic peptide hydrolysis. *Eur. J. Clin. Investig.* **1995**, *25*, 206–212. [CrossRef] [PubMed]
51. Ockner, R.K.; Weisiger, R.A.; Gollan, J.L. Hepatic uptake of albumin-bound substances: Albumin receptor concept. *Am. J. Physiol.* **1983**, *245*, G13–G18. [CrossRef] [PubMed]

Disclaimer/Publisher's Note: The statements, opinions and data contained in all publications are solely those of the individual author(s) and contributor(s) and not of MDPI and/or the editor(s). MDPI and/or the editor(s) disclaim responsibility for any injury to people or property resulting from any ideas, methods, instructions or products referred to in the content.

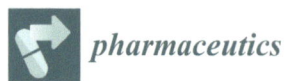 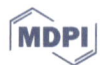

Article

Population Pharmacokinetic Analysis of Perampanel in Portuguese Patients Diagnosed with Refractory Epilepsy

Rui Silva [1,2], Helena Colom [3,4], Joana Bicker [1,2], Anabela Almeida [2,5], Ana Silva [6], Francisco Sales [6], Isabel Santana [6], Amílcar Falcão [1,2] and Ana Fortuna [1,2,*]

1. Laboratory of Pharmacology, Faculty of Pharmacy, University of Coimbra, 3000-548 Coimbra, Portugal; rui.freixo@gmail.com (R.S.)
2. CIBIT/ICNAS—Coimbra Institute for Biomedical Imaging and Translational Research, University of Coimbra, 3000-548 Coimbra, Portugal; almeida.anabela@gmail.com
3. Farmacoteràpia, Farmacogenètica i Tecnologia Farmacèutica, IDIBELL—Institut d'Investigació Biomèdica de Bellvitge, 08907 Hospitalet de Llobregat, Spain; helena.colom@ub.edu
4. Pharmacy and Pharmaceutical Technology and Physical Chemistry Department, Universitat de Barcelona, 08028 Barcelona, Spain
5. CIVG—Vasco da Gama Research Center, EUVG—Vasco da Gama University School, 3020-210 Coimbra, Portugal
6. Refractory Epilepsy Reference Centre, Centro Hospitalar e Universitário de Coimbra, EPE, 3004-561 Coimbra, Portugal; franciscosales@chuc.min-saude.pt (F.S.)
* Correspondence: anacfortuna@gmail.com or afortuna@ff.uc.pt; Tel.: +351-239488400; Fax: +351-239488503

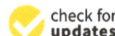

Citation: Silva, R.; Colom, H.; Bicker, J.; Almeida, A.; Silva, A.; Sales, F.; Santana, I.; Falcão, A.; Fortuna, A. Population Pharmacokinetic Analysis of Perampanel in Portuguese Patients Diagnosed with Refractory Epilepsy. *Pharmaceutics* 2023, 15, 1704. https://doi.org/10.3390/pharmaceutics15061704

Academic Editors: Cristina Manuela Drăgoi, Alina Crenguța Nicolae and Ion-Bogdan Dumitrescu

Received: 12 May 2023
Revised: 7 June 2023
Accepted: 8 June 2023
Published: 10 June 2023

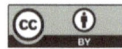

Copyright: © 2023 by the authors. Licensee MDPI, Basel, Switzerland. This article is an open access article distributed under the terms and conditions of the Creative Commons Attribution (CC BY) license (https://creativecommons.org/licenses/by/4.0/).

Abstract: Perampanel is a promising antiepileptic drug (AED) for refractory epilepsy treatment due to its innovative mechanism of action. This study aimed to develop a population pharmacokinetic (PopPK) model to be further used in initial dose optimization of perampanel in patients diagnosed with refractory epilepsy. A total of seventy-two plasma concentrations of perampanel obtained from forty-four patients were analyzed through a population pharmacokinetic approach by means of nonlinear mixed effects modeling (NONMEM). A one-compartment model with first-order elimination best described the pharmacokinetic profiles of perampanel. Interpatient variability (IPV) was entered on clearance (CL), while the residual error (RE) was modeled as proportional. The presence of enzyme-inducing AEDs (EIAEDs) and body mass index (BMI) were found as significant covariates for CL and volume of distribution (V), respectively. The mean (relative standard error) estimates for CL and V of the final model were 0.419 L/h (5.56%) and 29.50 (6.41%), respectively. IPV was 30.84% and the proportional RE was 6.44%. Internal validation demonstrated an acceptable predictive performance of the final model. A reliable population pharmacokinetic model was successfully developed, and it is the first enrolling real-life adults diagnosed with refractory epilepsy.

Keywords: perampanel; epilepsy; population pharmacokinetics; NONMEM; therapeutic drug monitoring

1. Introduction

Characterized by recurrent and unpredictable interruptions of normal brain function, epilepsy is an heterogeneous group of complex diseases and one of the most common neurological disorders worldwide [1,2]. The main therapeutic approach clinically applied for epileptic seizure control is pharmacological treatment with one or more antiepileptic drugs (AEDs) that restore the balance between cerebral excitation and inhibition through several pharmacological mechanisms, such as modulation of voltage-gated ion channels, potentiation of GABAergic activity, inhibition of glutamatergic processes, and modification of the neurotransmitter release [3–5]. Although epilepsy is one of the oldest diseases and more than twenty AEDs are currently used in clinical practice, one-third of adequately medicated patients remain with uncontrolled seizures, requiring a greater social interest and increasing awareness of epilepsy [6,7]. AEDs with innovative mechanisms of action seem to be a promising choice when other AEDs fail. However, they remain unable to provide an effective treatment in all patients with refractory epilepsy [8,9].

Personalizing the dose scheme for each patient in an attempt to improve the efficacy and tolerability of AEDs is hence emergent [10,11]. In this context, therapeutic drug monitoring (TDM) and population pharmacokinetic (PopPK) models are prominent decision-making support tools for the definition and optimization of pharmacological therapy through the design of pharmacotherapeutic schemes according to the specific characteristics of each patient [12–14]. Particularly, they have been applied to individualize AED dosing and promote seizure control without adverse effects that significantly affect the patient's quality of life [10,11,15–18]. TDM ensures optimal exposure to avoid treatment failures resulting from low concentrations and side effects that result from concentrations above the therapeutic window. Indeed, TDM is a clinical tool applied to improve drug efficacy through the individual adjustment of therapeutic dosing regimens. This has been applied in classic drugs, such as phenytoin or digoxin [19], as well as new drugs, such as tyrosine kinase inhibitors [20] or direct oral anticoagulants [21]. On the other hand, PopPK modeling has been ascribed as a robust tool for precision medication in comparison to classic pharmacokinetic analysis, which needs a complete set of concentrations at each time point [13,14,22]. Their combination quantitatively assesses the pharmacokinetic characteristics and interpatient variability (IPV), contributing to a personalized/precise pharmacotherapy. Their application is straightforward in drugs with narrow therapeutic range, IPV and when there is a relationship between drug pharmacokinetics and pharmacodynamics [23].

Perampanel is a third-generation AED, approved as adjunctive treatment of focal-onset seizures with or without secondarily generalization and for primary generalized tonic-clonic seizures in patients with idiopathic generalized epilepsy [24]. It meets the previously mentioned three criteria, making the development of PopPK models necessary to integrate TDM in clinical practice and individualize drug posology. Indeed, the efficacy and tolerability of perampanel are directly related to its systemic exposure. Based on a clinical study enrolling pharmacoresistant epileptic patients with focal-onset seizures [25], the narrow therapeutic window of perampanel was established by the International League Against Epilepsy as 0.180–0.980 mg/L [16]. However, a wider range of 0.1–1.0 mg/L has been applied until more clinical information is available [26]. Furthermore, multiple factors determine plasma drug exposure, resulting in large IPV of pharmacological effects. In spite of its rapid and complete intestinal absorption (bioavailability $\approx$ 100%) [27], perampanel is bound to plasma proteins, mainly albumin and α-1-acid glycoprotein, in the range between 95 and 97% [27,28]. Additionally, its volume of distribution is approximately 1.1 L/70 kg and it is extensively metabolized primarily by the cytochrome P450 3A4 (CYP3A4) isoenzyme, leading to various pharmacologically inactive metabolites [27]. These characteristics increase drug–drug interaction potential and the variability of its response.

To the best of our knowledge, there are currently only two published PopPK perampanel models, constructed with data from phase II and phase III clinical trials [29,30]. One enrolls adolescents, and none include patients with refractory epilepsy. Therefore, while covering every step of a modeling and simulation workflow, the present investigation aimed to develop a PopPK model to be further used in initial dose optimization of perampanel in adults diagnosed with refractory epilepsy.

2. Materials and Methods
2.1. Patients and Pharmacotherapy

A retrospective observational study was performed including 44 Portuguese refractory epileptic patients admitted to the Refractory Epilepsy Centre of the Coimbra Hospital and University Centre, EPE (CHUC, EPE, Coimbra, Portugal) between April 2019 and December 2022. The study was approved by the Ethics Committee of the Faculty of Medicine of the University of Coimbra, Coimbra, Portugal (CE-061/2018) and by the Ethics Committee of CHUC, EPE (CHUC-144-18). The anonymity of all patients was ensured. Inclusion criteria were: patients older than 18 years of age, diagnosis of refractory epilepsy, and perampanel treatment for seizure control for at least a month and submitted to TDM as part of their routine clinical management. Patients were considered refractory when two appropriate and tolerated AED schedules failed to achieve sustained seizure freedom [31]. Patients chronically prescribed with drugs other than AEDs were excluded, as well as those admitted to the intensive care unit or diagnosed with *status epilepticus*. The following data were collected: sex, age (years), weight (kg), height (cm), and the prescribed AED regimen (including drugs and respective posology). Body surface area (BSA, m^2) and body mass index (BMI, kg/m^2) were calculated.

2.2. Laboratory Testing

Blood samples were collected in tubes containing a clot activator and serum gel separator in order to quantify albumin (g/dL), total proteins (g/dL), alanine aminotransferase (U/L), alkaline phosphatase (U/L), aspartate aminotransferase (U/L), gamma-glutamyl transferase (U/L), lactate dehydrogenase (U/L), total bilirubin (mg/dL), C-reactive protein (mg/dL), and serum creatinine (mg/dL). Serum concentrations were determined through the integrated clinical chemistry and immunoassay equipment Alinity ci-series (Abbott Diagnostics). Glomerular filtration rate (eGFR, mL/min/1.73 m^2) was estimated by the Chronic Kidney Disease Epidemiology Collaboration equations [32].

2.3. Blood Sampling and Perampanel Quantification

A total of 72 plasma concentrations of perampanel were obtained at steady-state. Blood sample collection was performed according to the TDM protocol implemented in the Refractory Epilepsy Centre of CHUC, EPE. Since perampanel is once daily administered and at bedtime, blood samples were collected in the following morning (from 9.7 to 14 h after drug intake, $n = 42$) and before drug administration (from 20.5 to 24 h after drug intake, $n = 30$). Blood sampling was performed while avoiding meal times. The date and time of each sample collection were recorded. Blood samples were collected in heparin-lithium tubes and centrifuged at 4 °C and 2880 g for 10 min, followed by plasma collection for further sample treatment and drug quantification. Plasma samples were submitted to a double liquid-liquid extraction procedure with ethyl acetate and drug concentrations were determined by a validated high-performance liquid chromatography method with diode array detection, as previously described in Sabença et al. [33]. The method was linear in the concentration range of 0.03 to 4.50 mg/L.

2.4. Population Pharmacokinetic Analysis

Perampanel plasma concentration time data were analyzed through the PopPK approach by means of nonlinear mixed effects modeling resorting to the software NONMEM® version 7.4 (ICON Early Phase, San Antonio, TX, USA). The first-order conditional estimation method with interaction (FOCEI) was used for the parameter estimation and model construction process.

2.4.1. Base Model Development

One- and two-compartment with first-order elimination models were firstly used to fit the concentration-time data of perampanel. Since concentrations were obtained during the elimination phase, the absorption rate constant of perampanel could not be determined and, hence, the intravenous bolus administration was herein chosen, similarly to other published investigations [29,30]. IPV was evaluated for all pharmacokinetic parameters and modeled exponentially, assuming a log-normal distribution. Additive, proportional, and combined (additive + proportional) errors were tested and compared to assess the residual error (RE) associated with drug concentrations. The log-likelihood ratio test was used to compare nested models. A significance level of p-value < 0.005 corresponding to a difference in the minimum objective function value of 7.88 was adopted [34,35]. The physiological plausibility of the model parameters and its estimation precision, expressed as the relative standard error (RSE), were also considered.

2.4.2. Covariate Model Development

Demographic (gender, age), anthropometric (weight, height, BSA, BMI), clinical parameters (albumin, total proteins, alanine aminotransferase, alkaline phosphatase, aspartate aminotransferase, gamma-glutamyl transferase, lactate dehydrogenase and total bilirubin), and renal function (given by eGFR) were tested for inclusion as covariates in the model. Moreover, the influence of each concomitant AED was investigated as well as the impact of enzyme-inducing AEDs (EIAEDs) that include carbamazepine, oxcarbazepine, phenobarbital, and phenytoin, and the non-EIAEDs, which include clobazam, eslicarbazepine acetate, lacosamide, lamotrigine, levetiracetam, topiramate, valproic acid and zonisamide).

Firstly, covariates were investigated by a univariate approach, and secondly, by stepwise forward inclusion and stepwise backward elimination procedures. The effect of the inclusion of each covariate on the pharmacokinetic parameters of perampanel was considered significant when the minimum objective function value (MOFV) decreased by at least 3.84 ($p = 0.05$). The included covariates were retained if its elimination resulted in an increase in MOFV of at least 10.8 ($p = 0.001$) [34,35]. Furthermore, the inclusion of each covariate was also evaluated according to (i) the physiological plausibility of the pharmacokinetic parameter values, which had to be similar to the previous analysis, (ii) the precision of estimated parameters, expressed as RSE, (iii) significant clinical reduction in IPV associated to each pharmacokinetic parameter (10%), (iv) condition number, which is the square root of the ratio of the major to the minor eigenvalue, (v) the η- and ϵ-shrinkage values, as measures of model overparameterization [36], and (vi) the visual inspection of the goodness-of-fit plots which included: observed concentrations (OBS) versus typical population model predicted (PRED) or individual predicted concentrations (IPRED), individual weighted residuals (IWRES) versus IPRED and conditional weighted residuals (CWRES) versus time [37,38].

2.4.3. Model Evaluation

Internal validation of the final model was assessed using prediction-corrected visual predictive check (VPC) [39] and bootstrap methods [40–42]. Based on 1000 replicated data sets from the original data set, prediction-corrected VPC was assessed to investigate the predictive ability of the method. Median, 2.5th and 97.5th percentiles of the observations were checked whether they were within the non-parametric 95% confidence intervals of the median, 2.5th and 97.5th percentiles of the simulated profiles. The stability and precision of the final model were evaluated resorting to bootstrap method, using 50 resamplings from the initial data set. The fixed and random effect parameters were calculated as median and 95% confidence interval (2.5% and 97.5% percentiles). For each parameter, bias was determined as the percentage of the difference between median derived from bootstrap and the final population estimate.

2.5. Model-Based Simulations

From the final model, Monte Carlo simulations were carried out with NONMEM® software version 7.4 to evaluate the effect of the covariate combination in the relationship between perampanel dose and its plasma concentrations. In the present study, we found that BMI and concomitant EIAEDs affected perampanel clearance. Therefore, concentration-time profiles for different perampanel dosing regimens (2, 4, 6, 8, 10 and 12 mg once daily) were simulated according to BMI (18.5, 22.5, 27.5 and 32.5 kg/m^2) and the presence or absence of EIAEDs.

In addition, concentration-time profiles for the same daily doses of perampanel were divided in one or two daily administrations and simulated according to BMI in the presence of EIAEDs. Each simulation generated 1000 perampanel concentration-time profiles for of each combination of covariates using the final estimates of V and CL. Mean trough plasma concentrations were calculated for each combination of covariates. Considering the therapeutic plasma range for perampanel (0.1 to 1.0 mg/mL), trough plasma concentrations were classified as under, within and over the therapeutic range and compared between the several groups.

2.6. Statistical Analysis

R software version 4.1.3 (The R Foundation for Statistical Computing) was used for statistical analysis and nonlinear mixed effects model diagnostics. Descriptive statistics were stated as absolute and relative frequencies for categorical variables and as median (minimum–maximum) for continuous variables. The package xpose4 version 4.7.1 was used to guide the model building.

3. Results

A population pharmacokinetic model was developed resorting to seventy-two plasma concentrations of perampanel obtained from forty-four refractory epileptic patients. Patient characteristics are described in Table 1.

Table 1. Demographic and clinical characteristics of patients included in the study and their AED treatments.

Study Feature	Property Value
Patients, n	44
Sex, n (%) Males Females	 27 (61.40%) 17 (38.60%)
Age (years)	33.00 (19.00–76.00)
Weight (kg)	77.50 (45.00–99.00)
Height (cm)	168.50 (155.00–194.00)
BSA (m^2)	1.88 (1.48–2.27)
BMI (kg/m^2)	25.14 (15.76–36.20)
Albumin (g/dL)	4.40 (3.70–5.20)
Total proteins (g/dL)	7.00 (6.20–8.30)
Alanine aminotransferase (U/L)	20.00 (8.00–12.00)
Alkaline phosphatase (U/L)	71.00 (26.00–230.00)
Aspartate aminotransferase (U/L)	17.00 (12.00–73.00)
Gamma-glutamyl transferase (U/L)	36.50 (10.00–694.00)
Lactate dehydrogenase (U/L)	197.50 (138.00–260.00)
Total bilirubin (mg/dL)	0.45 (0.20–2.00)
eGFR (mL/min/1.73 m^2)	110.63 (49.31–134.90)
CRP (mg/dL) <0.5 0.6–1.0 1.1–3.0	 37 (84.0%) 3 (6.8.0%) 3 (6.8.0%)
Daily dose, n (%) 2 mg 4 mg 6 mg 8 mg 10 mg	 1 (2.30%) 14 (31.80%) 12 (27.30%) 11 (25.00%) 6 (13.60%)

Table 1. Cont.

Study Feature	Property Value
Co-administered AEDs per patient, n (%)	
0	1 (2.30%)
1	9 (20.50%)
2	16 (36.40%)
3	13 (29.50%)
4	5 (11.30%)
Concomitant AEDs, n (%)	
Carbamazepine	15 (34.10%)
Clobazam	11 (25.00%)
Eslicarbazepine acetate	10 (22.70%)
Lacosamide	5 (11.40%)
Lamotrigine	5 (11.40%)
Levetiracetam	28 (63.60%)
Oxcarbazepine	2 (4.50%)
Phenobarbital	3 (6.80%)
Phenytoin	2 (4.50%)
Topiramate	5 (11.40%)
Valproic acid	8 (18.20%)
Zonisamide	6 (13.60%)

AED, antiepileptic drug; BMI, body mass index; BSA, body surface area; CRP, C-reactive protein; eGFR, estimated glomerular filtration rate. Results are expressed as relative and absolute frequencies or median and range.

Most of the patients were men (61.4%) with a median of 38 years of age (19–76), while 38.60% were women with a median of 32 years of age (21–67). The observed median BMI in men (25.10 kg/m^2) and women (26.22 kg/m^2) corresponds to the overweight category. With the exception of alkaline phosphatase and gamma-glutamyl transferase, remaining clinical results were all within normal clinical ranges (Table 1). Median eGFR was 110.63 mL/min/1.73 m^2; however, it ranged from moderately decreased to normal values (49.31–134.90 mL/min/1.73 m^2). Perampanel dosing regimens ranged from 2 to 10 mg daily, although the most frequently administered daily doses ranged from 4 to 8 mg.

It should be noted that most patients were on polytherapy with two (36.4%) and three (29.5%) AEDs besides perampanel. Levetiracetam (63.6%) and carbamazepine (34.1%) were the most often co-prescribed AEDs. Twenty (45.5%) patients were co-prescribed with EIAEDs. More details can be seen in Table S1 (Supplementary Materials).

3.1. Population Pharmacokinetic Modeling

Plasma concentrations of perampanel were better described by a one-compartment model with first-order elimination parameterized by volume of distribution (V) and clearance (CL) than by a two-compartment model. IPV was entered on CL, while residual variability was modelled as proportional.

Inclusion of all the candidate covariates in the model, one at each step, identified BW, BSA, and BMI as covariates with statistically significant effects on V, and gamma-glutamyl transferase, the presence of carbamazepine, clobazam, lacosamide, phenytoin, and the group of EIAEDs as covariates significantly affecting the CL (Supplementary Materials: Tables S2–S5).

The final covariate model only retained the presence of EIAEDs and BMI as covariates for CL and V, respectively. Inclusion of EIAEDs resulted in a decrease in MOFV of −54.259 and IPV of −27.8%. The sequential inclusion of BMI in V resulted in a decrease in MOFV of −19.965. The proportional residual error decreased from 9.03% in the base model to 6.44% in the final covariate model.

Thus, in the final model, the presence of EIAEDs, which included carbamazepine, oxcarbazepine, phenobarbital, and phenytoin, increased the typical value of perampanel

CL 2.76-times. BMI normalized by its median value affected the V of perampanel directly and positively. The final model equations were as follows in Equations (1) and (2):

$$V(L) = 29.5 \times \left(\frac{BMI}{25.1}\right)^{2.12} \quad (1)$$

$$CL(L/h) = 0.419 \times 2.76^{IND} \quad (2)$$

in which, BMI is the body mass index, in kg/m^2, and IND is equal to 0 or 1 if EIAEDs are absent or present.

Parameter estimates of the base and final models as well as the bootstrap results are summarized in Table 2. The successful ratio of minimization runs was one. All pharmacokinetic parameters were estimated with adequate precision. Mean population values of model parameters were within the 95% confidence intervals estimated by the bootstrap method. The relative deviation between the true population value and the median value provided by bootstrap was lower than 10% for all pharmacokinetic parameters. The condition number of the model was 2.63, suggesting no notable collinearity. Acceptable values were found for the ε-shrinkage (36.1%) and η-shrinkage (0.01%) associated to the CL.

Table 2. Population parameter estimates for the base and final models and bootstrap results.

Parameter	Base Model		Final Model		Bootstrap		Bias (%)
	Estimate	RSE (%)	Estimate	RSE (%)	Median	95%CI	
TVCL (L/h)	0.672	9.30	0.419	5.56	0.417	0.372–0.470	0.45
TVV (L)	33.10	10.36	29.50	6.41	29.49	23.29–32.31	0.04
IND$_{CL}$	-	-	2.76	9.89	2.79	2.21–3.66	−1.27
BMI$_V$	-	-	2.12	1.37	2.02	1.38–2.87	4.63
IPV$_{CL}$ (%)	58.57	16.62	30.82	16.19	29.73	23.96–35.83	7.00
RE$_{proportional}$ (%)	9.03	20.10	6.44	24.81	6.16	3.95–7.80	8.43

BMI$_V$, body mass index effect on volume of distribution; IPV$_{CL}$, interpatient variability of clearance; IND$_{CL}$, EIAED effect on clearance; RE$_{proportional}$, proportional residual error; RSE, relative standard error; TVCL, typical value of clearance; TVV, typical value of volume of distribution. 95% CI; 95% confidence interval.

The main goodness-of-fit plots for the final model are depicted in Figure 1. The OBS concentration versus PRED concentrations spread randomly around the identity line (Figure 1a), while conditional weighted residuals (CWRES) vs. time (Figure 1d) uniformly spread around the zero line (Figure 1c), indicating no model misspecification. Furthermore, OBS concentrations versus IPRED concentrations scattered around the identity line (Figure 1b) as well as IWRES versus IPRED uniformly spread around zero (Figure 1c), suggesting an adequate description of IPV and RE, respectively.

Prediction-corrected VPC indicated that the final model could acceptably predict the distribution of the observed plasma concentrations of perampanel for patients not co-administered (Figure 2a) and administered EIAEDs (Figure 2b). The parameter estimates obtained with the final model are consistent with the median parameter estimates from the bootstrap and are within the 95% confidence intervals (Table 2).

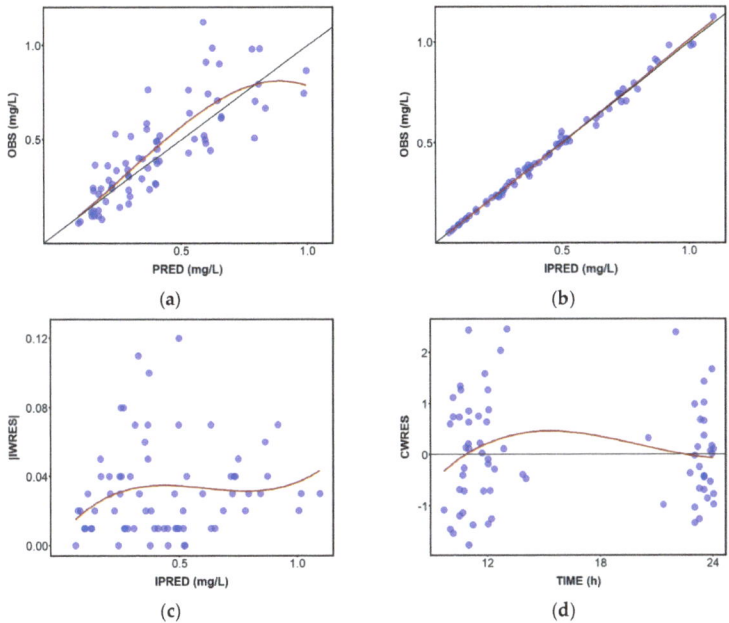

Figure 1. Goodness-of fit plots of the final model: (**a**) population predicted (PRED) concentrations vs. observed (OBS) concentrations, (**b**) individual predicted concentrations (IPRED) vs. OBS concentrations, (**c**) absolute individual weighted residuals (IWRES) vs. individual predicted concentrations, and (**d**) conditional weighted residuals (CWRES) vs. time after dose. OBS, observed concentrations (mg/L); IPRED, individual predicted concentrations (mg/L); PRED, population predicted concentrations (mg/L). Blue dots represent perampanel plasma concentrations; Black line, line of identity; Red line, data smoother.

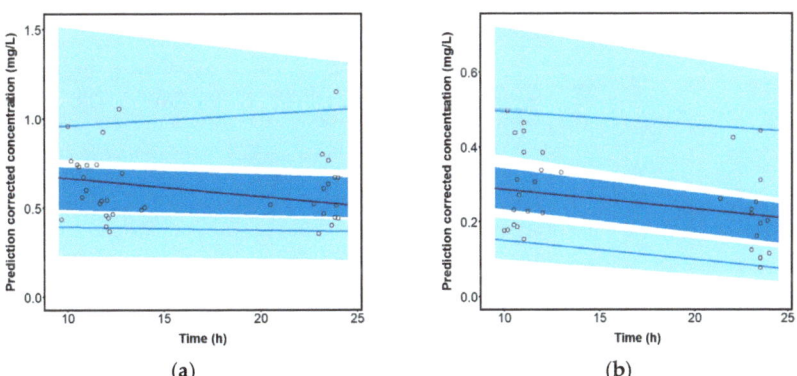

Figure 2. Prediction-corrected visual predictive check of the final model for (**a**) patients not taking and (**b**) patients taking EIAEDs. The dots represent the prediction-corrected concentrations of perampanel (mg/L) at the respective time after dose administration. The lines represent from top to bottom the 2.5th, 50th and 97.5th observed percentiles, respectively. Dark blue shading displays the simulated based 95% confidence intervals for the 50th percentile and light blue shading the 2.5th and 97.5th percentiles.

3.2. Model-Based Dosing Simulations

Table 3 displays the mean steady-state trough plasma concentrations of perampanel simulated for each daily dose according to BMI, and with or without EIAED co-administration. For each daily dose, mean trough plasma concentrations increased with BMI, and were higher in patients not co-administered with EIAEDs (0.151 to 1.145 mg/L) than in co-administered patients (0.030 to 0.347 mg/L).

Table 3. Mean steady-state trough plasma concentration (mg/L) from simulations of different daily doses of perampanel according to body mass index (BMI) and the co-administration of EIAEDs. Concentrations within the therapeutic range of perampanel (0.1–1.0 mg/L) are shaded in grey.

Daily Dose	Without EIAEDs				With EIAEDs			
	BMI 18.5 kg/m^2	BMI 22.5 kg/m^2	BMI 27.5 kg/m^2	BMI 32.5 kg/m^2	BMI 18.5 kg/m^2	BMI 22.5 kg/m^2	BMI 27.5 kg/m^2	BMI 32.5 kg/m^2
2 mg	0.151	0.170	0.182	0.193	0.030 [#]	0.041 [#]	0.051 [#]	0.058 [#]
4 mg	0.305	0.340	0.368	0.376	0.059 [#]	0.084 [#]	0.103	0.115
6 mg	0.447	0.508	0.550	0.567	0.091 [#]	0.126	0.152	0.174
8 mg	0.583	0.681	0.741	0.765	0.118	0.163	0.210	0.234
10 mg	0.764	0.847	0.909	0.941	0.144	0.208	0.260	0.287
12 mg	0.908	1.015 [##]	1.075 [##]	1.145 [##]	0.178	0.246	0.309	0.347

[#] Mean steady-state trough plasma concentration below the therapeutic range (<0.1 mg/L); [##] Mean steady-state trough plasma concentration above the therapeutic range (>1.0 mg/L).

In patients not co-administered with EIAEDs, mean steady-state trough plasma concentrations were within the therapeutic range (0.1 to 1.0 mg/L) when perampanel doses ranged from 2 to 10 mg/daily. When the dose was 12 mg/daily, mean steady-state trough plasma concentration remained within the therapeutic range only for the subpopulation with a BMI of 18.5 kg/m^2. In contrast, patients co-medicated with EIAEDs revealed mean steady-state trough plasma concentrations within the therapeutic range only when the dose of perampanel ranged from 6 to 12 mg/daily (Table 3). Doses of 2 and 4 mg/day revealed concentrations bellow the therapeutic range (<0.1 mg/L).

Figure 3 depicts the percentages of steady-state trough plasma concentrations simulated from different daily doses of perampanel within and outside the therapeutic range according to BMI and EIAED co-administration. Regarding patients not taking EIAEDs, daily doses ranging from 4 mg to 8 mg provided the highest proportions (>90%) of trough plasma concentrations within the therapeutic range. Significant percentages of trough plasma concentrations above the therapeutic range (>20%) were found among patients with daily doses of 10 and 12 mg. Considering patients co-medicated with EIAEDs, proportions higher than >90% were found in patients treated with perampanel doses of 8 to 12 mg/daily. Significant percentages (>20%) of trough plasma concentrations under the therapeutic range were found among patients under 2 and 8 mg/daily.

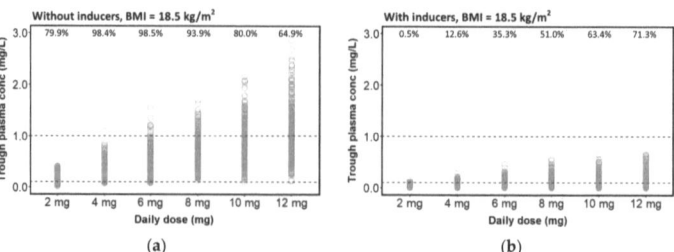

Figure 3. *Cont.*

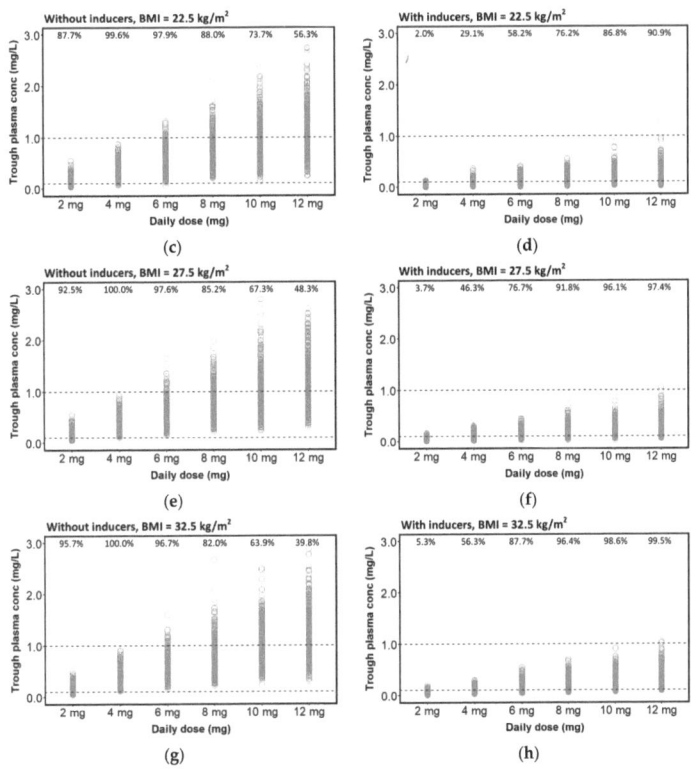

Figure 3. Plasma concentrations (mg/L) simulated for once-daily perampanel in patients not taking EIAEDs and (**a**) body mass index (BMI) = 18.5 kg/m², (**c**) BMI = 22.5 kg/m², (**e**) BMI = 27.5 kg/m² and (**g**) BMI = 32.5 kg/m² and in patients taking EIAEDs and (**b**) BMI = 18.5 kg/m², (**d**) BMI = 22.5 kg/m², (**f**) BMI = 27.5 kg/m² and (**h**) BMI = 32.5 kg/m². The percentages of perampanel plasma concentrations within the therapeutic range (0.1–1.0 mg/L) are displayed on top of the graph.

Due to the low trough plasma concentrations of perampanel observed in patients taking EIAEDs, a new set of simulations were performed considering a twice daily administration and the corresponding mean steady-state trough plasma concentrations are summarized in Table 4, while the percentages of steady-state trough plasma concentrations, within and outside the therapeutic range, are depicted in Figure 4.

Table 4. Mean steady-state trough plasma concentration (mg/L) from simulations of different twice-daily doses of perampanel according to BMI in patients co-administered with EIAEDs. The concentrations within the therapeutic range of perampanel (0.1–1.0 mg/L) are shaded in grey.

Daily Dose	With EIAEDs			
	BMI 18.5 kg/m²	BMI 22.5 kg/m²	BMI 27.5 kg/m²	BMI 32.5 kg/m²
2 mg	0.048 [#]	0.055 [#]	0.061 [#]	0.066 [#]
4 mg	0.097 [#]	0.116	0.124	0.131
6 mg	0.146	0.171	0.188	0.197
8 mg	0.189	0.228	0.257	0.268
10 mg	0.239	0.276	0.309	0.331
12 mg	0.288	0.340	0.370	0.402

[#] Mean steady-state trough plasma concentration below the therapeutic range (<0.1 mg/L).

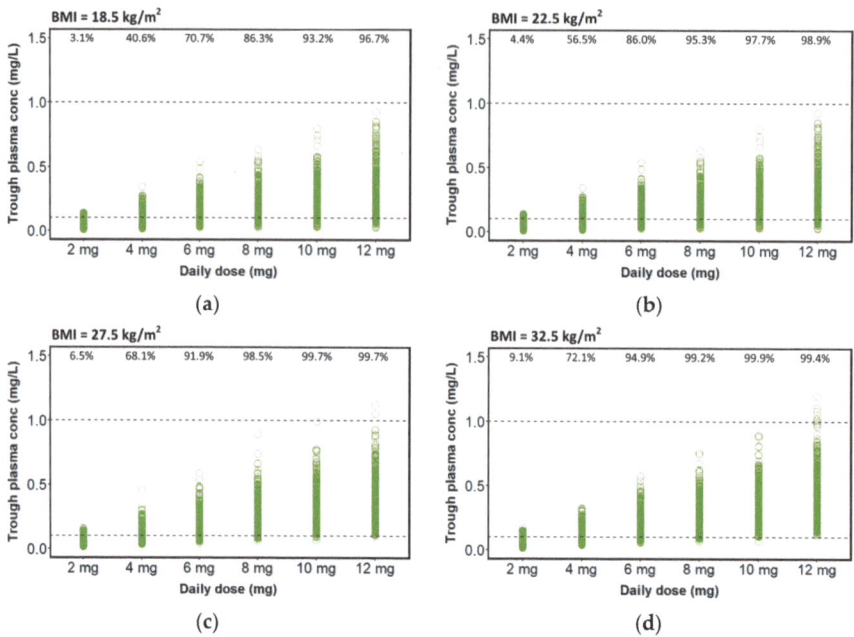

Figure 4. Plasma concentrations (mg/L) simulated for twice-daily perampanel in patients taking EIAEDs and (**a**) body mass index (BMI) = 18.5 kg/m^2, (**b**) BMI = 22.5 kg/m^2, (**c**) BMI = 27.5 kg/m^2 and (**d**) BMI = 32.5 kg/m^2. The percentages of perampanel plasma concentrations within the therapeutic range (0.1–1.0 mg/L) are displayed on top of the graph.

4. Discussion

Personalized medicine in pharmacotherapy, although not a new concept, is currently gaining interest not only by the medical community and other health professionals, but also by the scientific community and academic institutions [43]. TDM together with PopPK accurately support the design of pharmacotherapeutic schemes according to the specific characteristics of each patient and their pathological state. Therefore, model-informed precision dosing is an a priori TDM strategy based on the application of mathematical and statistical models developed for specific populations of patients. Furthermore, these models could be employed through a Bayesian approach to adjust dosing regimens a posteriori [14,44].

A PopPK model for perampanel was herein successfully developed in a population of Portuguese patients diagnosed with refractory epilepsy. There are currently two other PopPK models for perampanel; however, the model herein reported is the only model that includes data from adult refractory epileptic patients under real TDM processes instead of patients enrolled in clinical trials [29,30].

Consistent with the sparse nature of the data collected during the elimination phase and in accordance with the previous studies [29,30], the pharmacokinetics of perampanel in the present population was best described by a one-compartment model with first-order elimination. Herein, the typical estimated CL (0.419 L/h) for perampanel was approximately 50–60% lower than the typical CL estimated by Villanueva et al. [29] (0.729 L/h) and Takenaka et al. [30] (0.668 L/h). In the cited studies, it was not possible to estimate the V of perampanel and therefore it was fixed at 43.5 L. Herein, clinical data allowed an accurate estimation of V for perampanel (29.5 L), which is lower than those used in the literature (43.5 L). This can be attributed to the fact that the plasma concentrations were obtained after the distribution phase (9.7 to 24 h after drug intake). Importantly, we found lower proportional residual error (6.44%) and IPV associated to CL (30.82%) comparatively to already published models [29,30]. These findings highlight that the present model is clinically relevant and can be further used in drug individualization. Indeed, due to the small residual variability herein observed, the overall expected variation is mainly associated with CL, which is overcome when BMI and inducers are included to individualize the posology of perampanel.

To identify the factors affecting the pharmacokinetics of perampanel, several covariates were tested for inclusion in the model. In agreement with already published models [29,30], age did not affect the pharmacokinetic parameters of perampanel in our study. On the other hand, the same authors observed a significant difference between the CL of male and female patients, but in the real-life study presented by Patsalos et al. [45] there were no differences between perampanel pharmacokinetic parameters in women and men. Similarly, in our study, gender did not affect the pharmacokinetic parameters of perampanel. None of the analytical variables herein investigated revealed a significant impact on perampanel pharmacokinetics, probably because these characteristics were within normal clinical ranges for most patients (Table 1, Section 3). Ideally, patients with values out of the reference range should also be included and investigated.

The co-administration of EIAEDs and BMI were found as significant covariates that affect the CL and V of perampanel, respectively. The co-administration of EIAEDs increased the typical value of perampanel CL by two and seventy-six hundredths-fold, in accordance with reported models [29,30]. Indeed, it is well-known that perampanel is eliminated by hepatic CYP450 isoenzymes, mainly CYP3A4, and CYP3A5 to a minor extent [27,46,47]. Genetic polymorphisms in CYP3A4 do not influence perampanel CL [48]. However, EIAEDs enhance the metabolism of perampanel. Given that perampanel is approved as adjunctive therapy, co-prescription with EIAEDs may decrease its plasma concentrations, probably compromising drug efficacy [45,49]. The magnitude of the inducing effect of each of the EIAEDs has been reported to be different and dose dependent [27,45,49]. A study including data from phase III clinical trials showed that carbamazepine was the drug with the greatest inducing effect, causing a reduction of 67% in the area under the concentration-time curve of perampanel, compared with a reduction of 50% caused by oxcarbazepine and phenytoin [27]. These AEDs, particularly carbamazepine, continue to be used with considerable frequency in clinical practice [50].

In the present model, EIAEDs demonstrated the greatest impact on perampanel CL comparatively to each EIAEDs individually, probably due to the small sample when considering each EIAED and combination of EIAEDs. However, previous models [29,30] were developed resorting to large populations, whereby, it was possible to identify the effects of EIAEDs, separately. Carbamazepine was the main EIAED affecting the CL of perampanel, followed by oxcarbazepine/phenytoin. Carbamazepine is the EIAED with the highest effect, augmenting the CL of perampanel by two and sixty-four hundredths-fold [29] and two and ninety-five hundredths-fold [30]. The presence of oxcarbazepine/phenytoin showed an increase of one and seventy-eight hundredths-fold [29] and one and ninety-nine hundredths-fold [30] and topiramate/phenobarbital of one and twenty-one hundredths-fold [30].

On the other hand, BMI was identified as an individual characteristic that affected the V of perampanel in a direct relationship, probably because the extracellular water increases as the fat mass enhances [51] and the V of perampanel is closer to total body water [27]. Indeed, the patients herein enrolled encompassed a wide range of BMI (from 15.76 to 36.10 kg/m^2), allowing its association with V, which is a pharmacokinetic parameter useful for drug load definition. Regarding the effect of weight on perampanel pharmacokinetics, only Yamamoto et al. [49] suggested that, in addition to the effect of EIAEDs, age, sex, body weight, and CYP3A5 polymorphisms may contribute to fluctuations of perampanel plasma concentrations.

Importantly, the results found during the model internal validation showed an acceptable predictive performance (Table 2 and Figure 2), supporting its use in clinical practice to design effective and safe dose regimens of perampanel in patients diagnosed with refractory epilepsy. Thus, this model can be applied not only to design a priori dosing regimens, but also to design a posteriori adjustments of perampanel dosing regimens, employing a Bayesian approach.

After model development and validation, it was used to perform model-based simulations aiming to define the maintenance dosing posology of perampanel in patients diagnosed with refractory epilepsy. According to the summary of product characteristics, the maintenance dose of perampanel recommended for adults is 4 mg to 8 mg daily for patients diagnosed with focal-onset seizures, and up to 8 mg daily for patients diagnosed with primary generalized tonic-clonic seizures. In both cases, the maintenance dose must be titrated from 2 mg daily to the recommended dose, according to patient individual response. The drug should be taken orally, once daily and at bedtime to minimize its most common adverse events, namely dizziness, somnolence, and fatigue [24].

The efficacy and tolerability of perampanel is directly related with its systemic exposure [25]. Thus, applying the developed model, simulations of concentration-time profiles of perampanel were performed for doses ranging from 2 mg to 12 mg according to various scenarios, combining the absence or presence of EIAEDs with BMI. Then, trough plasma concentrations were evaluated according to the therapeutic range established for perampanel (0.1 to 1.0 mg/L). As V affects mainly the maximum concentrations, a great effect of BMI on trough plasma concentrations was not expected.

More than 90% of the patients not co-administered with EIAEDs were expected to exhibit trough plasma concentrations within the therapeutic range when daily doses ranging from 2 to 8 mg once daily were administered (Figure 3). On the other hand, patients co-administered with EIAEDs had lower trough plasma concentrations (Table 3). The highest rates (>90%) of trough plasma concentrations within the therapeutic range were observed with daily doses up to 8 mg once daily (Figure 3). Since the efficacy and tolerability of perampanel is directly related with its systemic exposure [25], it is interesting to comment on the study carried out by Gidal et al. [52]. Accordingly, the magnitude of the therapeutic efficacy of perampanel is influenced by concomitant therapy. Therapeutic response was significantly greater in patients not taking EIAEDs and receiving 8 and 12 mg/daily. The occurrence of adverse events was also greater in these patients, leading to discontinuation. In contrast, the co-administration of EIAEDs reduced the incidence of adverse events, which is consistent with the reduction in exposure caused by these drugs.

Currently, there are no recommendations for a dosing adjustment in patients co-prescribed with EIAEDs [24]. Therefore, aiming to explore the most appropriate dosing regimens of perampanel in patients taking EIAEDs, a set of simulations was herein tested for twice daily administrations (Table 4 and Figure 4). We demonstrated that patients taking EIAEDs are highly probable to obtain perampanel trough plasma concentrations within the therapeutic range if under a twice daily dosing regimen, rather than if administered with once daily dose regimen. Regarding patients not administered with EIAEDs, BMI had a greater effect, mainly when higher doses (10 to 12 mg/daily) were administered, while the greater effect of BMI in co-administered patients was found when doses ranged from 2 to 8 mg/daily (Table 3 and Figure 3). Interestingly, in patients not administered with EIAEDs and taking doses ranging from 2 to 4 mg/day, the percentage of trough plasma concentrations within the therapeutic range increased with BMI. Nonetheless, this percentage decreased when the daily drug dose ranged from 6 to 12 mg. In patients taking EIAEDs, the percentage of trough plasma concentrations within the therapeutic range increased with BMI, independently of daily perampanel dose.

This study presented some limitations, namely the relatively small number of patients that did not allow the performance of an external validation. Moreover, the variety and complexity of concomitant antiepileptic therapy hampered the comparison between groups of patients taking perampanel and each AED. Nonetheless, the pharmacokinetic data enabled an accurate estimation of all model parameters (Table 2).

5. Conclusions

A population pharmacokinetic model of perampanel was successfully developed for patients diagnosed with refractory epilepsy. BMI and the co-prescription of EIAEDs were identified as covariates that significantly affect the V and CL of perampanel, respectively.

The model was able to predict pharmacokinetic parameters and subsequently the plasma concentrations of perampanel with accuracy and precision. Thus, it could be applied in clinical practice to individualize the dosing regimens of perampanel, either through an a priori model-informed strategy or an a posteriori Bayesian adjustment.

To achieve plasma concentrations within the therapeutic range, maintenance doses ranging from 4 to 6 mg once daily are recommended for patients not co-administered with perampanel and EIAEDs. On the other hand, maintenance daily doses ranging from 4 to 6 mg twice daily are recommended for patients taking EIAEDs.

These findings highlight the importance of TDM of new generation AEDs and underline the value of model-informed dosing to personalize AED treatment. Due to its pharmacokinetic properties and narrow therapeutic window, TDM is recommended for perampanel, especially in patients also treated with other drugs that induce its metabolism.

Supplementary Materials: The following supporting information can be downloaded at: https://www.mdpi.com/article/10.3390/pharmaceutics15061704/s1, Table S1: Demographic and pharmacotherapeutic characteristics of the patients included in the study; Table S2: Covariates tested for volume of distribution; Table S3: Covariates tested for clearance; Table S4: Antiepileptic drugs tested for clearance; Table S5: Covariates tested for final model. At bold is the final model.

Author Contributions: Conceptualization, A.F. (Ana Fortuna); formal analysis, R.S., H.C. and A.F. (Amílcar Falcão); investigation, R.S., H.C., A.F. (Ana Fortuna), I.S., J.B. and A.S.; writing—original draft preparation, R.S.; writing—review and editing, A.F. (Ana Fortuna), H.C., A.A., J.B. and F.S.; supervision, A.F. (Ana Fortuna), A.F. (Amílcar Falcão) and A.A.; project administration, A.F. (Ana Fortuna); funding acquisition, A.F. (Ana Fortuna), A.F. (Amílcar Falcão) and F.S. All authors have read and agreed to the published version of the manuscript.

Funding: This research was funded by FEDER funds through Portugal 2020 in the scope of the Operational Programme for Competitiveness and Internationalization, and Fundação para a Ciência e Tecnologia (FCT), Portuguese Agency for Scientific Research, within the scope of the research project POCI-01-0145-FEDER-030478.

Institutional Review Board Statement: The study was conducted in accordance with the Declaration of Helsinki, and approved by the Ethics Committee of Faculty of Medicine of University of Coimbra, Coimbra, Portugal (CE-061/2018) on the 23 July 2018 and by the Ethics Committee of CHUC, EPE (CHUC-144-18) on the 3 July 2019.

Informed Consent Statement: Informed consent was obtained from all subjects involved in the study.

Data Availability Statement: Not applicable.

Acknowledgments: The authors thank the nurses and the doctors of the Refractory Epilepsy Centre and the technicians of the Laboratory of Neurochemistry for their collaboration.

Conflicts of Interest: The authors declare no conflict of interest.

References

1. Fisher, R.S.; Van Emde Boas, W.; Blume, W.; Elger, C.; Genton, P.; Lee, P.; Engel, J. Epileptic seizures and epilepsy: Definitions proposed by the International League Against Epilepsy (ILAE) and the International Bureau for Epilepsy (IBE). *Epilepsia* **2005**, *46*, 470–472. [CrossRef]
2. Fisher, R.S.; Acevedo, C.; Arzimanoglou, A.; Bogacz, A.; Cross, J.H.; Elger, C.E.; Engel, J.; Forsgren, L.; French, J.A.; Glynn, M.; et al. ILAE Official Report: A practical clinical definition of epilepsy. *Epilepsia* **2014**, *55*, 475–482. [CrossRef] [PubMed]
3. Rogawski, M.A.; Löscher, W. The neurobiology of antiepileptic drugs. *Nat. Rev. Neurosci.* **2004**, *5*, 553–564. [CrossRef] [PubMed]
4. Sills, G.J.; Rogawski, M.A. Mechanisms of action of currently used antiseizure drugs. *Neuropharmacology* **2020**, *168*, 107966. [CrossRef] [PubMed]
5. Brodie, M.J. Antiepileptic drug therapy the story so far. *Seizure Eur. J. Epilepsy* **2010**, *19*, 650–655. [CrossRef]
6. Kwan, P.; Brodie, M. Early identification of refractory epilepsy. *N. Engl. J. Med.* **2000**, *342*, 314–319. [CrossRef]

7. Chen, Z.; Brodie, M.J.; Liew, D.; Kwan, P. Treatment outcomes in patients with newly diagnosed epilepsy treated with established and new antiepileptic drugs a 30-year longitudinal cohort study. *JAMA Neurol.* **2018**, *75*, 279–286. [CrossRef]
8. Löscher, W.; Potschka, H.; Sisodiya, S.M.; Vezzani, A. Drug resistance in epilepsy: Clinical impact, potential mechanisms, and new innovative treatment options. *Pharmacol. Rev.* **2020**, *72*, 606–638. [CrossRef]
9. Riva, A.; Golda, A.; Balagura, G.; Amadori, E.; Vari, M.S.; Piccolo, G.; Iacomino, M.; Lattanzi, S.; Salpietro, V.; Minetti, C.; et al. New Trends and Most Promising Therapeutic Strategies for Epilepsy Treatment. *Front. Neurol.* **2021**, *12*, 753753. [CrossRef]
10. Johannessen Landmark, C.; Johannessen, S.I.; Patsalos, P.N. Therapeutic drug monitoring of antiepileptic drugs: Current status and future prospects. *Expert Opin. Drug Metab. Toxicol.* **2020**, *16*, 227–238. [CrossRef]
11. Landmark, C.J.; Johannessen, S.I.; Tomson, T. Dosing strategies for antiepileptic drugs: From a standard dose for all to individualised treatment by implementation of therapeutic drug monitoring. *Epileptic Disord.* **2016**, *18*, 367–383. [CrossRef]
12. IATDMCT, E.C. Definitions of TDM & CT. Available online: https://www.iatdmct.org/about-us/about-association/about-definitions-tdm-ct.html (accessed on 1 February 2023).
13. Donagher, J.; Martin, J.H.; Barras, M.A. Individualised medicine: Why we need Bayesian dosing. *Intern. Med. J.* **2017**, *47*, 593–600. [CrossRef]
14. Pérez-Blanco, J.S.; Lanao, J.M. Model-Informed Precision Dosing (MIPD). *Pharmaceutics* **2022**, *14*, 4–7. [CrossRef]
15. Patsalos, P.N.; Berry, D.J.; Bourgeois, B.F.D.; Cloyd, J.C.; Glauser, T.A.; Johannessen, S.I.; Leppik, I.E.; Tomson, T.; Perucca, E. Antiepileptic drugs—Best practice guidelines for therapeutic drug monitoring: A position paper by the subcommission on therapeutic drug monitoring, ILAE Commission on Therapeutic Strategies. *Epilepsia* **2008**, *49*, 1239–1276. [CrossRef] [PubMed]
16. Patsalos, P.N.; Spencer, E.P.; Berry, D.J. Therapeutic drug monitoring of antiepileptic drugs in epilepsy: A 2018 update. *Ther. Drug Monit.* **2018**, *40*, 526–548. [CrossRef] [PubMed]
17. Johannessen, S.I.; Landmark, C.J. Value of therapeutic drug monitoring in epilepsy. *Expert Rev. Neurother.* **2008**, *8*, 929–939. [CrossRef]
18. Jacob, S.; Nair, A.B. An Updated Overview on Therapeutic Drug Monitoring of Recent Antiepileptic Drugs. *Drugs R&D* **2016**, *16*, 303–316.
19. Zhao, W.; Jacqz-aigrain, E. Principles of Therapeutic Drug Monitoring. *Pediatr. Clin. Pharmacol.* **2011**, *205*, 77–90.
20. Menz, B.D.; Stocker, S.L.; Verougstraete, N.; Kocic, D.; Galettis, P.; Stove, C.P.; Reuter, S.E. Barriers and opportunities for the clinical implementation of therapeutic drug monitoring in oncology. *Br. J. Clin. Pharmacol.* **2021**, *87*, 227–236. [CrossRef]
21. Hu, K.; Ertl, G.; Nordbeck, P. Therapeutic Monitoring of Direct Oral Anticoagulants-Back to the Future? *J. Cardiovasc. Pharmacol.* **2020**, *76*, 374–375. [CrossRef]
22. Neely, M. Scalpels not hammers: The way forward for precision drug prescription. *Clin. Pharmacol. Ther.* **2017**, *101*, 368–372. [CrossRef]
23. Guidi, M.; Csajka, C.; Buclin, T. Parametric Approaches in Population Pharmacokinetics. *J. Clin. Pharmacol.* **2022**, *62*, 125–141. [CrossRef]
24. European Medicines Agency FYCOMPA. Summary of Product Characteristics. Available online: https://www.ema.europa.eu/en/documents/product-information/fycompa-epar-product-information_en.pdf (accessed on 1 February 2023).
25. Gidal, B.E.; Ferry, J.; Majid, O.; Hussein, Z. Concentration-effect relationships with perampanel in patients with pharmacoresistant partial-onset seizures. *Epilepsia* **2013**, *54*, 1490–1497. [CrossRef]
26. Reimers, A.; Berg, J.A.; Burns, M.L.; Brodtkorb, E.; Johannessen, S.I.; Landmark, C.J. Reference ranges for antiepileptic drugs revisited: A practical approach to establish national guidelines. *Drug Des. Devel. Ther.* **2018**, *12*, 271–280. [CrossRef]
27. Patsalos, P.N. The clinical pharmacology profile of the new antiepileptic drug perampanel: A novel noncompetitive AMPA receptor antagonist. *Epilepsia* **2015**, *56*, 12–27. [CrossRef]
28. Patsalos, P.N.; Zugman, M.; Lake, C.; James, A.; Ratnaraj, N.; Sander, J.W. Serum protein binding of 25 antiepileptic drugs in a routine clinical setting: A comparison of free non–protein-bound concentrations. *Epilepsia* **2017**, *58*, 1234–1243. [CrossRef]
29. Villanueva, V.; Majid, O.; Nabangchang, C.; Yang, H.; Laurenza, A.; Ferry, J.; Hussein, Z. Pharmacokinetics, exposure–cognition, and exposure–efficacy relationships of perampanel in adolescents with inadequately controlled partial-onset seizures. *Epilepsy Res.* **2016**, *127*, 126–134. [CrossRef] [PubMed]
30. Takenaka, O.; Ferry, J.; Saeki, K.; Laurenza, A. Pharmacokinetic/pharmacodynamic analysis of adjunctive perampanel in subjects with partial-onset seizures. *Acta Neurol. Scand.* **2018**, *137*, 400–408. [CrossRef] [PubMed]
31. Kwan, P.; Brodie, M.J. Definition of refractory epilepsy: Defining the indefinable? *Lancet Neurol.* **2010**, *9*, 27–29. [CrossRef] [PubMed]
32. Palacio-Lacambra, M.E.; Comas-Reixach, I.; Blanco-Grau, A.; Suñé-Negre, J.M.; Segarra-Medrano, A.; Montoro-Ronsano, J.B. Comparison of the Cockcroft–Gault, MDRD and CKD-EPI equations for estimating ganciclovir clearance. *Br. J. Clin. Pharmacol.* **2018**, *84*, 2120–2128. [CrossRef] [PubMed]
33. Sabença, R.; Bicker, J.; Silva, R.; Carona, A.; Silva, A.; Santana, I.; Sales, F.; Falcão, A.; Fortuna, A. Development and application of an HPLC-DAD technique for human plasma concentration monitoring of perampanel and lamotrigine in drug-resistant epileptic patients. *J. Chromatogr. B Anal. Technol. Biomed. Life Sci.* **2021**, *1162*, 122491. [CrossRef] [PubMed]
34. Yamaoka, K. Application of Akaike's Information Criterion (AIC) in the Evaluation of Linear Pharmacokinetic Equations. *J. Pharmacokinet. Biopharm.* **1978**, *6*, 165–175. [CrossRef] [PubMed]

35. Olofsen, E.; Dahan, A. Using Akaike's information theoretic criterion in mixed-effects modeling of pharmacokinetic data: A simulation study [version 2; peer review: 1 approved, 1 approved with reservations, 1 not approved]. *F1000Research* **2014**, *2*, 71. [CrossRef] [PubMed]
36. Savic, R.M.; Karlsson, M.O. Importance of shrinkage in empirical bayes estimates for diagnostics: Problems and solutions. *AAPS J.* **2009**, *11*, 558–569. [CrossRef]
37. Ette, E.I.; Ludden, T.M. Population Pharmacokinetic Modeling: The Importance of Informative Graphics. *Pharm. Res.* **1995**, *12*, 1845–1855. [CrossRef]
38. Karlsson, M.O.; Savic, R.M. Diagnosing Model Diagnostics. *Clin. Pharm. Ther.* **2007**, *82*, 1507–1514. [CrossRef]
39. Bergstrand, M.; Hooker, A.C.; Wallin, J.E.; Karlsson, M.O. Prediction-corrected visual predictive checks for diagnosing nonlinear mixed-effects models. *AAPS J.* **2011**, *13*, 143–151. [CrossRef]
40. Ette, E.I. Stability and performance of a population pharmacokinetic model. *J. Clin. Pharmacol.* **1997**, *37*, 486–495. [CrossRef]
41. Ette, E.I.; Williams, P.J.; Kim, Y.H.; Lane, J.R.; Liu, M.J.; Capparelli, E.V. Model appropriateness and population pharmacokinetic modeling. *J. Clin. Pharmacol.* **2003**, *43*, 610–623. [CrossRef]
42. Efron, B. Bootstrap methods: Another look at the jackknife. *Ann. Stat.* **1979**, *7*, 1–26. [CrossRef]
43. Brew-Sam, N.; Parkinson, A.; Lueck, C.; Brown, E.; Brown, K.; Bruestle, A.; Chisholm, K.; Collins, S.; Cook, M.; Daskalaki, E.; et al. The current understanding of precision medicine and personalised medicine in selected research disciplines: Study protocol of a systematic concept analysis. *BMJ Open* **2022**, *12*, e060326. [CrossRef]
44. Keizer, R.J.; ter Heine, R.; Frymoyer, A.; Lesko, L.J.; Mangat, R.; Goswami, S. Model-Informed Precision Dosing at the Bedside: Scientific Challenges and Opportunities. *CPT Pharmacomet. Syst. Pharmacol.* **2018**, *7*, 785–787. [CrossRef] [PubMed]
45. Patsalos, P.N.; Gougoulaki, M.; Sander, J.W. Perampanel Serum Concentrations in Adults With Epilepsy: Effect of Dose, Age, Sex, and Concomitant Anti-epileptic Drugs. *Ther. Drug Monit.* **2016**, *38*, 358–364. [CrossRef] [PubMed]
46. de Biase, S.; Gigli, G.L.; Nilo, A.; Romano, G.; Valente, M. Pharmacokinetic and pharmacodynamic considerations for the clinical efficacy of perampanel in focal onset seizures. *Expert Opin. Drug Metab. Toxicol.* **2019**, *15*, 93–102. [CrossRef]
47. Meirinho, S.; Rodrigues, M.; Fortuna, A.; Falcão, A.; Alves, G. Study of the metabolic stability profiles of perampanel, rufinamide and stiripentol and prediction of drug interactions using HepaRG cells as an in vitro human model. *Toxicol. Vitr.* **2022**, *82*, 105389. [CrossRef] [PubMed]
48. Ohkubo, S.; Akamine, Y.; Ohkubo, T.; Kikuchi, Y.; Miura, M. Quantification of the Plasma Concentrations of Perampanel Using High-Performance Liquid Chromatography and Effects of the CYP3A4* 1G Polymorphism in Japanese Patients. *J. Chromatogr. Sci.* **2020**, *58*, 915–921. [CrossRef]
49. Yamamoto, Y.; Usui, N.; Nishida, T.; Takahashi, Y.; Imai, K.; Kagawa, Y.; Inoue, Y. Therapeutic Drug Monitoring for Perampanel in Japanese Epilepsy Patients: Influence of Concomitant Antiepileptic Drugs. *Ther. Drug Monit.* **2017**, *39*, 446–449. [CrossRef]
50. Grześk, G.; Stolarek, W.; Kasprzak, M.; Grześk, E.; Rogowicz, D.; Wiciński, M.; Krzyżanowski, M. Therapeutic drug monitoring of carbamazepine: A 20-year observational study. *J. Clin. Med.* **2021**, *10*, 5396. [CrossRef]
51. Brunani, A.; Perna, S.; Soranna, D.; Rondanelli, M.; Zambon, A.; Bertoli, S.; Vinci, C.; Capodaglio, P.; Lukaski, H.; Cancello, R. Body composition assessment using bioelectrical impedance analysis (BIA) in a wide cohort of patients affected with mild to severe obesity. *Clin. Nutr.* **2021**, *40*, 3973–3981. [CrossRef]
52. Gidal, B.E.; Laurenza, A.; Fain, R. Perampanel efficacy and tolerability with enzyme-inducing AEDs in patients with epilepsy. *Neurology* **2015**, *12*, 1972–1980. [CrossRef]

Disclaimer/Publisher's Note: The statements, opinions and data contained in all publications are solely those of the individual author(s) and contributor(s) and not of MDPI and/or the editor(s). MDPI and/or the editor(s) disclaim responsibility for any injury to people or property resulting from any ideas, methods, instructions or products referred to in the content.

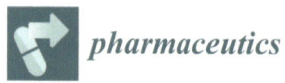 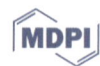

Article

Angiotensin II Receptor Blockers Reduce Tau/Aß42 Ratio: A Cerebrospinal Fluid Biomarkers' Case-Control Study

Gemma García-Lluch [1,2], Carmen Peña-Bautista [1], Lucrecia Moreno Royo [2,3], Miguel Baquero [1,2,4], Antonio José Cañada-Martínez [5] and Consuelo Cháfer-Pericás [1,2,*]

[1] Research Group in Alzheimer Disease, Instituto de Investigación Sanitaria La Fe, 46026 Valencia, Spain
[2] Cátedra DeCo MICOF-CEU UCH, Universidad Cardenal Herrera-CEU, 46115 Valencia, Spain
[3] Department of Pharmacy, Universidad Cardenal Herrera-CEU, CEU Universities, 46115 Valencia, Spain
[4] Neurology Unit, Hospital Universitari i Politècnic La Fe, 46026 Valencia, Spain
[5] Data Science and Biostatistics Unit, Health Research Institute La Fe, 46026 Valencia, Spain
* Correspondence: m.consuelo.chafer@uv.es

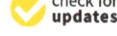

Citation: García-Lluch, G.; Peña-Bautista, C.; Royo, L.M.; Baquero, M.; Cañada-Martínez, A.J.; Cháfer-Pericás, C. Angiotensin II Receptor Blockers Reduce Tau/Aß42 Ratio: A Cerebrospinal Fluid Biomarkers' Case-Control Study. *Pharmaceutics* 2023, 15, 924. https://doi.org/10.3390/pharmaceutics15030924

Academic Editors: Cristina Manuela Drăgoi, Alina Crenguța Nicolae and Ion-Bogdan Dumitrescu

Received: 14 February 2023
Revised: 3 March 2023
Accepted: 3 March 2023
Published: 12 March 2023

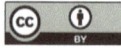

Copyright: © 2023 by the authors. Licensee MDPI, Basel, Switzerland. This article is an open access article distributed under the terms and conditions of the Creative Commons Attribution (CC BY) license (https://creativecommons.org/licenses/by/4.0/).

Abstract: (1) Background: The role of antihypertensives in Alzheimer's Disease (AD) prevention is controversial. This case-control study aims to assess whether antihypertensive medication has a protective role by studying its association with amyloid and tau abnormal levels. Furthermore, it suggests a holistic view of the involved pathways between renin-angiotensin drugs and the tau/amyloidß42 ratio (tau/Aß42 ratio); (2) Methods: The medical records of the participant patients were reviewed, with a focus on prescribed antihypertensive drugs and clinical variables, such as arterial blood pressure. The Anatomical Therapeutic Chemical classification was used to classify each drug. The patients were divided into two groups: patients with AD diagnosis (cases) and cognitively healthy patients (control); (3) Results: Age and high systolic blood pressure are associated with a higher risk of developing AD. In addition, combinations of angiotensin II receptor blockers are associated with a 30% lower t-tau/Aß42 ratio than plain angiotensin-converting enzyme inhibitor consumption; (4) Conclusions: Angiotensin II receptor blockers may play a potential role in neuroprotection and AD prevention. Likewise, several mechanisms, such as the PI3K/Akt/GSK3ß or the ACE1/AngII/AT1R axis, may link cardiovascular pathologies and AD presence, making its modulation a pivotal point in AD prevention. The present work highlights the central pathways in which antihypertensives may affect the presence of pathological amyloid and tau hyperphosphorylation.

Keywords: Alzheimer's disease; antihypertensives; amyloid; tau; angiotensin-converting enzyme inhibitor; angiotensin II receptor blockers; therapeutic strategies; personalized medicine

1. Introduction

Alzheimer's Disease (AD) is associated with alterations in the amyloid beta peptide (Aß) and tau proteins, as well as changes in cholinergic function [1–3]. The main AD cerebrospinal fluid (CSF) biomarkers are amyloid -ß42- (Aß42), total tau (t-tau), hyperphosphorylated tau (p-tau), and the tau/Aß42 ratio [4]. First, CSF Aß42 levels decrease in the development of the disease [5], which represents a reduced clearance from the brain into the blood, resulting in a higher accumulation of Aß plaques in the brain [6]. Second, the tau protein stabilizes microtubules in normal conditions as a compensatory mechanism against oxidative stress and Aß toxicity, and GSK3ß regulates its phosphorylation [7]. Elevated CSF tau levels are associated with neurodegeneration and are statistically associated with the progression from mild cognitive impairment to AD, and p-tau elevation reflects the formation of neurofibrillary tangles in the brain [8].

Since AD has a long asymptomatic period, risk factors such as hypertension are involved in its progression [1,9,10]. Hypertension is associated with a doubling in the likelihood of developing AD [2,9,11,12], and this risk increases if hypertension persists over the years [13]. In addition, hypertension causes oxidative stress and endothelial dysfunction, leading to blood vessel atrophy, which becomes particularly important with aging and is associated with cognitive impairment and increased Aß deposition in the brain [12].

Antihypertensives are of interest in dementia prevention due to their cerebrovascular structure protection and other mechanisms besides blood pressure control [13–16]. Nevertheless, not all antihypertensives have the same influence on AD, as their mechanisms of action differ. Antiadrenergic agents, such as the α-1-adrenoceptor antagonists, decrease peripheral vascular resistance [17] and are associated with (Aß) modulation [15,18]. On the other hand, diuretics may minimize cerebrovascular events and act on Aß peptides [15]. Vasodilator drugs enhance nitric oxide (NO), the role of which in AD is controversial [19]. Otherwise, diosmin stands out among the vascular vasoprotective agents because it reduces Aß and p-tau formation in mouse models [20], and ß-blockers may have the same effect on AD hallmarks [15]. Finally, calcium channel blockers (CCB) are highlighted due to their neuroprotective properties [15,21–24] and, along with the renin-angiotensin system (RAS)-acting agents, they both appear to be the most effective option in AD risk modulation [16]. In this sense, the angiotensin-converting enzyme inhibitors (ACEi) and the angiotensin II receptor blockers (ARBs) stand out as the main drugs acting on the RAS system. They both are associated with AD risk reduction, but their mechanisms of action differ. While the ACEi prevent the inactivation of bradykinin and the formation of Angiotensin II (1–8), affecting AT1R and AT2R [25,26], ARBs are AT1 receptor antagonists, and, therefore, they enhance AT2, Ang IV, and Ang (1–7) receptors [3,25–29].

For all the above, the present study aims to evaluate the associations between antihypertensive treatments and AD CSF biomarkers.

2. Materials and Methods

2.1. Participants and Study Design

The present work is a retrospective case-control study conducted at the Neurology Unit of the University and Polytechnic Hospital La Fe (Valencia, Spain). The Ethics Committee for Biomedical Research at CEU Cardenal Herrera University and the Medicaments Research Ethics Committee at the Health Research Institute Hospital La Fe have approved this study (CEI21/052 and 202-705-1).

The participants were recruited through a medical interview between January 2017 and December 2020. The enrolled patients received information and signed the informed consent, following the Declaration of Helsinki, the Good Clinical Practices, and local regulations.

The inclusion criteria for this study were to be between 50 and 80 years old, sign the informed consent, and have medical records of CFS biomarkers (Aβ42, t-tau, p-tau), neuropsychological evaluation, and medication intake. The exclusion criteria for the present study were not to meet the inclusion criteria, be enrolled in a clinical trial, have other neurological diseases such as epilepsy, multiple sclerosis, or brain damage, or have psychiatric disorders, such as depression (major disorder) or bipolar disorder. In addition, patients with severe dementia or previous disabilities were excluded.

The patients' diagnoses were based on The National Institute on Aging-Alzheimer's Association clinical criteria [30]. Therefore, a neuropsychological evaluation based on the Clinical Dementia Rating (CDR) [31], the Repeatable Battery for the Assessment of Neuropsychological Status-Delayed Memory (RBANS.DM) [32], the Mini-Mental State Examination (MMSE) [33], the Functionality Assessment Questionnaire (FAQ) [34], and the AD Cooperative Study ADL Scale for Mild Cognitive Impairment (SDCS-ADL-MCI) [35] were performed. In addition, neuroimaging and CFS biomarkers (ß42, t-tau, p-tau, tau/Aß42 ratio) were assessed. Patients were "and tau/Aß42 ratio were found. Neuropsychological evaluation was considered to optimize a patient's diagnosis and establish a patient's cognitive decline stage. Patients with normal CSF levels and who were cognitively healthy were classified as control participants. All efforts were made to include a biologically defined control group (CSF biomarkers) in the study.

2.2. Data Source and Variables

The patients were anonymized, and the electronic health system was used to perform an exhaustive review of their medical records at the Polytechnic University Hospital La Fe (Valencia). Thus, age, sex, smoking history, and comorbidities such as hypertension were registered. Furthermore, total and high-density lipoprotein (HDL) cholesterol, as well as blood pressure levels, were calculated from the average of two or more measurements, preferably within six months before or after diagnosis. Those variables were gathered at the participant's hospital and related healthcare centers.

CSF samples were obtained as part of the diagnosis protocol at the Polytechnic University Hospital La Fe (Valencia). From 5 to 10 mL of CSF was collected and stored at $-80\ °C$ until analysis. Biochemical determinations (Aβ42, t-tau, p-tau) were carried out by a chemiluminescence immunoassay [36]. Specifically, the CSF biomarker cut-off established for t-tau/Aβ42 was >0.51 and was >485, >56, and <725 pg/mL for t-tau, p-tau, and Aβ42, respectively [37].

An antihypertensive treatment prescription was acquired by a medical history review, and it was registered by Yes/No using the Anatomical Therapeutical Chemical (ATC) code of the WHO Collaborating Centre for Drug Statistics Methodology (WHO) "https://www.whocc.no/atc_ddd_index/ (accessed on 1 May 2021)". ATCs were firstly regrouped and analyzed by therapeutic subgroup (2nd ATC level) and, secondly, by introducing agents acting on the RAS as their pharmacological subgroup (3rd level). As for the C02 ATC group, only doxazosin was found. Thus, for greater clarity, reference to this group will be made directly to this active ingredient. The same situation was performed with vasoprotective medication, with calcium dobesilate as the representative drug. Finally, the duration of treatment was represented in months.

2.3. Statistical Analysis

The data were summarized using the median (1st and 3rd quartiles) for the numeric variables and the absolute frequency (%) for the qualitative variables. The biomarkers were log-transformed to avoid skewed data.

On the one hand, logistic regression models were performed to assess the relationship between clinical classification attending to CSF biomarkers (AD group, control group) and age, gender, and systolic and diastolic blood pressure. In addition, 2-way interactions with systolic blood pressure (SBP) X "antihypertensives", diastolic blood pressure (DBP) X "antihypertensives", and hypertension X "antihypertensives" were explored. Finally, conditional effects with their 95% CI were depicted.

On the other hand, elastic net linear regression models were adjusted for each biomarker (β42 amyloid, t-tau, p-tau, and t-tau/β42 ratio) to select their associated characteristics. The general model included the following variables: age, sex, SBP, DBP, diabetes mellitus type 2, total cholesterol, smoking habit, number of chronic treatments, and antihypertensive drugs intake (doxazosin, diuretics, peripheral vasodilators, calcium dobesilate, beta-blocking agents, calcium channel blockers, plain ACEI, combinations of ACEi, plain ARBs, and combinations of ARBs).

The elastic net regularization method of the estimated beta coefficients improves upon ordinary least squares. It linearly combines the L1 and L2 penalties of the lasso and ridge methods. The regularization parameter λ determines the amount of regularization. An optimal value for λ was determined by performing a 10-fold cross-validation, which yielded the minimum cross-validated mean-squared error (CVM). A median of 1000 repetitions of the cross-validation was calculated to improve lambda's robustness.

The ARBs and ACEi and their relation to t-tau/β42 amyloid were analyzed by multivariable logistic regression. Multiple comparisons were performed to assess the differences in the before-mentioned groups. The goodness of fit for the adjusted model was carried out using simulated scale residual diagnostics.

All the statistical analyses were performed using R (V. 4.0.3.) and the packages glmnet (V.4.1-3), click (V.0.8.0), ggeffects (V.1.1.1), ggplot2 (V.3.3.5), and DHARMa (V. 0,4.4).

3. Results

3.1. Participants

Seven hundred and forty-six participants were enrolled in the present study. From these, duplicated records due to follow-up ($n = 31$), patients without CSF biomarkers (n = 143), those diagnosed with other dementias (non-AD), or those with moderate or severe dementia due to AD ($n= 273$) were not included. Finally, the patients without medical records of total cholesterol levels or blood pressure ($n = 17$) or with the simultaneous prescription of ARBs or ACEi ($n = 2$) were excluded (see Figure 1).

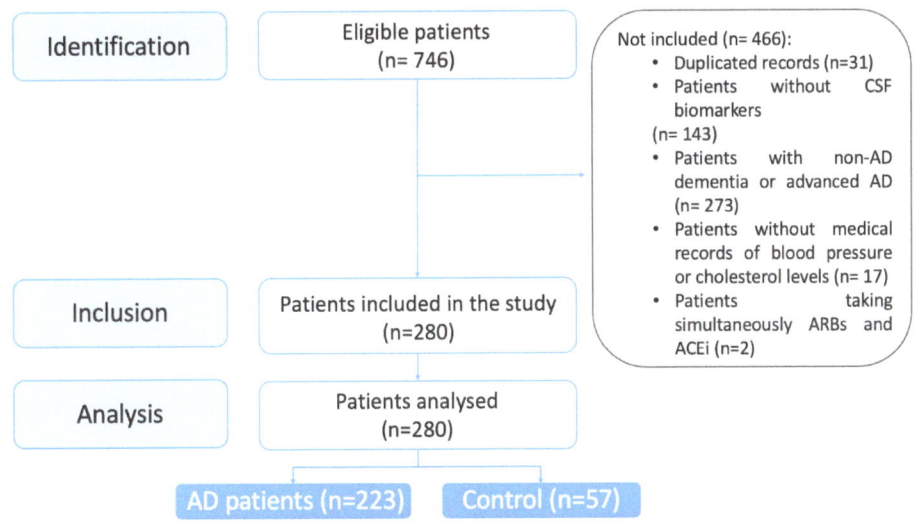

Figure 1. STROBE participant's selection flow chart. ACEi= angiotensin-converting enzyme inhibitor; AD = Alzheimer's Disease; ARBs = angiotensin II receptor blockers; CSF = cerebrospinal fluid.

From the initial cohort, 280 patients were included. They were classified as AD and cognitively healthy patients, according to their CSF levels. Thus, 57 participants were considered cognitively healthy patients (controls) and 223 were considered AD patients (cases), of whom 160 patients (71.75%) had mild cognitive impairment due to AD and 63 patients (28.25%) had mild dementia due to AD.

3.2. Demographic and Clinical Data of Participants

Table 1 shows the demographic and clinical variables for each group of participants. As can be seen, the AD patients were older than the controls, were predominantly female, and had more chronic concomitant medications prescribed.

Table 1. Demographic and clinical variables for the participants' groups.

Variable	AD (n = 223)	Control (n = 57)
Age (years, median (IQR))	71 (67.5, 74)	65 (62, 69)
Sex (female, n (%))	135 (60.54%)	25 (43.86%)
CSF biomarkers		
Aß42 levels (pg/mL, median (IQR))	600 (468.04, 702.1)	1206.15 (996, 1472)
t-tau levels (pg/mL, median (IQR))	586 (414, 837)	240 (182, 313)
p-tau levels (pg/mL, median (IQR))	92 (72.5, 131)	42 (32, 56)
Ratio t-tau/Aß42 (median (IQR))	0.94 (0.68, 1.43)	0.19 (0.14, 0.24)

Table 1. Cont.

Variable	AD (n = 223)	Control (n = 57)
Smoking history		
No (n, %)	145 (65.02%)	34 (59.65%)
No (Ex-smoker), (n, %)	45 (20.18%)	10 (17.54%)
Yes (n, %)	33 (14.8%)	13 (22.81%)
Number of concomitant medications	5 (3, 7)	3 (2, 5)
Total cholesterol (mg/dL, median (IQR))	189 (165.25, 212)	196 (170, 222)
HDL cholesterol (mg/dL, median (IQR))	55.5 (47, 66.25)	55 (44, 67.6)
Lipid-modifying agents (n, %)	123 (55.16%)	28 (49.12%)
Antidiabetic drugs (n, %)	36 (16.14%)	11 (19.3%)
Systolic blood pressure (mmHg, median (IQR))	135 (124.58, 143.42)	130 (118, 139)
Diastolic blood pressure (DBP) (mmHg, median (IQR))	75 (70, 81)	78 (71, 82.5)
Hypertension (n, %)	122 (54.71%)	30 (52.63%)

Aß42 = ß amyloid 42; CSF = cerebrospinal fluid; dL = deciliter; IQR = interquartile range; mg = milligrams; mL = milliliters; mmHg = millimeters of mercury; n = number of patients; pg = picograms; p-tau = phosphorylated tau; t-tau = total tau.

Regarding cardiovascular risk factors, the patients with AD were predominantly non-smokers and had lower total cholesterol levels. In contrast, they had a greater rate of lipid-modifying prescription, SBP levels, and hypertension than the control patients. However, the control patients were more prone to taking antidiabetic drugs and having higher DBP than the case group (Table 1).

3.3. Hypertension and Alzheimer's Disease

Multivariate logistic regression was performed. In addition, age, gender, and blood pressure levels were analyzed and compared to the presence of AD. SBP and antihypertensive prescription statistical interaction were explored without significant differences. Thus, the [SBP x antihypertensive intake] interaction was removed.

A positive association was found between the likelihood of suffering from AD and age (OR = 1.174, IC95% [1.105; 1.255], p-value < 0.001) and higher SBP (OR = 1.036, IC95% [1.004; 1.071], p-value = 0.033). On the contrary, men seemed less likely to develop AD than women despite the result being non-significant (OR = 0.513, IC95% [0.246; 1.051], p-value = 0.07). No differences were found regarding diastolic blood pressure and antihypertensive intake (see Table S1 of Supplementary Information).

3.4. Antihypertensive Drugs and Alzheimer's Disease Biomarkers

Each therapeutic subgroup prescription was examined to assess whether antihypertensive drugs are associated with AD (Table 2). As can be seen, the AD patients were older when the first antihypertensive drug was prescribed and took the medication for more years. In addition, ß-blocking agents and CCB were consumed more among the AD patients, whereas diuretics and agents acting on RAS were the most common drugs among the control patients.

Moreover, all the models associated older age with impaired CFS biomarkers levels (Table 3). Additionally, a trend was observed between antidiabetic consumption and higher Aß42 and lower t-tau/Aß42, whereas being male seemed to be linked to lower t-tau levels. CCB seemed to be associated with a higher t-tau/ß42 amyloid ratio. Finally, plain ACEi drugs were associated with higher t-tau and t-tau/ß42 amyloid levels, whereas combinations of ARBs were related to lower levels of this biomarker.

Table 2. Antihypertensive prescription for the participants' groups.

Variable	AD (n = 223)	Control (n = 57)
Antihypertensive drugs prescription (n, %)	116 (52.02%)	29 (50.88%)
Age at first prescribed antihypertensive treatment (years, median (IQR))	61 (58, 65)	56 (53, 62)
Years since 1st antihypertensive treatment prescription (years, median (IQR))	7 (0, 11)	2 (0, 10)
Number of antihypertensives daily intake (n, %)		
0	107 (47.98%)	28 (49.12%)
1	59 (26.46%)	11 (19.3%)
2	40 (17.94%)	11 (19.3%)
3	16 (7.17%)	6 (10.53%)
4	1 (0.45%)	0 (0%)
5	0 (0%)	1 (1.75%)
Doxazosin prescription (n, %)	2 (0.9%)	2 (3.51%)
Diuretics prescription (n, %)	9 (4.04%)	3 (5.26%)
Peripheral vasodilators (n, %)	3 (1.35%)	1 (1.75%)
Calcium dobesilate prescription (n, %)	0 (0%)	1 (1.75%)
Beta-blocking agents prescription (n, %)	20 (8.97%)	1 (1.75%)
Calcium channel blockers prescription (n, %)	36 (16.14%)	8 (14.04%)
Agents acting on the renin-angiotensin system (n, %)	90 (40.36%)	25 (43.86%)

IQR = Interquartile range; n = number of patients.

Table 3. Elastic net model for CSF biomarkers (Aß-42, p-tau, t-tau, ratio t-tau/Aß42) from antihypertensive variables.

Variable	Aß42 Model (Estimate)	p-tau Model (Estimate)	t-tau Model (Estimate)	Ratio tau/Aß42 Amyloid Model (Estimate)
Sex (male)	-	-	−0.087	−0.1
Age	−0.015	0.015	0.024	0.047
Antidiabetic drugs	0.043	-	-	−0.035
Total cholesterol (mg/dL)	-	-	−0.001	−0.001
Diastolic blood pressure	-	-	−0.002	-
Number of antihypertensives	0	-	-	-
Doxazosin prescription	0.123	-	−0.107	−0.481
Calcium dobesilate prescription	0.175	-	-	−0.421
Calcium channel blockers	-	-	-	0.053
ACEi, plain	-	-	0.059	0.05
ARBs, combinations	-	-	−0.041	−0.206
lambda	0.067	0.123	0.069	0.075

Alpha = 0.5. ACEi = Angiotensin-converting enzyme inhibitors; ARBs = Angiotensin receptor blockers; Aß42 = ß amyloid 42; dL = deciliter; p-tau = phosphorylated tau; t-tau = total tau.

3.5. ACEi and ARBs Pharmacological Subgroups

Since ARBs and ACEi showed opposite t-tau/Aß42 ratio effects (Table 3), a deeper analysis was performed (Table 4). As a result, it was observed that a significant proportion of the patients with AD were taking ACEi, whereas ARBs were the most consumed drugs among the control patients. Moreover, almost all the control patients were taking plain ACEi.

Table 4. Renin-angiotensin drugs subgroups consumption between AD and control patients.

Variable	AD	Control
Angiotensin-converting enzyme inhibitors prescription (n, (%))	40 (17.94)	5 (8.77)
Angiotensin-converting enzyme inhibitors prescription duration (months, median (IQR))	42 (11, 106)	19 (1, 48)
Plain angiotensin-converting enzyme inhibitors prescription prescription (n, (%))	30 (13.45)	1 (1.75)
Combinations of angiotensin-converting enzyme inhibitors prescription prescription (n, (%))	10 (4.48%)	4 (7.02%)
Angiotensin-converting enzyme inhibitors prescription without medical records of angiotensin II receptor blockers prescription (n, (%))	33 (14.8%)	4 (7.02%)
Angiotensin II receptor blockers prescription (n, (%))	50 (22.42%)	20 (35.09%)
Angiotensin II receptor blockers duration (months, median (IQR))	83 (56.75, 118.75)	69 (39, 95)
Plain angiotensin II receptor blockers (n, (%))	21 (9.42%)	7 (12.28%)
Combinations of angiotensin II receptor blockers (n, (%))	29 (13%)	12 (21.05%)
Angiotensin II receptor blockers prescription without medical records of angiotensin-converting enzyme inhibitors prescription (n, (%))	43 (19.28)	18 (31.58)

IQR = Interquartile range; n = number of patients.

Firstly, it was observed that the consumption of ARBs was significantly associated with a lower t-tau/Aß42 ratio when compared to ACEi (see Figure 2).

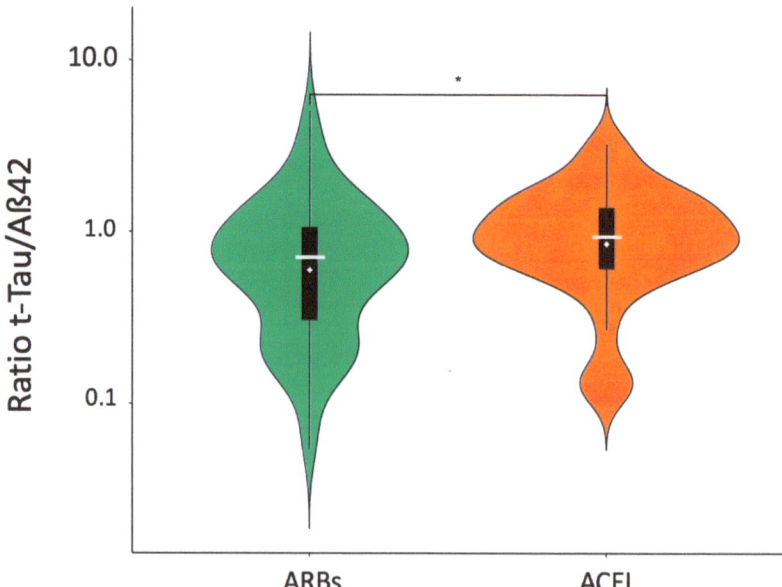

Figure 2. Comparison of ARBs and ACEi consumption with t-tau/Aß42 ratio values using violin model. * = Level of significance is provided by Wilcox Test. Aß42 = Amyloid beta 42; ACEi = Angiotensin-converting enzyme inhibitors; ARBs = Angiotensin receptor blockers; t-tau = total CSF tau levels; t-tau = total tau.

Secondly, multivariable logistic regression was performed to confirm the abovementioned results and predict the t-tau/Aß42 ratio association with ARBs and ACEi (see Table S2). The model included sex and age as covariables because they seemed to be the variables with the strongest association with AD. It was observed that combinations of ARBs consumption were associated with a 30% lower t-tau/Aß42 ratio than plain ACEi consumption (estimate = −0.334, IC95%, [−0.613, −0.055], p-value = 0.019).

Thirdly, statistical differences in the t-tau/Aß42 ratio between patients taking combinations of ARBs and patients consuming plain ACEi were observed (estimate = −0.5242, IC95% (−0.1984; −2.643), p-value = 0.026), as well as between patients taking combinations of ARBs and those not taking plain ACEi or combinations of ARBs (estimate = −0.3339, IC95% (0.1418; −2.354), p-value = 0.0485) (Figure 3).

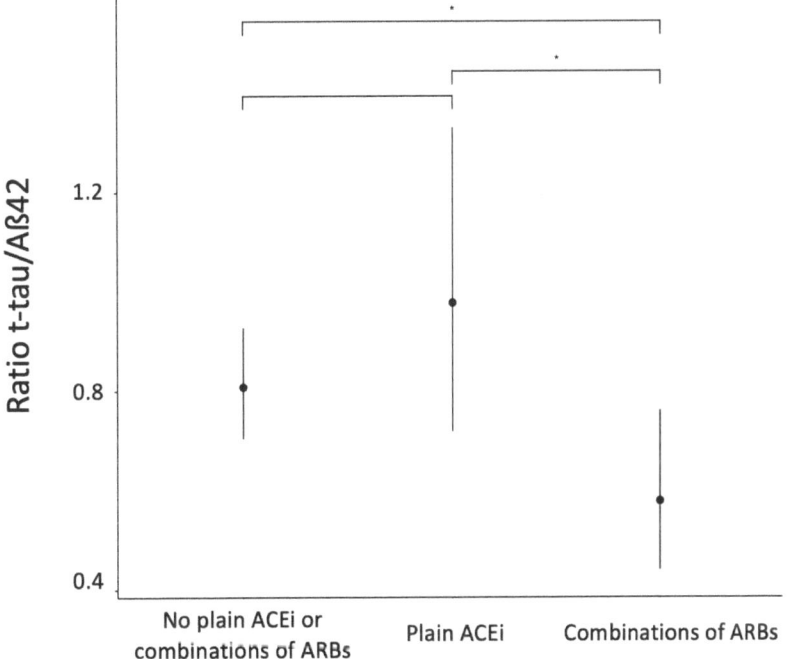

Figure 3. Conditional effects of t-tau/Aß42 ratio to combination ARBs and plain ACEi and Tukey multiples comparisons. Adjusted for age = 69 years, female. (*) = p-value <0.05. ß42 = Amyloid beta 42; ACEi = Angiotensin-converting enzyme inhibitors; ARBs = Angiotensin receptor blockers; t-tau = total tau.

4. Discussion

The present study compares the differences between the different antihypertensive treatments and the alteration of fluid biomarkers for AD. Previous studies point out that antihypertensive medication is associated with AD risk reduction, but they are mainly based on cognitive test evolution or dementia diagnosis conversion [22,38,39]. In order to follow a standardized biological criterion, CSF biomarkers were used in AD diagnosis. To our knowledge, this is one of the few antihypertensive studies in AD that defines case and control groups based on CSF biomarker levels. For instance, a clinical trial performed in 2012 about ACEi modulation of ACEs activity in CSF included fourteen volunteers [40]. Moreover, the study of Hestad and co-workers included eight patients with subjective memory complaints as a control group out of 72 subjects [8]. Finally, Nation et al. performed a study of antihypertensives based on CSF AD biomarkers in 2016, but it just included 124 patients [41].

This study shows that high SBP and AD are associated, which is consistent with the recent findings of Hestad et al. who found an association between SBP and CSF t-tau concentrations with lower delayed memory [8,41]. In addition, Affleck and co-workers showed in 2020 that the amyloid brain burden was lower in normotensive AD patients than in hypertense AD patients [2]. Hypertension seems to be associated with an increase in ß-secretase, the enzyme responsible for activating the amyloidogenic pathway of Aß production, and an increase in the Aß42/Aß40 ratio [12]. In addition, several studies affirm that the association between SBP and dementia is significant in midlife but not later life [13]. Altogether, it seems that vascular damage is associated with AD. Due to the long period that elapses from when the pathological pathways begin to be altered until the first symptoms appear, it is possible in middle age when this factor becomes especially important.

Furthermore, this study compares the association between antihypertensive use and abnormal AD CSF biomarkers. A previous study performed by Affleck and co-workers in 2020 revealed that patients who take this medication have lower neurofibrillary tangle formation [2]. Nevertheless, when Hestad et al. compared antihypertensive consumption and cognitive functions, they showed worse cognitive function in the antihypertensive consumption group [8].

We did not observe AD diagnosis or CSF biomarker differences in our group compared to antihypertensive consumption per se. Nevertheless, it was observed that the AD patients received their first antihypertensive drug at an older age and for more years in our cohort than the control patients. Therefore, antihypertensives may not avoid AD development, but they may affect mild cognitive impairment or progression by minimizing vascular damage at the early stages and through mechanisms other than blood pressure control [16]. As a result, each antihypertensive class was analyzed separately and compared in four AD-biomarker models.

First, doxazosin prescription was associated with higher CSF Aß42 concentrations and lower t-tau and a lower tau/Aß42 ratio. In addition, despite scarce literature about doxazosin and AD biomarkers, a recent study showed that doxazosin prevented Akt reduction, avoiding tau phosphorylation in an in vitro model of organotypic hippocampal cultures exposed to Aß [18]. However, our results must be taken carefully due to the reduced number of patients taking this drug in our cohort.

Regarding vasoprotective medication, calcium dobesilate releases NO, producing vasodilation [42,43]. The role of NO with biomarkers is controversial since it is involved in GSK-3ß activation and the consequent tau phosphorylation [19], as well as with Akt and cyclic-AMP-response-element-binding protein (CREB), which promotes cell survival and neuroprotection [44]. Recent studies indicate that an NO neuroprotective or neurotoxic effect depends on its concentration. It modulates heme-metals-Aß binding and plays a key role in Aß toxic effects [45]. In our cohort, calcium dobesilate seemed to be associated with higher CSF amyloid concentrations and a lower tau/Aß42 ratio. Nevertheless, only one patient was taking this antihypertensive in our sample, so further studies are needed to obtain conclusions.

As for beta-blocking agents, we did not observe any statistical difference between their consumption and AD hallmark alteration, which is consistent with previously published research [16]

In other matters, CCB highlights promising results in dementia prevention [15,22–24]. Intracellular calcium is elevated in elderly patients and plays a part in neurodegeneration, amyloid production enhancement, and tau hyperphosphorylation [15,16,23,46]. Thus, CCB may downregulate intracellular calcium levels and slow amyloid production [16,23]. In addition, CCB can enhance cerebral vascularization [15] and, in the case of nimodipine, can act as a cerebral vasodilator [46]. Among CCB, the dihydropyridine compounds stand out with promising results in Aß42 clearance [21,23]. Nevertheless, as shown in the work of Bachmeier et al., not all the dihydropyridines have the same effect on brain vasculature, and their effect on Aß42 clearance may not depend on blood–brain barrier (BBB) penetration. Whereas drugs such as nimodipine or nitrendipine are likely to enhance Aß clearance from the blood to the brain; others, such as amlodipine or nifedipine, do not seem to facilitate Aß42 transcytosis across the BBB in in vivo models, despite the fact that all of them can cross the BBB [21].

When we analyzed our cohort, we noticed that CCB was associated with a higher tau/Aß42 ratio and that the most CCB consumed was amlodipine. Moreover, just one patient took nimodipine when the lumbar puncture was performed. A recent study by Sadleir Id and colleagues aimed to explore whether nimodipine could modify amyloid pathogenesis when it begins in mouse models, but it did not show any changes in the Aß42 or total Aß levels nor amyloid plaque deposition [46]. In addition, it was shown in work performed by Murray and colleagues in 2002 that CCBs were not associated with dementia prevention. Most of the prescribed dihydropyridines in our study were the same that did not boost Aß42 clearance in a study performed by Bachmeier and colleagues in 2011 [21,39]. Moreover, in the Baltimore Longitudinal Study of Aging, CCB did not reduce the incidence risk of AD [47], an effect that was neither observed in the Gingko Evaluation of Memory Study [48] nor the NIVALD study, the phase III clinical trial that tested nivaldipine vs. placebo in AD patients [49].

Altogether, it could explain why we did not observe a protective effect in our sample, although further studies are needed to elucidate the exact mechanism by which amlodipine may increase the tau/Aß42 ratio.

Lastly, RAS drugs stand out among the antihypertensive drugs thanks to their potential ability to limit Aß plaques [14] and neurofibrillary tangle formation [2,14]. There is evidence of a dysregulation of endogenous RAS activity in AD patients, which has been confirmed in post-mortem brain tissue [14,27]. As recently reviewed by Gouveia and colleagues, ARBs and ACEi may be more effective at preventing AD than other antihypertensives [14,16,24,29]. Nevertheless, the bibliography suggests that certain ACEi are associated with the risk of dementia [12], whereas ARBs may act as neuroprotectors [16,29]. As a result, studying the effects of both drugs and their influence on CSF AD biomarkers is of interest.

The ACEi mechanism of action prevents the formation of Angiotensin II (1–8) and the degradation of plasma bradykinin through ACE inhibition, thus, contributing to inflammation, vascular and blood–brain barrier permeability, and impaired cerebral flow [50–54].

Moreover, ACE1 degrades Aß-42 into Aß40, its soluble form [3,55], and studies show that ACEi can modify ACEs activity in CSF [40]. As a result, if ACE becomes blocked by ACEi, the clearance of Aß42 may not succeed, and plaques may accumulate in the brain [41].

Conversely, ACE inhibition may enhance the bradykinin concentrations in plasma and B1R and B2R activity in microglial cells [56]. B2R expresses constitutively under normal conditions, is activated in acute inflammation [51,53,57–59], and has a higher affinity for bradykinin and Lys-bradykinin peptides [53,58]. However, B1R is upregulated by chronic inflammation [53,58,60] and has a higher affinity for Lys-des-Arg9-BK and des-Arg9-BK [50,51,53,57,58,61]. Moreover, the B1R-derived pro-inflammatory cytokine release may contribute to BBB permeability and its disruption [58], being an essential pathophysiological mediator of cerebrovascular dysfunction, neuroinflammation, and Aß pathology in AD [62].

Furthermore, higher bradykinin levels are linked to Aß deposition, and its presence may enhance B1R, accentuating amyloid toxicity. In addition, the Aß42-amyloid peptide can induce the plasma contact system and activate the kallikrein-kinin system (KKS) because of its negative charge [51,52,56]. As a result, an increase in bradykinin production takes place, enhancing cerebral inflammation and vascular permeability [50–54] and up-regulating bradykinin receptors again (Figure 4).

On the contrary, there is evidence that ARBs reduce the Aß burden in mice models and can reduce p-tau and neurofibrillary tangles in the hippocampus [29]. Their neuroprotector effect is attributed, in part, to AT1R blockade while stimulating AT2R, AT4R, and MasR [63].

AT1R can release aldosterone and cause vasoconstriction, fluid retention, and the M1 phenotype of microglial cell activation, which releases pro-inflammatory cytokines [29,63].

In addition, AT1R is related to hypertension, heart dysfunction, brain ischemia, abnormal stress responses, BBB breakdown, and inflammation [64]. Thus, the AT1R/Ang II axis links to pro-inflammatory and prooxidant effects, increasing BBB permeability [3,29], as well as cognitive impairment and tau hyperphosphorylation through the activation of GSK3ß [14], which has an essential role in the modulation of insulin [7]. Moreover, microglial activation is higher in elderly patients, and Aß pathogenesis may exacerbate this process [3].

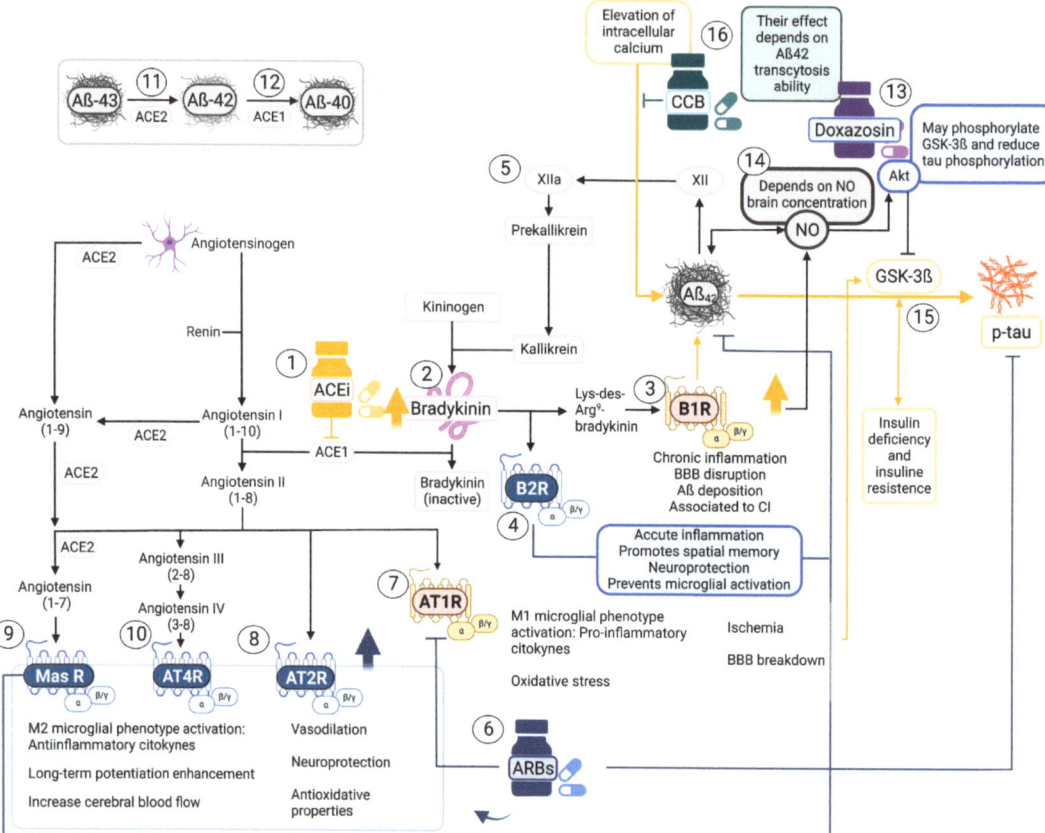

Figure 4. Proposed mechanism of action among antihypertensive drugs and CSF amyloid and tau alterations. Pathological processes are represented in yellow, whereas neuroprotective mechanisms appear in blue. Created with BioRender.com. Aß40 = Amyloid beta 40; Aß42 = Amyloid beta 42; ACEi = Angiotensin-converting enzyme inhibitors; ACE1 = Angiotensin-converting enzyme 1; ACE2 = Angiotensin-converting enzyme 2; Akt = Protein kinase B; ARBs = Angiotensin receptor blockers; AT1 = Angiotensin 1 Receptor; AT2 = Angiotensin 2 Receptor; AT4R = Angiotensin 4 Receptor; B1R = Bradykinin 1 receptor; B2R = Bradykinin 2 receptor; CCB = Calcium Channel Blocker; GSK-3ß = Glycogen synthase kinase 3ß; MasR = Mitochondrial Assembly Receptor; NO = nitric oxide; p-tau = phosphorylated tau.

Conversely, AT2R causes angiogenesis, an NO increase, vasodilation, and the activation of the M2 phenotype of microglial cells, thereby releasing anti-inflammatory cytokines [29,63].

MasR produces anti-inflammatory, anti-oxidative, anti-fibrotic, vasodilation, and M2 activation effects [27,63], improving memory, learning, and long-period potentiation in mouse models [27]. Finally, insulin-regulated aminopeptidase is associated with vasodilation and long-term potentiation enhancement [3,28].

Interestingly, AT1R is expressed more in the brain than AT2R [29]. As a result, drugs acting as AT1R antagonists may promote AT2R, MasR, and insulin-regulated activation, which may become significant in cognitive abilities. Other described mechanisms of action by which ARBs may have a protector role in AD are neuronal differentiation, DNA repair, the modulation of the cerebral microvasculature, the reversion of oxidative stress and inflammation, and ischemic brain injury prevention [41].

This work shows a positive association between the tau/Aß42 ratio and the use of ACEi, with an opposite effect when compared to using ARBs in combination (Figure 4). These findings are broadly consistent with slower Aß [28,65] and tau progression when ARBs are consumed instead of ACEi.

The previously described mechanisms may explain why we observed a higher t-tau/Aß42 ratio in patients taking ACEi and its contrary effect in patients taking ARBs. Compared to published work, metanalysis shows similar results in dementia risk prevention with ARBs consumption, whereas ACEi does not seem to reduce the risk of dementia [16,25] or reduce its risk less than ARBs [26]. In addition, the longitudinal study by Nation et el. in 2016 showed higher CSF Aß42 levels and lower p-tau levels over time when ARBs treated patients were compared to patients not taking antihypertensives. This study showed that Aß42 reduction was independent of age, the most influential risk factor of AD [41]. Finally, a metanalysis performed by D'Silva et al. in 2022 shows how other clinical trials in which ARBs were compared to a placebo obtained conflicting results. One trial showed less deterioration in episodic memory and attention, whereas others did not show differences. Moreover, when compared to CBB, cognitive improvements were not observed, but an increase in cerebral blood flow in several brain regions, including the parietal lobe, was observed [26].

Finally, it must be noted that in our study, ARBs showed a protective effect in combination with diuretics, which is the most prescribed combination. In this sense, several studies pointed out the possible role of diuretics in AD risk reduction [38,48]. Their possible role may be due to the effect of these drugs on reducing cerebrovascular events, such as silent vascular lesions, that are involved in white matter changes, a common hallmark in AD and other dementias [38]. In addition, diuretics may act as AD risk reducers by their vasorelaxant effect, which may counteract the vasoconstriction produced by amyloid pathogenesis [38,48]. Among them, thiazide diuretics and potassium-sparing diuretics stand out as AD risk reducers in the Cache County study [22]. Thus, the protective role of ARBs could be enhanced by the neuroprotector properties that diuretics seem to have.

Strengths and Limitations

A strength of the present study is that the medications were registered according to exact dates and exact doses. In addition, the participants were classified as attending to CSF biomarkers levels, while most antihypertensive studies that correlate this medication with AD are based only on cognitive tests. In this sense, the present study provides an objective and accurate AD diagnosis.

It should be considered that the inclusion criteria for this study were to consent to a lumbar puncture, which is an invasive intervention that dissuades potential participants, especially cognitively healthy adults. In spite of the required invasive sampling with some adverse side effects (headaches, pain), a relevant number of cognitively healthy participants was included in the present study. This is a strength because, to our knowledge, there are few studies about antihypertensives with a control sample based on CSF biomarkers, and published work has a few participants. On the contrary, this fact is also a limitation, and future studies including more participants are needed.

Lastly, it must be considered that the study was performed at an outpatient consultation center of the Cognitive Disorders Unit, where other healthcare professionals refer patients due to pathological suspicion or memory complaints. Moreover, adherence has not been verified, and genetic risk factors such as APOE e4 have not been analyzed.

5. Conclusions

High SBP, elderly age, and female gender are variables associated with a higher risk of AD diagnosis. In addition, calcium channel blockers and plain ACEi consumption are associated with a higher tau/Aß42 ratio, whereas consuming ARBs is associated with a lower tau/Aß42 ratio. Thus, ARBs should be considered a primary antihypertensive option for patients at risk of AD.

Supplementary Materials: The following supporting information can be downloaded at https://www.mdpi.com/article/10.3390/pharmaceutics15030924/s1, Table S1: Multivariate logistic regression to obtain the risk of AD from SBP and DBP and controlled by age, sex and antihypertensive intake; Table S2: Association between t-tau/Aß42 ratio and sex, age, ARBs and ACEi drugs:ç; Table S3: Relationship between renin-angiotensin-system- acting agents and Alzheimer's Disease biomarkers.

Author Contributions: Conceptualization, C.C.-P., L.M.R., M.B. and G.G.-L.; methodology, G.G.-L., C.P.-B., M.B. and A.J.C.-M.; formal analysis, A.J.C.-M.; investigation and data curation, G.G.-L.; writing—original draft preparation, G.G.-L.; writing—review and editing, C.C.-P., L.M.R., M.B. and G.G.-L.; supervision, C.C.-P., L.M.R. and M.B.; funding acquisition, Catedra DeCo. All authors have read and agreed to the published version of the manuscript.

Funding: This research was funded by Cathedra DeCo Micof-UCH and by Instituto de Salud Carlos III through the project PI19/00570 (Co-funded by European Union, "A way to make Europe").

Institutional Review Board Statement: The study was conducted in accordance with the Declaration of Helsinki and was approved by the Ethics Committee for Biomedical Research at CEU Cardenal Herrera University and the Medicaments Research Ethics Committee at the Health Research Institute Hospital La Fe (CEI21/052, 26MAY2021 and 202-705-1, 27JAN2021).

Informed Consent Statement: Informed consent was obtained from all the subjects involved in the study.

Data Availability Statement: The data presented in this study are available on request from the corresponding author.

Acknowledgments: C.C.-P. acknowledges a postdoctoral "Miguel Servet" grant CPII21/00006 and a FIS PI19/00570 grant from the Health Institute Carlos III (Spanish Ministry of Economy, Industry and Innovation) and a predoctoral "PFIS" grant FI20/00022 from the Health Institute Carlos III. The authors are grateful to Cathedra DeCo Micof-UCH, GINEA's team, and all the participants and caregivers of the study participants.

Conflicts of Interest: The authors declare no conflict of interest.

References

1. Breijyeh, Z.; Karaman, R. Comprehensive Review on Alzheimer's Disease: Causes and Treatment. *Molecules* **2020**, *25*, 5789. [CrossRef] [PubMed]
2. Affleck, A.J.; Sachdev, P.S.; Stevens, J.; Halliday, G.M. Antihypertensive medications ameliorate Alzheimer's disease pathology by slowing its propagation. *Alzheimer's Dement.* **2020**, *6*, e12060. [CrossRef]
3. Ribeiro, V.T.; de Souza, L.C.; Simões e Silva, A.C. Renin-Angiotensin System and Alzheimer's Disease Pathophysiology: From the Potential Interactions to Therapeutic Perspectives. *Protein Pept. Lett.* **2020**, *27*, 484–511. [CrossRef] [PubMed]
4. Álvarez, I.; Diez-Fairen, M.; Aguilar, M.; González, J.M.; Ysamat, M.; Tartari, J.P.; Carcel, M.; Alonso, A.; Brix, B.; Arendt, P.; et al. Added value of cerebrospinal fluid multimarker analysis in diagnosis and progression of dementia. *Eur. J. Neurol.* **2021**, *28*, 1142–1152. [CrossRef]
5. Peña-Bautista, C.; Roca, M.; López-Cuevas, R.; Baquero, M.; Vento, M.; Chafer-Pericas, C. Metabolomics study to identify plasma biomarkers in alzheimer disease: ApoE genotype effect. *J. Pharm. Biomed. Anal.* **2020**, *180*, 113088. [CrossRef] [PubMed]
6. Uddin, M.S.; Kabir, M.T.; Rahman, M.S.; Behl, T.; Jeandet, P.; Ashraf, G.M.; Najda, A.; Bin-Jumah, M.N.; El-Seedi, H.R.; Abdel-Daim, M.M. Revisiting the Amyloid Cascade Hypothesis: From Anti-Aβ Therapeutics to Auspicious New Ways for Alzheimer's Disease. *Int. J. Mol. Sci.* **2020**, *21*, 5858. [CrossRef]
7. Zhang, Y.; Huang, N.Q.; Yan, F.; Jin, H.; Zhou, S.Y.; Shi, J.S.; Jin, F. Diabetes mellitus and Alzheimer's disease: GSK-3β as a potential link. *Behav. Brain Res.* **2018**, *339*, 57–65. [CrossRef]

8. Hestad, K.A.; Horndalsveen, P.O.; Engedal, K. Blood Pressure and T-Tau in Spinal Fluid Are Associated With Delayed Recall in Participants With Memory Complaints and Dementia of the Alzheimer's Type. *Front. Aging Neurosci.* **2021**, *13*, 685. [CrossRef]
9. Hahad, O.; Lelieveld, J.; Birklein, F.; Lieb, K.; Daiber, A.; Münzel, T. Ambient air pollution increases the risk of cerebrovascular and neuropsychiatric disorders through induction of inflammation and oxidative stress. *Int. J. Mol. Sci.* **2020**, *21*, 4306. [CrossRef]
10. Ramos, H.; Moreno, L.; Gil, M.; García-Lluch, G.; Sendra-Lillo, J.; Alacreu, M. Pharmacists' Knowledge of Factors Associated with Dementia: The A-to-Z Dementia Knowledge List. *Int. J. Environ. Res. Public Health* **2021**, *18*, 9934. [CrossRef]
11. Organización Mundial de la Salud. Envejecimiento y salud. *Cent Prensa OMS.* 2018, pp. 1–2. Available online: https://www.who.int/es/news-room/fact-sheets/detail/envejecimiento-y-salud (accessed on 5 May 2020).
12. Wahidi, N.; Lerner, A.J. Blood Pressure Control and Protection of the Aging Brain. *Neurotherapeutics* **2019**, *16*, 569–579. [CrossRef]
13. Livingston, G.; Huntley, J.; Sommerlad, A.; Ames, D.; Ballard, C.; Banerjee, S.; Brayne, C.; Burns, A.; Cohen-Mansfield, J.; Cooper, C.; et al. Dementia prevention, intervention, and care: 2020 report of the Lancet Commission. *Lancet* **2020**, *396*, 413–446. [CrossRef]
14. Wharton, W.; Zhao, L.; Steenland, K.; Goldstein, F.C.; Schneider, J.A.; Barnes, L.L.; Gearing, M.; Yasar, S. Neurofibrillary Tangles and Conversion to Mild Cognitive Impairment with Certain Antihypertensives. *J. Alzheimers Dis.* **2019**, *70*, 153–161. [CrossRef] [PubMed]
15. Lebouvier, T.; Chen, Y.; Duriez, P.; Pasquier, F.; Bordet, R. Antihypertensive agents in Alzheimer's disease: Beyond vascular protection. *Expert Rev. Neurother.* **2020**, *20*, 175–187. [CrossRef]
16. den Brok, M.G.; van Dalen, J.W.; Abdulrahman, H.; Larson, E.B.; van Middelaar, T.; van Gool, W.A.; van Charante, E.P.; Richard, E. Antihypertensive Medication Classes and the Risk of Dementia: A Systematic Review and Network Meta-Analysis. *J. Am. Med. Dir. Assoc.* **2021**, *22*, 1386–1395. [CrossRef] [PubMed]
17. Carretero, M. Doxazosina | Offarm. *Doxazosina.* 2002, pp. 176–178. Available online: https://www.elsevier.es/es-revista-offarm-4-articulo-doxazosina-13035880 (accessed on 24 April 2022).
18. Coelho, B.P.; Gaelzer, M.M.; dos Santos Petry, F.; Hoppe, J.B.; Trindade, V.M.; Salbego, C.G.; Guma, F.T. Dual Effect of Doxazosin: Anticancer Activity on SH-SY5Y Neuroblastoma Cells and Neuroprotection on an In Vitro Model of Alzheimer's Disease. *Neuroscience* **2019**, *404*, 314–325. [CrossRef]
19. Zhang, Y.-J.; Xu, Y.-F.; Liu, Y.-H.; Yin, J.; Wang, J.-Z. Nitric oxide induces tau hyperphosphorylation via glycogen synthase kinase-3b activation. *FEBS Lett.* **2005**, *579*, 6230–6236. [CrossRef]
20. Sawmiller, D.; Habib, A.; Li, S.; Darlington, D.; Hou, H.; Tian, J.; Shytle, R.D.; Smith, A.; Giunta, B.; Mori, T.; et al. Diosmin reduces cerebral Aβ levels, tau hyperphosphorylation, neuroinflammation, and cognitive impairment in the 3xTg-AD Mice. *J. Neuroimmunol.* **2016**, *299*, 98. [CrossRef]
21. Bachmeier, C.; Beaulieu-Abdelahad, D.; Mullan, M.; Paris, D. Selective dihydropyiridine compounds facilitate the clearance of β-amyloid across the blood-brain barrier. *Eur. J. Pharmacol.* **2011**, *659*, 124–129. [CrossRef]
22. Chuang, Y.F.; Breitner, J.C.; Chiu, Y.L.; Khachaturian, A.; Hayden, K.; Corcoran, C.; Tschanz, J.; Norton, M.; Munger, R.; Welsh-Bohmer, K.; et al. Use of diuretics is associated with reduced risk of Alzheimer's disease: The Cache County Study. *Neurobiol. Aging* **2014**, *35*, 2429–2435. [CrossRef] [PubMed]
23. Hwang, D.; Kim, S.; Choi, H.; Oh, I.H.; Kim, B.S.; Choi, H.R.; Kim, S.Y.; Won, C.W. Calcium-Channel Blockers and Dementia Risk in Older Adults—National Health Insurance Service—Senior Cohort (2002–2013). *Circ. J.* **2016**, *80*, 2336–2342. [CrossRef]
24. Barus, R.; Béné, J.; Deguil, J.; Gautier, S.; Bordet, R. Drug interactions with dementia-related pathophysiological pathways worsen or prevent dementia. *Br. J. Pharmacol.* **2019**, *176*, 3413–3434. [CrossRef]
25. Scotti, L.; Bassi, L.; Soranna, D.; Verde, F.; Silani, V.; Torsello, A.; Parati, G.; Zambon, A. Association between renin-angiotensin-aldosterone system inhibitors and risk of dementia: A meta-analysis. *Pharmacol. Res.* **2021**, *166*, 105515. [CrossRef] [PubMed]
26. D'Silva, E.; Meor Azlan, N.F.; Zhang, J. Angiotensin II Receptor Blockers in the Management of Hypertension in Preventing Cognitive Impairment and Dementia—A Systematic Review. *Pharmaceutics* **2022**, *14*, 2123. [CrossRef]
27. Evans, C.E.; Miners, J.S.; Piva, G.; Willis, C.L.; Heard, D.M.; Kidd, E.J.; Good, M.A.; Kehoe, P.G. ACE2 activation protects against cognitive decline and reduces amyloid pathology in the Tg2576 mouse model of Alzheimer's disease. *Acta Neuropathol.* **2020**, *139*, 485. [CrossRef] [PubMed]
28. Ouk, M.; Wu, C.Y.; Rabin, J.S.; Edwards, J.D.; Ramirez, J.; Masellis, M.; Swartz, R.H.; Herrmann, N.; Lanctôt, K.L.; Black, S.E.; et al. Associations between brain amyloid accumulation and the use of angiotensin-converting enzyme inhibitors versus angiotensin receptor blockers. *Neurobiol. Aging* **2021**, *100*, 22–31. [CrossRef] [PubMed]
29. Gouveia, F.; Camins, A.; Ettcheto, M.; Bicker, J.; Falcão, A.; Cruz, M.T.; Fortuna, A. Targeting brain Renin-Angiotensin System for the prevention and treatment of Alzheimer's disease: Past, present and future. *Ageing Res. Rev.* **2022**, *77*, 101612. [CrossRef]
30. Albert, M.S.; DeKosky, S.T.; Dickson, D.; Dubois, B.; Feldman, H.H.; Fox, N.C.; Gamst, A.; Holtzman, D.M.; Jagust, W.J.; Petersen, R.C.; et al. The diagnosis of mild cognitive impairment due to Alzheimer's disease: Recommendations from the National Institute on Aging-Alzheimer's Association workgroups on diagnostic guidelines for Alzheimer's disease. *Alzheimers Dement.* **2011**, *7*, 270–279. [CrossRef]
31. Hughes, C.P.; Berg, L.; Danziger, W.L.; Coben, L.A.; Martin, R.L. A new clinical scale for the staging of dementia. *Br. J. Psychiatry* **1982**, *140*, 566–572. [CrossRef]
32. Randolph, C.; Tierney, M.C.; Mohr, E.; Chase, T.N. The Repeatable Battery for the Assessment of Neuropsychological Status (RBANS): Preliminary clinical validity. *J. Clin. Exp. Neuropsychol.* **1998**, *20*, 310–319. [CrossRef]

33. Folstein, M.F.; Folstein, S.E.; McHugh, P.R. "Mini-mental state". A practical method for grading the cognitive state of patients for the clinician. *J. Psychiatr. Res.* **1975**, *12*, 189–198. [CrossRef]
34. Pfeffer, R.I.; Kurosaki, T.T.; Harrah, C.H.; Chance, J.M.; Filos, S. Measurement of functional activities in older adults in the community. *J. Gerontol.* **1982**, *37*, 323–329. [CrossRef] [PubMed]
35. Galasko, D.; Bennett, D.; Sano, M.; Ernesto, C.; Thomas, R.; Grundman, M.; Ferris, S. An inventory to assess activities of daily living for clinical trials in Alzheimer's disease. *Alzheimer Dis. Assoc. Disord.* **1997**, *11*, 33–39. [CrossRef]
36. Peña-Bautista, C.; López-Cuevas, R.; Cuevas, A.; Baquero, M.; Cháfer-Pericás, C. Lipid peroxidation biomarkers correlation with medial temporal atrophy in early Alzheimer Disease. *Neurochem. Int.* **2019**, *129*, 104519. [CrossRef]
37. Peña-Bautista, C.; Álvarez-Sánchez, L.; Ferrer, I.; López-Nogueroles, M.; Cañada-Martínez, A.J.; Oger, C.; Galano, J.M.; Durand, T.; Baquero, M.; Cháfer-Pericás, C. Lipid Peroxidation Assessment in Preclinical Alzheimer Disease Diagnosis. *Antioxidants* **2021**, *10*, 1043. [CrossRef]
38. Guo, Z.; Fratiglioni, L.; Zhu, L.; Fastbom, J.; Winblad, B.; Viitanen, M. Occurrence and Progression of Dementia in a Community Population Aged 75 Years and Older Relationship of Antihypertensive Medication Use. *Arch. Neurol.* **1999**, *56*, 991–996. [CrossRef] [PubMed]
39. Murray, M.D.; Lane, K.A.; Gao, S.; Evans, R.M.; Unverzagt, F.W.; Hall, K.S.; Hendrie, H. Preservation of cognitive function with antihypertensive medications: A longitudinal analysis of a community-based sample of African Americans. *Arch. Intern. Med.* **2002**, *162*, 2090–2096. [CrossRef]
40. Wharton, W.; Stein, J.H.; Korcarz, C.; Sachs, J.; Olson, S.R.; Zetterberg, H.; Dowling, M.; Ye, S.; Gleason, C.E.; Underbakke, G.; et al. The Effects of Ramipril in Individuals at Risk for Alzheimer's Disease: Results of a Pilot Clinical Trial NIH Public Access. *J. Alzheimers. Dis.* **2012**, *32*, 147–156. [CrossRef] [PubMed]
41. Nation, D.A.; Ho, J.; Yew, B. Older Adults Taking AT1-Receptor Blockers Exhibit Reduced Cerebral Amyloid Retention. *J. Alzheimer's Dis.* **2016**, *50*, 779–789. [CrossRef]
42. Angulo, J.; Cuevas, P.; Fernández, A.; Gabancho, S.; Videla, S.; Sáenz De Tejada, I. Calcium dobesilate potentiates endothelium-derived hyperpolarizing factor-mediated relaxation of human penile resistance arteries. *Br. J. Pharmacol.* **2003**, *139*, 854. [CrossRef]
43. Ruiz, E.; Lorente, R.; Tejerina, T. Effects of calcium dobesilate on the synthesis of endothelium-dependent relaxing factors in rabbit isolated aorta. *Br. J. Pharmacol.* **1997**, *121*, 711–716. [CrossRef] [PubMed]
44. Siciliano, R.; Barone, E.; Calabrese, V.; Rispoli, V.; Allan Butterfield, D.; Mancuso, C. Experimental research on nitric oxide and the therapy of Alzheimer disease: A challenging bridge. *CNS Neurol. Disord. Drug Targets* **2011**, *10*, 766–776. [CrossRef] [PubMed]
45. Kumar Nath, A.; Ghosh Dey, S. Dalton Transactions FRONTIER Simultaneous binding of heme and Cu with amyloid β peptides: Active site and reactivities. *Dalton Trans.* **2022**, *51*, 4986–4999. [CrossRef] [PubMed]
46. Sadleir Id, K.R.; Popovic, J.; Khatri, A.; Vassar, R. Oral nimodipine treatment has no effect on amyloid pathology or neuritic dystrophy in the 5XFAD mouse model of amyloidosis. *PLoS ONE* **2022**, *17*, e0263332. [CrossRef]
47. Yasar, S.; Corrada, M.; Brookmeyer, R.; Kawas, C. Calcium channel blockers and risk of AD: The Baltimore Longitudinal Study of Aging. *Neurobiol. Aging* **2005**, *26*, 157–163. [CrossRef]
48. Yasar, S.; Xia, J.; Yao, W.; Furberg, C.D.; Xue, Q.L.; Mercado, C.I.; Fitzpatrick, A.L.; Fried, L.P.; Kawas, C.H.; Sink, K.M.; et al. Antihypertensive drugs decrease risk of Alzheimer disease. *Neurology* **2013**, *81*, 896–903. [CrossRef] [PubMed]
49. Lawlor, B.; Segurado, R.; Kennelly, S.; Olde Rikkert, M.G.; Howard, R.; Pasquier, F.; Börjesson-Hanson, A.; Tsolaki, M.; Lucca, U.; Molloy, D.W.; et al. Nilvadipine in mild to moderate Alzheimer disease: A randomised controlled trial. *Fani Tsolaki-TagarakiID* **2018**, *25*, 39. [CrossRef]
50. Viel, T.; Buck, S.H. Kallikrein-kinin system mediated inflammation in Alzheimer's disease in vivo. *Curr. Alzheimer Res.* **2011**, *8*, 59–66. [CrossRef] [PubMed]
51. Asraf, K.; Torika, N.; Danon, A.; Fleisher-Berkovich, S. Involvement of the bradykinin B1 Receptor in microglial activation: In vitro and in vivo studies. *Front. Endocrinol. (Lausanne)* **2017**, *8*, 82. [CrossRef]
52. Chen, Z.L.; Singh, P.; Wong, J.; Horn, K.; Strickland, S.; Norris, E.H. An antibody against HK blocks Alzheimer's disease peptide β-amyloid-induced bradykinin release in human plasma. *Proc. Natl. Acad. Sci. USA* **2019**, *116*, 22921–22923. [CrossRef]
53. Dutra, R.C. Kinin receptors: Key regulators of autoimmunity. *Autoimmun. Rev.* **2017**, *16*, 192–207. [CrossRef]
54. Vivek Kumar, S.; Thakur Gurjeet, S. Navigating Alzheimer's Disease via Chronic Stress: The Role of Glucocorticoids. *Curr. Drug Targets* **2020**, *21*, 433–444. [CrossRef]
55. Gebre, A.K.; Altaye, B.M.; Atey, T.M.; Tuem, K.B.; Berhe, D.F. Targeting Renin-Angiotensin System Against Alzheimer's Disease. *Front. Pharmacol.* **2018**, *9*, 440. [CrossRef]
56. Singh, P.K.; Chen, Z.L.; Strickland, S.; Norris, E.H. Increased Contact System Activation in Mild Cognitive Impairment Patients with Impaired Short-Term Memory. *J. Alzheimers Dis.* **2020**, *77*, 59–65. [CrossRef] [PubMed]
57. Bitencourt, R.M.; de Souza, A.C.; Bicca, M.A.; Pamplona, F.A.; de Mello, N.; Passos, G.F.; Medeiros, R.; Takahashi, R.N.; Calixto, J.B.; Prediger, R.D. Blockade of hippocampal bradykinin B1 receptors improves spatial learning and memory deficits in middle-aged rats. *Behav. Brain Res.* **2017**, *316*, 74–81. [CrossRef]
58. Mugisho, O.O.; Robilliard, L.D.; Nicholson, L.F.B.; Graham, E.S.; O'Carroll, S.J. Bradykinin receptor-1 activation induces inflammation and increases the permeability of human brain microvascular endothelial cells. *Cell Biol. Int.* **2019**, *44*, 343–351. [CrossRef]

59. Zhong, K.L.; Chen, F.; Hong, H.; Ke, X.; Lv, Y.G.; Tang, S.S.; Zhu, Y.B. New views and possibilities of antidiabetic drugs in treating and/or preventing mild cognitive impairment and Alzheimer's Disease. *Metab. Brain Dis.* **2018**, *33*, 1009–1018. [CrossRef]
60. Ji, B.; Wang, Q.; Xue, Q.; Li, W.; Li, X.; Wu, Y. The Dual Role of Kinin/Kinin Receptors System in Alzheimer's Disease. *Front. Mol. Neurosci.* **2019**, *12*, 234. [CrossRef]
61. Vipin, A.; Ng, K.K.; Ji, F.; Shim, H.Y.; Lim, J.K.; Pasternak, O.; Zhou, J.H.; Alzheimer's Disease Neuroimaging Initiative. Amyloid burden accelerates white matter degradation in cognitively normal elderly individuals. *Hum. Brain Mapp.* **2019**, *40*, 2065. [CrossRef]
62. Zhang, X.; Yu, R.; Wang, H.; Zheng, R. Effects of rivastigmine hydrogen tartrate and donepezil hydrochloride on the cognitive function and mental behavior of patients with Alzheimer's disease. *Exp. Ther. Med.* **2020**, *20*, 1789–1795. [CrossRef]
63. Urmila, A.; Rashmi, P.; Nilam, G.; Subhash, B. Recent Advances in the Endogenous Brain Renin-Angiotensin System and Drugs Acting on It. *J. Renin Angiotensin Aldosterone Syst.* **2021**, *2021*, 9293553. [CrossRef] [PubMed]
64. Naffah-Mazzacoratti M da, G.; Gouveia, T.L.F.; Simões, P.S.R.; Perosa, S.R. What have we learned about the kallikrein-kinin and renin-angiotensin systems in neurological disorders? *World J. Biol. Chem.* **2014**, *5*, 130–140. [CrossRef] [PubMed]
65. Hajjar, I.; Brown, L.; Mack, W.J.; Chui, H. Impact of Angiotensin Receptor Blockers on Alzheimer Disease Neuropathology in a Large Brain Autopsy Series. *Arch. Neurol.* **2012**, *69*, 1632–1638. [CrossRef] [PubMed]

Disclaimer/Publisher's Note: The statements, opinions and data contained in all publications are solely those of the individual author(s) and contributor(s) and not of MDPI and/or the editor(s). MDPI and/or the editor(s) disclaim responsibility for any injury to people or property resulting from any ideas, methods, instructions or products referred to in the content.

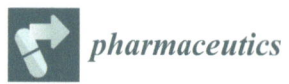

Article

Kinin B_1 and B_2 Receptors Contribute to Cisplatin-Induced Painful Peripheral Neuropathy in Male Mice

Gabriela Becker, Maria Fernanda Pessano Fialho, Indiara Brusco and Sara Marchesan Oliveira *

Graduate Program in Biological Sciences: Biochemical Toxicology, Center of Natural and Exact Sciences, Federal University of Santa Maria, Camobi, Santa Maria 97105-900, RS, Brazil
* Correspondence: saramarchesan@hotmail.com or saramarchesan@ufsm.br; Tel.: +55-55-3220-8053; Fax: +55-55-3220-8756

Abstract: Cisplatin is the preferential chemotherapeutic drug for highly prevalent solid tumours. However, its clinical efficacy is frequently limited due to neurotoxic effects such as peripheral neuropathy. Chemotherapy-induced peripheral neuropathy is a dose-dependent adverse condition that negatively impacts quality of life, and it may determine dosage limitations or even cancer treatment cessation. Thus, it is urgently necessary to identify pathophysiological mechanisms underlying these painful symptoms. As kinins and their B_1 and B_2 receptors contribute to the development of chronic painful conditions, including those induced by chemotherapy, the contribution of these receptors to cisplatin-induced peripheral neuropathy was evaluated via pharmacological antagonism and genetic manipulation in male Swiss mice. Cisplatin causes painful symptoms and impaired working and spatial memory. Kinin B_1 (DALBK) and B_2 (Icatibant) receptor antagonists attenuated some painful parameters. Local administration of kinin B_1 and B_2 receptor agonists (in sub-nociceptive doses) intensified the cisplatin-induced mechanical nociception attenuated by DALBK and Icatibant, respectively. In addition, antisense oligonucleotides to kinin B_1 and B_2 receptors reduced cisplatin-induced mechanical allodynia. Thus, kinin B_1 and B_2 receptors appear to be potential targets for the treatment of cisplatin-induced painful symptoms and may improve patients' adherence to treatment and their quality of life.

Keywords: bradykinin; neuropathic pain; chemotherapy; allodynia; CIPN

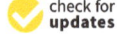

Citation: Becker, G.; Fialho, M.F.P.; Brusco, I.; Oliveira, S.M. Kinin B_1 and B_2 Receptors Contribute to Cisplatin-Induced Painful Peripheral Neuropathy in Male Mice. *Pharmaceutics* **2023**, *15*, 852. https://doi.org/10.3390/pharmaceutics15030852

Academic Editors: Cristina Manuela Drăgoi, Alina Crenguța Nicolae and Ion-Bogdan Dumitrescu

Received: 10 January 2023
Revised: 2 March 2023
Accepted: 3 March 2023
Published: 6 March 2023

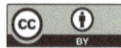

Copyright: © 2023 by the authors. Licensee MDPI, Basel, Switzerland. This article is an open access article distributed under the terms and conditions of the Creative Commons Attribution (CC BY) license (https://creativecommons.org/licenses/by/4.0/).

1. Introduction

Cancer incidence is increasing yearly, with an expected expansion rate of approximately 50% by 2040 [1]. Concomitantly, remarkable improvements in the survival rates of cancer patients have been observed due to advances in early detection and available treatments [2–4]. With the increasing number of cancer survivors, more attention must be given to the potential risk of developing severe adverse effects associated with therapy, such as chemotherapy-induced peripheral neuropathy (CIPN) [3,5,6].

CIPN is the most frequent and potentially permanent neurological complication of cancer treatment [5,7,8]. Platinum-based chemotherapeutics, such as cisplatin, are associated with a high incidence of CIPN and may affect up to 85% of treated patients [5,7–11].

Cisplatin treats highly prevalent tumours such as those of bladder, ovarian, testicular, lung, and head and neck cancers, as well as sarcomas [12]. However, cisplatin accumulation in the dorsal root ganglia neurons causes neuronal dysfunction and apoptosis, often resulting in irreversible changes in the peripheral nervous system, leading to peripheral neuropathy [7,9,13]. The incidence and severity of cisplatin-induced peripheral neuropathy are dose-dependent, and the symptoms appear during or after treatment [6–8]. Consequently, this condition can lead to dose reduction and treatment discontinuation, affecting overall patient survival [6,8,9,14].

Clinically, CIPN sensory symptoms are predominant in patients and can persist for months after completion of chemotherapy [7,8,14,15]. They usually develop first in the feet and hands; however, prolonged treatment may aggravate the signs and symptoms and extend to more proximal limb areas [6,8,9,16]. Patient symptoms manifest as spontaneous or evoked abnormal sensations such as paraesthesia, dysesthesias, numbness, and tingling. In addition, neuropathic-like painful sensations are frequently reported, such as mechanical or thermal allodynia or hyperalgesia, burning pain, and shooting or electric shock-like pain [6,8,16]. An essential aspect of platinum-based CIPN is the "coasting" phenomenon, whereby the signs and symptoms may worsen months after the discontinuation of chemotherapy [9,12,16].

Currently, there are no preventive strategies to attenuate this painful condition, and treatment is limited and commonly ineffective in many patients [14,15]. Although various pharmacologic agents have been evaluated for the treatment of CIPN, only duloxetine has been moderately recommended by the American Society of Clinical Oncology [14,15]. Given the limited treatment options for CIPN, it is necessary to identify efficacious and well-tolerated novel pharmacological strategies for CIPN symptoms without affecting cancer treatment regimens.

In this sense, kinin B_1 and B_2 receptors activated by kinins have attracted attention due to their involvement in nociceptive processes and different painful conditions [17–23]. Bradykinin (Bk) and kallidin target the B_2 receptor, while the B_1 receptor has a higher affinity for the active metabolites of kinins, namely des-Arg^9-Bk (DABk) and des-Arg^{10}-kallidin. Nociceptive neurons express kinin B_1 and B_2 receptors [21,24–26], which, when activated, cause painful nociceptive responses in humans and experimental animals [20,27–29]. Kinin B_1 and B_2 receptors mediate the acute and chronic pain induced by various pain models [17,18,20–23,30], including chemotherapy drugs such as paclitaxel and vincristine [27,31–33]. Furthermore, kinin B_1 and B_2 receptors are involved in cisplatin-induced nephrotoxicity since the pharmacological blockade and knockout animals of kinin receptors attenuate acute kidney injury [34,35].

Due to the significant implications for cancer survivors, it is important to gain an understanding of the principal pathophysiological mechanisms involved in chemotherapy-induced painful symptoms to aid in the search for potential therapies to prevent or minimize these pain symptoms. In this respect, using a model of cisplatin-induced painful neuropathy in mice, we evaluated the involvement of the kinin B_1 and B_2 receptors in the pain symptoms induced by cisplatin.

2. Materials and Methods

2.1. Drugs and Reagents

Cisplatin (cis-diamminedichloridoplatinum II, C-Platin®; Blau, SP, Brazil), bradykinin (Bk; kinin B_2 receptor agonist), Icatibant (peptide kinin B_2 receptor antagonist), des-Arg^9-bradykinin (DABk; kinin B_1 receptor agonist), and des-Arg^9-[Leu^8]-bradykinin (DALBK; peptide kinin B_1 receptor antagonist) were purchased from Sigma Chemical Company (St. Louis, MO, USA). FR173657 (non-peptide kinin B_2 receptor antagonist) and SSR240612 (non-peptide kinin B_1 receptor antagonist) were obtained from Sanofi-Aventis (Berlin, Germany). Antisense oligonucleotides targeting the kinin B_1 receptor (5'-AGG TTC CTG TGG ATG GCG TCCC-3'), kinin B_2 receptor (5'-AGA ATT CTG TTC ACT GTT TCT TCC CTG-3'), and nonsense oligonucleotides (5'-GGT GGA T TTG AGG ATT TCG GC-3') were acquired from GenOne Biotechnologies (Rio de Janeiro, Brazil). Cisplatin and antagonists were prepared in a saline solution (0.9%). Phosphate-buffered saline (PBS; 10 mM) was used to dilute reagents administered via the intraplantar route (kinin B_1 and B_2 receptor agonists). The control groups (vehicles) received the vehicles where the treatments were solubilized. All the intraperitoneal treatments were administered in mice in a volume of 10 mL/kg, while intraplantar injections were administered in a volume of 20 µL.

2.2. Animals

The experiments were conducted using adult male Swiss mice (25–30 g; 4–5 weeks of age) produced and provided by the Federal University of Santa Maria. The animals were maintained in a temperature-controlled room (22 ± 1 °C) under a 12 h light/12 h dark cycle with free access to food and water. Experimental protocols were performed with the approval of the Institutional Animal Care and Use Committee of the Federal University of Santa Maria (approval processes #7152261119/2020 and #6380261021/2022). Experimental protocols were conducted according to the guidelines for investigation of experimental pain in conscious animals [36,37], the Animal Research: Reporting in vivo Experiments ARRIVE guidelines [38], and national and international legislation (guidelines of the Brazilian Council of Animal Experimentation Control (CONCEA) and the U.S. Public Health Service's Policy on Humane Care and Use of Laboratory Animals (PHS policy)). The number of animals and the intensities of noxious stimuli used were the minimum necessary to demonstrate the consistent effects of the treatments. Behavioural experiments were conducted in a quiet, temperature-controlled room (20 °C to 22 °C) between 9 a.m. and 5 p.m. and were performed by investigators blinded to the treatment conditions. The group size for each experiment was based on studies with protocols similar to ours [27,39,40], which were confirmed by power calculations (G*Power version 3.1.9.7).

2.3. Cisplatin-Induced Peripheral Neuropathy Model

To establish the cisplatin-induced peripheral neuropathy model, the mice were treated with intraperitoneal (i.p.) injections of cisplatin at a dose of 2.3 mg/kg administered every 48 h for 10 days (days 0, 2, 4, 6, 8, and 10), totalling 6 doses of cisplatin [41,42]. The control group received the vehicle (10 mL/kg, i.p.; saline solution [0.9%]), employing the same administration schedule. Mannitol (125 mg/kg, intraperitoneal) was administered 1 h before cisplatin to avoid renal toxicity [43]. After the first cisplatin or vehicle injection, the animals were subjected to behavioural assessments. The experimental design is represented in Figure 1A.

2.4. Study Design for Behavioural Assessment

Mechanical paw withdrawal threshold (PWT) and cold sensitivity were evaluated before the cisplatin administration protocol (baseline, B1). Next, the mice received vehicle (control group; 10 mL/kg, i.p.) or cisplatin (2.3 mg/kg, i.p.). The PWT was continuously assessed 24 h after each cisplatin or vehicle administration up to 30 days after the first administration [following the protocol described below (2.6.1 Mechanical allodynia assessment)]. Cold sensitivity was evaluated on days 5, 11, 18, and 25 after the first cisplatin or vehicle administration [following the protocol described below (2.6.2 Cold sensitivity)]. The locomotor activity of the animals was evaluated in an open field on the 11th and 30th days after the first administration of cisplatin or vehicle [following the protocol described below (2.7.2 Locomotor Activity)].

Spontaneous pain was assessed by the voluntary wheel activity and nesting behaviour [following the protocols described below (2.6.3 Voluntary wheel activity and 2.6.4 Nesting behaviour test)]. Anxiety and depressive-like behaviours, as well as cognitive function, were assessed by thigmotaxis behaviour and a forced swimming test, as well as a novel object/place recognition test, respectively [following the protocols described below (2.6.5 Thigmotaxis behaviour, 2.6.6 Forced swimming test, and 2.6.7 Novel object place recognition test)].

2.5. Study Design for the Assessment of Kinin B_1 and B_2 Receptor Involvement in Cisplatin-Induced Painful Behaviours

A therapeutic and preventive protocol using kinin B_1 and B_2 receptor antagonists was performed to evaluate their contribution to the mechanical and cold painful hypersensitivity induced by cisplatin. Agonists and antisense oligonucleotides for the kinin B_1 and B_2 receptors were also used.

2.5.1. Therapeutic Protocol

The therapeutic protocol was designed to evaluate the effect of kinin B_1 and B_2 receptor antagonists in mice with mechanical and cold allodynia previously established by cisplatin.

The mechanical PWT and cold sensitivity of animals were measured before the cisplatin (2.3 mg/kg, i.p.) administrations (baseline values; B1) and 24 h after the last injection (11th day) (baseline values; B2). Next, the mice received a single intraperitoneal (i.p.) administration of the peptide kinin B_1 or B_2 receptor antagonist, i.e., DALBK (150 nmol/kg, i.p.) or Icatibant (100 nmol/kg, i.p.), respectively. The mechanical PWT and cold sensitivity were evaluated at different time points following the treatments (from 0.5 h up to 4 h). The mechanical PWT and cold sensitivity were also evaluated after treatments (from 0.5 to 24 h) with non-peptide kinin B_1 (SSR240612, 150 nmol/kg, i.p.) or B_2 (FR173657; 100 nmol/kg, i.p.) receptor antagonists. The experimental design is represented in Figure 3A.

2.5.2. Preventive Protocol

The preventive protocol was delineated to evaluate the capacity of the kinin B_1 and B_2 receptor antagonists to prevent the development of cisplatin-induced mechanical allodynia and cold sensitivity. Mechanical PWT and cold sensitivity were measured before cisplatin and treatments (baseline values; B1). After baseline measurements, the mice were treated concomitantly every 48 h for 10 days with cisplatin (2.3 mg/kg, i.p.) + vehicle (10 mL/kg, i.p.), cisplatin (2.3 mg/kg, i.p.) + kinin B_1 receptor antagonist (DALBK, 150 nmol/kg, i.p.), or cisplatin (2.3 mg/kg, i.p.) + kinin B_2 receptor antagonist (Icatibant, 100 nmol/kg, i.p.). Mechanical PWT and cold sensitivity were assessed 24 h after each administration up to 14 days after the first cisplatin administration. The experimental design is represented in Figure 4A.

2.5.3. Effects of Sub-Nociceptive Doses of Kinin B_1 and B_2 Receptor Agonists on Mechanical Allodynia in Mice with Cisplatin-Induced Peripheral Neuropathy

We examined whether low doses of kinin B_1 and B_2 receptor agonists could enhance the mechanical nociception of cisplatin-treated mice. The animals were previously treated with cisplatin (2.3 mg/kg, i.p.) or vehicle (10 mL/kg, i.p.). Twenty-four hours after the last cisplatin administration (11th day), the animals received an intraplantar (i.pl.) injection of DABk (3 nmol/paw, kinin B_1 receptor agonist) or Bk (1 nmol/paw, kinin B_2 receptor agonist), all in sub-nociceptive doses, or their vehicles (20 μL PBS/paw, i.pl.), and the mechanical PWT was evaluated again from 0.5 up to 3 h and from 0.5 up to 2 h after the agonist injections, respectively. The experimental design is represented in Figure 5A.

To confirm the involvement of kinin B_1 and B_2 receptors in mechanical allodynia, the mice were treated with DALBK (150 nmol/kg, i.p.) or Icatibant (100 nmol/kg, i.p.) 24 h after the last cisplatin dose (11th day). After 0.5 h, the same animals were treated with sub-nociceptive doses of the respective kinin B_1 and B_2 receptor agonists—DABk or Bk—by the intraplantar route. Next, the PWT was assessed until treatments with the antagonists showed an effect. The experimental design is represented in Figure 6A.

2.5.4. Effects of Antisense Oligonucleotides for Kinin B_1 and B_2 Receptors on Cisplatin-Induced Mechanical and Cold Sensitivity in Mice

To confirm the contribution of kinin B_1 and B_2 receptors to cisplatin-induced painful behaviours, mice were treated with intrathecal injections of an antisense oligonucleotide for kinin B_1 and B_2 receptors or their control. First, baseline (B1) mechanical PWT and cold sensitivity were measured. Then, the animals were treated with 6 doses of cisplatin (2.3 mg/kg, i.p.). Twenty-four h after the last cisplatin administration (11th day), mechanical and cold sensitivity were evaluated again (baseline values; B2). Next, the animals were treated intrathecally (5 μL; between L5 and L6) twice a day (12/12 h) for three consecutive days with antisense oligonucleotides targeting the kinin B_1 receptor (antisense B_1; 5 μg/site) and the kinin B_2 receptor (antisense B_2; 5 μg/site) or the control oligonucleotide (nonsense, 5 μL/site) [18]. On the fourth day, the animals received one last administration of antisense or nonsense oligonucleotides 1 h before evaluating mechanical PWT and cold sensitivity. The experimental design is represented in Figure 7A.

2.6. Behavioural Experiments

2.6.1. Mechanical Allodynia Assessment

Mechanical allodynia was assessed using flexible nylon filaments (von Frey) of increasing stiffness (0.02–10 g) by the up-and-down method [44,45]. The mechanical PWT response, expressed in grams (g), was calculated from the resulting scores using von Frey filaments, according to previous studies [23,27,45]. Mechanical allodynia was considered a decrease in the PWT compared with the baseline values (B1) before cisplatin administration.

2.6.2. Cold Sensitivity

Cold sensitivity was assessed with the acetone drop method as previously described [23,46]. The mice were placed on a wire mesh floor, and a drop of acetone (20 µL) was applied three times on the plantar surface of the right hind paw. The behavioural response was analysed for 30 s and recorded in scores. The scores were: 0 = no response; 1 = quick withdrawal, flick, or stamp the paw; 2 = prolonged withdrawal or repeated paw flicking; and 3 = repeated paw flicking with licking directed at the ventral side of the paw. The sum of the three scores was used for data analysis. Cold sensitivity was considered an increase in the scores compared with the baseline values before cisplatin administration.

2.6.3. Voluntary Wheel Activity

The running activity is a simple, observer-independent objective measure and provides a measure of spontaneous activity in a known environment, potentially reflecting whether the activity is painful [47]. The voluntary wheel activity was assessed in polycarbonate cages with free access to stainless steel activity wheels (Wheel activity EP 172—Insight, Ribeirão Preto, SP, Brazil). The wheel could be turned in either direction. The wheels were connected to a digit counter that automatically recorded the number of turns. First, mice were habituated in individual activity cages for three sessions over at least three days. The distance travelled by each animal on the wheel during each 1 h evaluation session was obtained by multiplying the number of turns by the wheel diameter (30 cm). The mice that refused to run on the wheels during the baseline measurement (travelled a distance <150 m) were excluded from further evaluation [47].

2.6.4. Nesting Behaviour Test

Nesting is an innate behaviour in mice that may be sensitive to pain conditions [48]. Mice were habituated to the nesting cage for 48 h before testing. As nesting material, one 5×5 cm^2 nestlet consisting of pressed virgin cotton was cut into six roughly equal pieces (~1.7×2.5 cm^2). The nest pieces were evenly placed in the four corners and the middle of each long side of the cage ($49 \times 34 \times 16$ cm^2), and the cage space was divided into six equal zones for nesting assessment. The nesting quality score ranged from 0.5 to 6 points and was measured as follows: 0.5 points were assigned to the mouse if it cleared one zone, and 0.5 points were assigned if the mouse shredded the nestlet. The nesting score ranged from 0.5 to 6 points. The nesting behaviour was scored after 120 min of exposure to the initial nesting material [48,49]. A decrease in the nesting score indicates pain-depressed nesting behaviour, suggesting one useful spontaneous nociception behaviour.

2.6.5. Thigmotaxis Behaviour

Thigmotaxis behaviour was evaluated using an open field (40 cm $\times$ 30 cm $\times$ 18 cm) with a delimited inner zone (12 $\times$ 12 cm). Each mouse was transferred to the apparatus and observed for 15 min [46,50]. The number of entries into the inner zone and the total immobility time were analysed by ANY-maze Software (7.0 version, Stoelting Co., Wood Dale, IL, USA). Thigmotaxis behaviour corresponds to a decreased exploration of the inner zone of the open field and indicates anxiety-like behaviour [50].

2.6.6. Forced Swimming Test

Forced swimming is a commonly used assay to study depressive-like behaviour in rodents [51]. The forced swimming test was performed using a cylinder (20 cm diameter and 45 cm height) filled with water (23–25 °C) at a height of 30 cm. Mice were placed in the water, and the time for which the mice remained immobile was quantified in seconds over a period of 2–6 min using a chronometer [46,50]. Immobility was defined as the absence of all movements except those required to maintain the head above water.

2.6.7. Novel Object/Place Recognition Test

To assess cognitive function, we subjected mice to a novel object/place recognition test (NOPRT). NOPRT measures the spatial and working memory of mice using the innate preference of mice for novelty [52,53] and was performed as previously described [52,54]. One day after administration of the last dose of cisplatin, mice were habituated to the test arena (40 cm × 30 cm × 18 cm), with two identical objects placed on the same side of the arena for 5 min (training phase), after which the mouse was returned to its home cage. Thirty minutes later, the mice were transferred back to the arena, which now contained one familiar object placed at the same location as in training and one novel object placed on the opposite end of the arena (testing phase), and they were allowed to explore for another 5 min. Sniffing, climbing, and touching the objects were regarded as exploration behaviour. The exploration time of the familiar and novel object was scored manually. The discrimination index was determined as *[time with the novel object − time with the familiar object]/total exploration time of both objects*.

2.7. Evaluation of Other Possible Adverse Effects

2.7.1. Physical and Behavioural Changes

Physical (body weight verified through a scale and hair appearance) and behavioural (irritability, salivation, and tremors) changes were visually evaluated before and throughout the experimental period (during and after cisplatin administration) by the experimenter.

2.7.2. Locomotor Activity

We assessed the effect of cisplatin on the locomotor activity of animals one day after the last cisplatin (2.3 mg/kg, i.p.) or vehicle (control group; 10 mL/kg, i.p.) administration (11th day). The spontaneous locomotor activity was recorded for 15 min in an open-field apparatus (40 cm × 30 cm × 18 cm), and the results of the total distance travelled were obtained by automated analysis ANY-maze™ software (7.0 version, Stoelting Co., Wood Dale, IL, US). The spontaneous locomotor activity was also evaluated on the 30th day after the first cisplatin or vehicle administration by an open-field test [55]. The open-field apparatus consists of a glass box (28 × 18 × 12 cm) divided into nine squares. On the 30th day after the first cisplatin or vehicle administration, each mouse was placed in the apparatus, and the number of squares crossed with all paws and rearing was counted in a 5 min session. The forced locomotor activity was evaluated using the rotarod test. Before the first cisplatin or vehicle dose, all the animals were trained in the rotarod (3.7 cm in diameter, 8 rpm) until they could remain in the apparatus for 60 s without falling. On the 30th day after the first cisplatin (2.3 mg/kg, i.p.) or vehicle (control group; 10 mL/kg, i.p.) dose, the number of falls from the apparatus was recorded for up to 240 s [55].

2.7.3. Biochemical Analysis

The mice received the cisplatin (2.3 mg/kg, i.p.) or vehicle (10 mL/kg, i.p.) administrations. On the 30th day after the first cisplatin dose, they were deeply anaesthetized, and blood was collected by heart puncture. The obtained serum was used for a biochemical assay to assess serum urea nitrogen and serum creatinine levels, as well as the activities of aspartate aminotransferase (AST) and alanine aminotransferase (ALT) enzymes.

2.8. Statistical Analysis

Statistical analyses were performed using Graph Pad Prism 8.0 software (Graph Pad, San Diego, CA, USA). Results were expressed as the mean ± standard error of the mean (SEM). The significance of differences between groups was evaluated with a Student's *t*-test and one-way or two-way analysis of variance (ANOVA) followed by Bonferroni's post hoc test. To meet the parametric assumptions, the data on the mechanical threshold were log-transformed before analyses. The nesting test scores are reported as medians followed by their 25th and 75th percentiles (interquartile range). The percentages of maximum effect were calculated for the maximal developed responses compared to baseline values or the control group. p-values less than 0.05 ($p < 0.05$) were considered statistically significant.

3. Results

3.1. Cisplatin Induces Prolonged Painful Peripheral Neuropathy in Mice

First, we explored whether the treatment regimen used to induce the peripheral neuropathy model (Figure 1A) causes mechanical allodynia and cold sensitivity. Cisplatin reduced the mechanical PWT of mice from the third cisplatin dose (5th day) until 30 days after the first cisplatin administration, indicating the development of mechanical allodynia (Figure 1B). A PWT reduction of 72 ± 7% was observed on the 11th day after the first cisplatin administration. Mice treated with cisplatin also developed cold sensitivity after the final dose of cisplatin (11th day) compared to the vehicle group (Figure 1C), which remained until the 18th day. Thus, the 11th day after the first cisplatin administration was chosen for subsequent experiments.

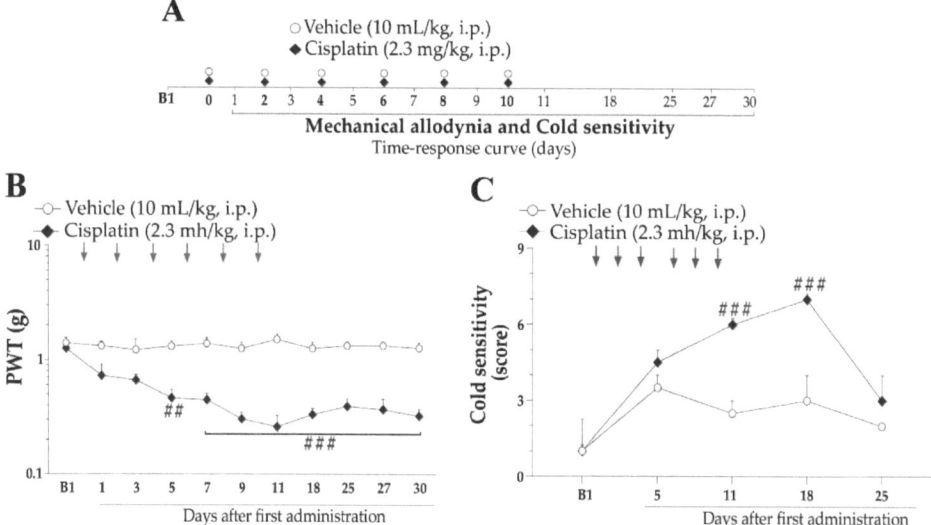

Figure 1. Characterization of cisplatin-induced painful peripheral neuropathy. (**A**) Male Swiss mice were treated intraperitoneally (i.p.) with cisplatin (2.3 mg/kg) or its vehicle (10 mL/kg) from day 0 onwards every other day (days 0, 2, 4, 6, 8, and 10) for a total of 10 days to induce the peripheral neuropathy experimental model. The mice's mechanical PWT was assessed between the treatment days until 30 days after the first cisplatin administration (**B**). Cold sensitivity was evaluated on the 5th, 11th, 18th, and 25th days after the first cisplatin administration (**C**). B1 denotes baseline values measured before the first cisplatin or vehicle dose. Data are expressed as the mean + SEM (n = 6/group) and were analysed by two-way ANOVA followed by Bonferroni post hoc test. ## $p < 0.01$ and ### $p < 0.001$ when compared to the vehicle group. The arrows represent the days of cisplatin or vehicle administration. PWT: paw withdrawal threshold.

Measurements of spontaneous pain were performed one day after the last cisplatin dose. Cisplatin partially decreased the distance travelled in the voluntary activity in the wheel test (Figure 2A) and reduced nesting behaviour compared to the vehicle group (Figure 2B). Mice treated with cisplatin showed a decreased preference for the novel object when compared to vehicle-treated mice, indicating impairment in cognitive function (Figure 2C). No differences were observed in the total time the animals interacted with objects, indicating that the decreased discrimination index of cisplatin-treated mice was not due to reduced interest (Figure 2D). Moreover, cisplatin did not cause anxiety and depressive-like behaviour, as evaluated by the number of entries to the inner zone and total immobility time in the open-field apparatus, and it did not increase the immobility time in the forced swimming test (Table S1).

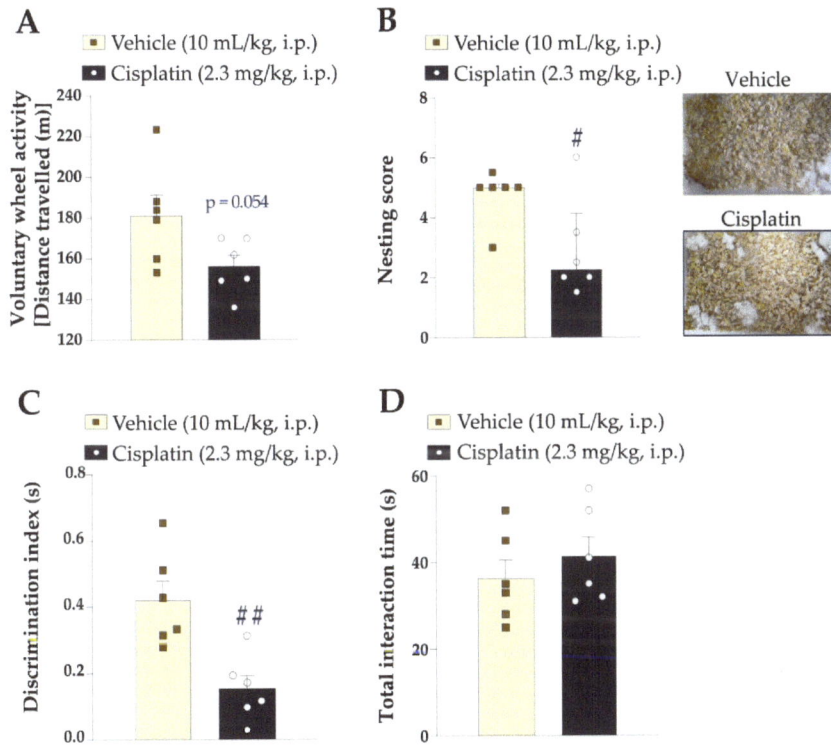

Figure 2. Treatment with cisplatin induced spontaneous nociceptive behaviours and impaired working and spatial memory in mice. Male Swiss mice were treated intraperitoneally (i.p.) with cisplatin (2.3 mg/kg) or its vehicle (10 mL/kg) from day 0 onwards every other day for a total of 10 days to induce the peripheral neuropathy experimental model. On the 11th day, the mice were subjected to behavioural tests. Spontaneous nociception was evaluated by voluntary wheel activity (**A**) and nesting behaviour (**B**). The cognitive function was evaluated by NORPT. The discrimination index demonstrates the preference for the novel object (**C**) and the total interaction time with the novel or familiar object (**D**). The symbols on the bars indicate individual values for each animal. $^{\#}\ p < 0.05$ and $^{\#\#}\ p < 0.01$ vs. vehicle group. Data are expressed as the mean + SEM (n = 6/group) and were analysed by an unpaired two-tailed Student's t-test, except (**B**) nesting score (n = 6/group) data, which are expressed as 25th and 75th percentiles (interquartile range) and were analysed by one-tailed Mann–Whitney test.

Furthermore, cisplatin neither changed the body weight (Table S2) nor caused behavioural alterations (e.g., irritability, salivation, or tremors) compared with the vehicle group. Cisplatin treatment also did not affect the locomotor function of mice, as demonstrated by the total distance travelled (m) in the open-field apparatus on the 11th day (Table S2). In addition, cisplatin treatment affected neither the mice's spontaneous locomotor function evaluated on the 30th day, as demonstrated by crossing and rearing numbers (Table S2), nor the forced locomotor activity, as shown by the mice's number of falls in the rotarod test (Table S2). The treatment with cisplatin that induced peripheral neuropathy did not cause changes in the urea and creatinine levels or ALT and AST enzyme activities (Table S3).

3.2. Kinin B_1 and B_2 Receptors Contribute to Mechanical Allodynia in Cisplatin-Induced Peripheral Neuropathy in Mice

First, utilizing a therapeutic protocol, we evaluated whether pharmacological blockade using the kinin B_1 and B_2 receptor antagonists reduces the cisplatin-induced mechanical allodynia (Figure 3A). The peptide antagonists for kinin B_1 (DALBK, 150 nmol/kg, i.p.) and B_2 (Icatibant, 100 nmol/kg, i.p.) receptors reduced cisplatin-induced mechanical allodynia from 0.5 up to 2 h after their administration (Figure 3B), with reductions of $52 \pm 7\%$ and $57 \pm 5\%$ at 2 h after treatments, respectively. Similar effects were observed for non-peptide kinin B_1 and B_2 receptor antagonists. Non-peptide antagonists for kinin B_1 (SSR240612, 150 nmol/kg, i.p.) and B_2 (FR173657, 100 nmol/kg, i.p.) receptors decreased the cisplatin-induced mechanical allodynia from 0.5 up to 4 h (reduction of $31 \pm 8\%$ at 0.5 h) and from 0.5 up to 6 h (reduction of $34 \pm 9\%$ at 2 h) after their treatments (Figure 3C), respectively. Peptide and non-peptide antagonists for kinin B_1 or B_2 receptors failed to reduce cisplatin-induced cold sensitivity.

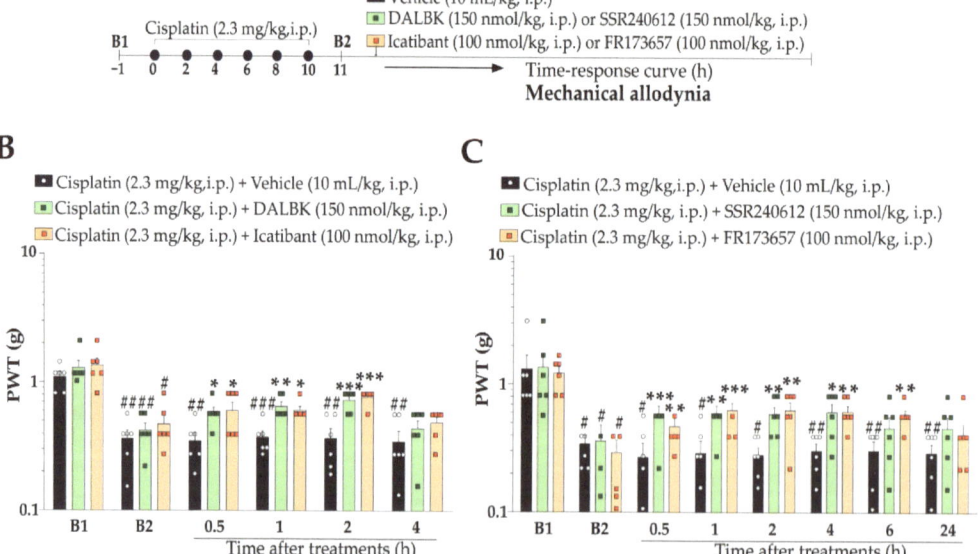

Figure 3. Therapeutic effect of kinin B_1 and B_2 receptor antagonists on cisplatin-induced mechanical allodynia. (**A**) *Therapeutic protocol*: Male Swiss mice were treated intraperitoneally (i.p.) with cisplatin (2.3 mg/kg) every 48 h for 10 days. On the 11th day after the first cisplatin dose, the animals received a single administration of DALBK or SSR240612 (150 nmol/kg, i.p., peptide and non-peptide kinin B_1 receptor antagonist, respectively), Icatibant or FR173657 (100 nmol/kg, i.p., peptide and non-peptide kinin B_2 receptor antagonist, respectively), or vehicle (10 mL/kg, i.p.). Time–response curve for mechanical allodynia after treatment with DALBK or Icatibant (**B**) and SSR240612 or FR173657 (**C**).

Baseline 1 (B1) values were measured before the first cisplatin dose. Baseline 2 (B2) values were measured on the 11th day after the first cisplatin dose and before the treatments. The symbols on the bars indicate individual values for each animal. $^{\#}$ $p < 0.05$, $^{\#\#}$ $p < 0.01$ and $^{\#\#\#}$ $p < 0.001$ vs. B1 values. * $p < 0.05$, ** $p < 0.01$, and *** $p < 0.001$ vs. cisplatin plus vehicle group. Data are expressed as the mean + SEM (n = 6/group) and were analysed by two-way ANOVA followed by the Bonferroni post hoc test. PWT: paw withdrawal threshold.

Next, we assessed the effect of peptide antagonists for kinin B_1 and B_2 receptors in preventing the mechanical allodynia development induced by cisplatin (Figure 4A). DALBK (150 nmol/kg, i.p.) effectively prevented mechanical allodynia development when administered concomitantly with cisplatin until the 12th day, with prevention of $55 \pm 21\%$ on the 5th day after the first treatment. Similarly, Icatibant (100 nmol/kg, i.p.) also prevented mechanical allodynia development when administered concomitantly with cisplatin until the 11th day after the first treatment, with prevention of $43 \pm 16\%$ on the 5th day (Figure 4B). Peptide kinin B_1 or B_2 receptor antagonists did not prevent cisplatin-induced cold sensitivity.

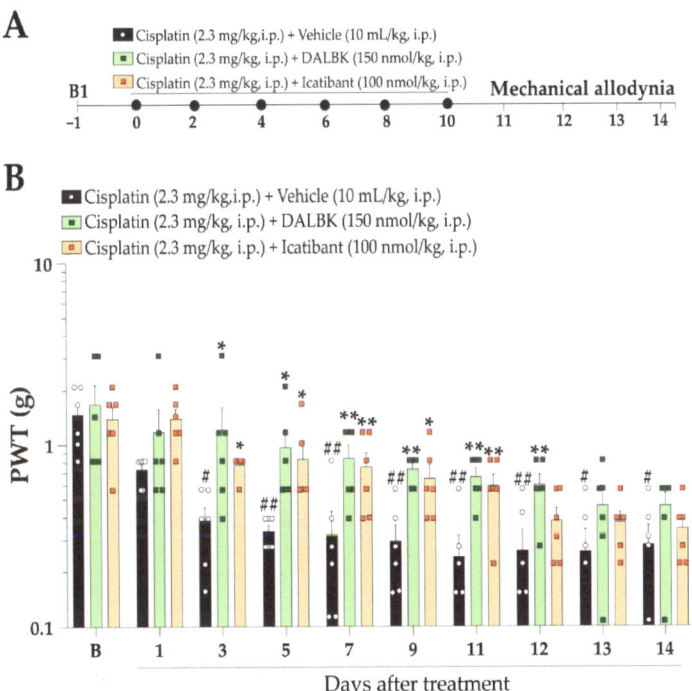

Figure 4. Preventive effect of kinin B_1 and B_2 receptor antagonists on cisplatin-induced mechanical allodynia. (**A**) *Preventive protocol*: Male Swiss mice were treated concomitantly by intraperitoneal (i.p.) injections with cisplatin (2.3 mg/kg) plus peptide kinin B_1 (DALBK, 150 nmol/kg, i.p.) or B_2 (Icatibant, 100 nmol/kg, i.p.) receptor antagonists or vehicle (10 mL/kg, i.p.) every 48 h for 10 days. Time–response curve for PWT throughout the treatment with cisplatin plus DALBK or Icatibant (**B**). Baseline (B) values were measured before the first cisplatin dose. The symbols on the bars indicate individual values for each animal. $^{\#}$ $p < 0.05$ and $^{\#\#}$ $p < 0.01$ vs. B1 values. * $p < 0.05$ and ** $p < 0.01$ vs. cisplatin plus vehicle group. Data are expressed as the mean + SEM (n = 6/group) and were analysed by two-way ANOVA followed by the Bonferroni post hoc test. PWT: paw withdrawal threshold.

3.3. Kinin B_1 and B_2 Receptor Agonists Enhanced Cisplatin-Induced Mechanical Nociception, Which Was Reversed by B_1 and B_2 Receptor Antagonists

First, we evaluated whether low doses of kinin B_1 and B_2 receptor agonists could enhance cisplatin-induced nociceptive behaviour (Figure 5A). Intraplantar (i.pl.) DABk (3 nmol/paw; a sub-nociceptive dose of kinin B_1 receptor agonist) enhanced cisplatin-induced mechanical nociception 2 h after its administration when compared to the cisplatin plus vehicle group (Figure 5B). Likewise, i.pl. Bk (1 nmol/paw; a sub-nociceptive dose of kinin B_2 receptor agonist) enhanced cisplatin-induced mechanical nociception 1 h after its administration when compared to the cisplatin plus vehicle group (Figure 5C). As expected, sub-nociceptive doses of the Bk and DABk agonists did not alter the mechanical sensitivity in animals previously treated with vehicle (Figure 5B,C).

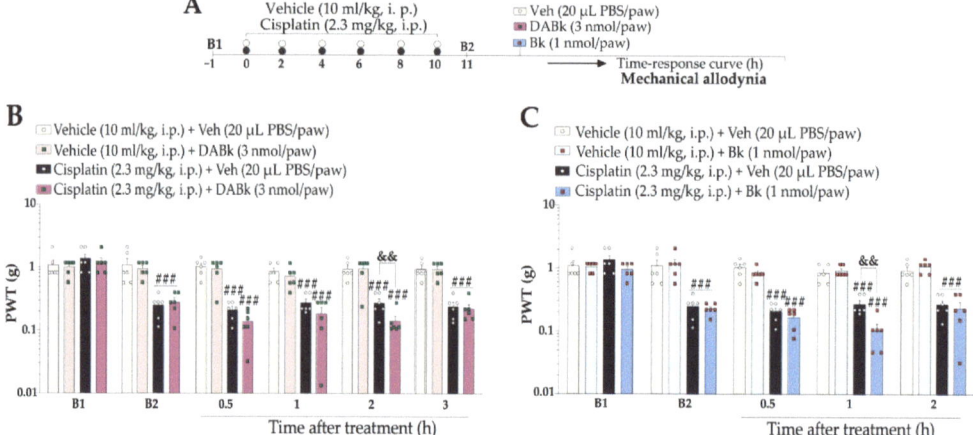

Figure 5. Sub-nociceptive doses of B_1 and B_2 receptor agonists intensified cisplatin-induced mechanical nociception. (**A**) Male Swiss mice were treated intraperitoneally (i.p.) with cisplatin (2.3 mg/kg) every 48 h for 10 days. On the 11th day after the first cisplatin injection, the animals were treated with sub-nociceptive doses of agonists kinin B_1 (DABk; 3 nmol/paw, i.pl.) or B_2 (Bk; 1 nmol/paw, i.pl.) receptor or vehicle (20 µL PBS/paw, intraplantar, i.pl.) via the intraplantar route. PWT (**B**,**C**) was assessed from 0.5 h up to 3 h after injection of sub-nociceptive doses of the agonists. Baseline 1 (B1) values were measured before cisplatin or vehicle administration. Baseline 2 (B2) values were measured on the 11th day after the first cisplatin dose and before the treatments. The symbols on the bars indicate individual values for each animal. ### $p < 0.001$ vs. Veh plus Veh group. && $p < 0.01$ vs. cisplatin plus Veh. Data are expressed as the mean + SEM (n = 6/group) and were analysed by two-way ANOVA followed by the Bonferroni post hoc test, except for the DABk effect on mechanical allodynia enhanced (Student's t-test). Veh: vehicle; PBS: phosphate-buffered saline; PWT: paw withdrawal threshold.

Since low doses of kinin B_1 and B_2 receptor agonists intensified the cisplatin-induced mechanical nociception, we evaluated whether kinin receptor antagonists prevented this behaviour (Figure 6A). The kinin B_1 receptor antagonist DALBK (150 nmol/kg, i.p., 0.5 h prior agonist injection) prevented the enhancement of mechanical nociception, with an effect of $31 \pm 4\%$ 2 h after its administration (Figure 6B). Icatibant (100 nmol/kg, i.p., 0.5 h prior to agonist injection), a kinin B_2 receptor antagonist, markedly prevented the enhancement of mechanical nociception, with an effect of $75 \pm 11\%$ at 1 h after its administration (Figure 6C).

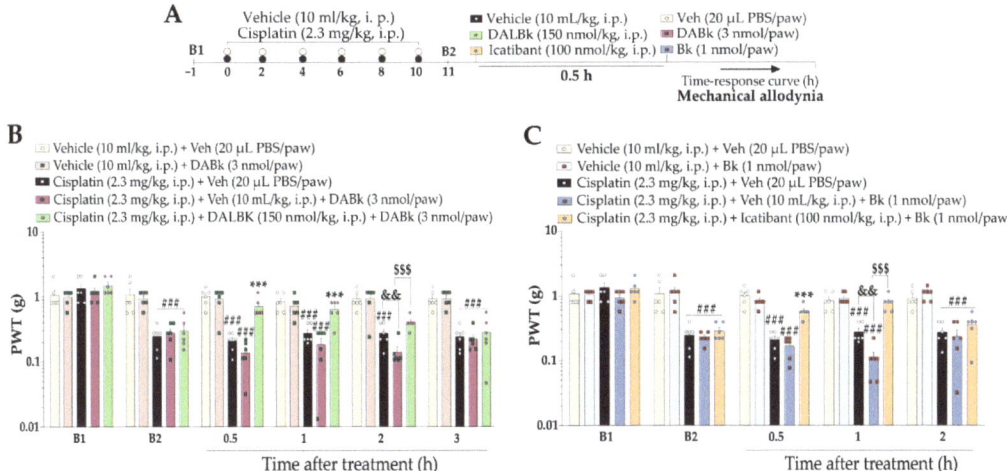

Figure 6. Kinin B_1 and B_2 receptor antagonists prevent the enhancement of B_1 and B_2 receptor agonist-induced mechanical nociception in cisplatin-treated mice. (**A**) Male Swiss mice were treated intraperitoneally (i.p.) with cisplatin (2.3 mg/kg) every 48 h for 10 days. On the 11th day after the first cisplatin injection, the animals received a single administration of DALBK (150 nmol/kg, i.p.), Icatibant (100 nmol/kg, i.p.), or vehicle (10 mL/kg, intraperitoneal, i.p.). After 0.5 h, sub-nociceptive doses of the respective agonists, i.e., DABk (3 nmol/paw, i.pl.) or Bk (1 nmol/paw, i.pl.), or vehicle (20 µL PBS/paw, intraplantar, i.pl.) were administered via the intraplantar route. PWT (**B**,**C**) was assessed from 0.5 h up to 3 h after the treatments. Baseline 1 (B1) values were measured before cisplatin or vehicle administration. Baseline 2 (B2) values were measured on the 11th day after the first cisplatin dose and before the treatments. The symbols on the bars indicate individual values for each animal. ### $p < 0.001$ vs. Veh plus Veh group. && $p < 0.01$ vs. cisplatin plus Veh. *** $p < 0.001$ vs. cisplatin plus Veh. \$\$\$ $p < 0.001$ vs. cisplatin plus DABk/Bk group. Data are expressed as the mean + SEM (n = 6/group) and were analysed by two-way ANOVA followed by the Bonferroni post hoc test, except for the DABk effect on mechanical allodynia (Student's *t*-test). Veh: vehicle; PBS: phosphate-buffered saline; PWT: paw withdrawal threshold.

3.4. Antisense Oligonucleotides for Kinin B_1 or B_2 Receptors Attenuated the Cisplatin-Induced Mechanical Allodynia

To reinforce the involvement of kinin B_1 and B_2 receptors in cisplatin-induced mechanical allodynia, we silenced the gene expression of the kinin B_1 or B_2 receptor using antisense oligonucleotides (Figure 7A). Antisense oligonucleotides for kinin B_1 and B_2 receptors attenuated cisplatin-induced mechanical allodynia, with inhibition of 57 ± 8% and 33 ± 7%, respectively (Figure 7B). On the other hand, control oligonucleotide injection (nonsense) did not affect the cisplatin-induced mechanical allodynia. Antisense oligonucleotides did not attenuate cisplatin-induced cold sensitivity.

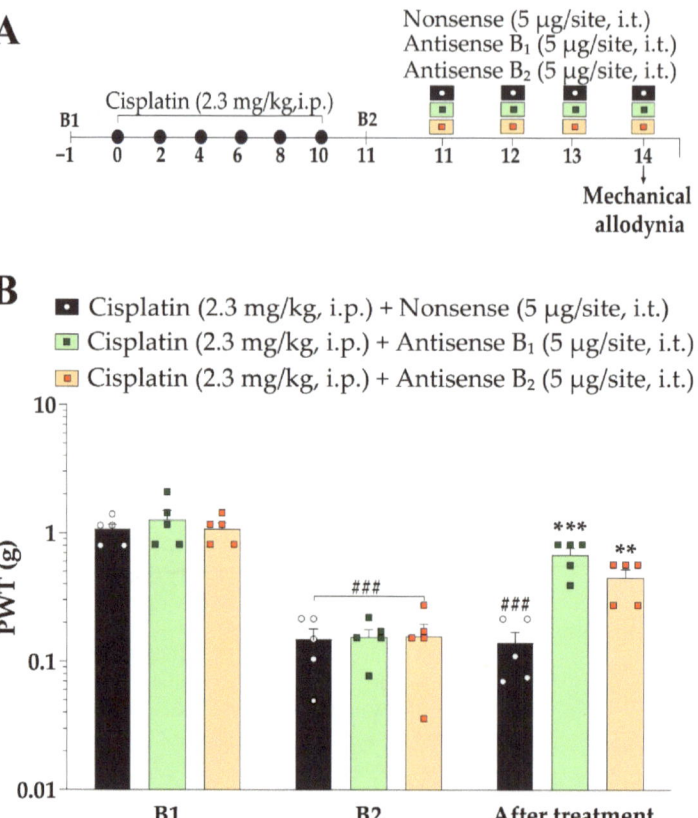

Figure 7. Antisense oligonucleotides for kinin B_1 and B_2 receptors relieved cisplatin-caused mechanical allodynia. (**A**) Male Swiss mice were treated by intraperitoneal (i.p.) injections with cisplatin (2.3 mg/kg) every 48 h for 10 days. Mice were treated with antisense oligonucleotides targeting kinin B_1 and B_2 receptors, and nonsense control was administered via the intrathecal (i.t.) route for three consecutive days every 12 h and 1 h before assessment of mechanical allodynia on the 14th day after induction of peripheral neuropathy by cisplatin. (**B**) Mechanical allodynia was evaluated on the 14th day after cisplatin-induced peripheral neuropathy. B1 values were measured before the first cisplatin dose. B2 values were measured on the 11th day after the first cisplatin dose and before the treatments. Results are presented as mean + SEM (n = 5–6/group). The symbols on the bars indicate individual values for each animal. ### $p < 0.001$ compared to baseline threshold (B1). ** $p < 0.01$; *** $p < 0.001$ compared to the nonsense group. Two-way ANOVA repeated measures followed by Bonferroni's post hoc test. PWT: paw withdrawal threshold.

4. Discussion

Peripheral neuropathy is one of the most common adverse effects of platinum-based chemotherapy drugs such as cisplatin. CIPN considerably impacts cancer treatment strategies, leading to a dose reduction or treatment discontinuation and negatively affecting the patients' quality of life [9,11,56]. The increasing number of cancer survivors and the lack of treatment to prevent or manage CIPN emphasizes the urgent need to unveil the pathophysiological mechanisms of CIPN to develop effective therapeutic strategies. This study provided the first evidence of the involvement of the kinin B_1 and B_2 receptors in cisplatin-induced painful peripheral neuropathy using pharmacological and genetic tools. Therefore, kinin receptors seem crucial to mediating mechanical nociception in cisplatin-induced peripheral neuropathy, suggesting that these receptors may also be critical in a clinical setting. Moreover, we demonstrated that kinin B_1 and B_2 receptor antagonists have therapeutic potential to relieve cisplatin-associated pain symptoms.

Clinically, cisplatin dose is a determinant for peripheral neuropathy development [11,12,57,58]. CIPN commonly manifests as an increased perception of innocuous (allodynia) or noxious (hyperalgesia) stimuli, which are hallmark symptoms of neuropathic pain [6,8,56]. In the present study, cisplatin treatment resulted in prominent and persistent mechanical allodynia lasting at least 30 days. This result agrees with previous data demonstrating the development of mechanical allodynia after the third cisplatin dose in a different strain of mice [41,42,59].

Changes in peripheral sensory sensations concerning cold stimuli are commonly associated with neuronal toxicity caused by antineoplastic agents such as platinum-based agents [11,12,56]. Here, we observed that six doses of cisplatin increased cold sensitivity. Although our results are consistent with previous studies [60–62], the changes in thermal hypersensitivity (cold and heat) caused by cisplatin are controversial [56] and seem to be more associated with oxaliplatin use—another platinum-based agent. Since literature data demonstrate no differences in the onset or severity of CIPN between male and female mice, we evaluated the cisplatin effects only on male but not female mice [56,63–65].

In this study, we demonstrated that cisplatin treatment induced spontaneous pain-like behaviours. The reduction in the spontaneous wheel-running activity and nesting performance reflects depressed pain behaviours typical during painful conditions in rodents [47,48,66]. Reductions in these behaviours were previously described for different pain models [47,49,67]. Nonetheless, these are the first data showing the effects of cisplatin on nest building and wheel running, indicating spontaneous pain development, that is, pain in the absence of a stimulus.

In addition to painful symptoms observed in CIPN, after undergoing cancer chemotherapy, patients also present a high risk of cognitive impairment—another neurotoxic condition of chemotherapy agents [53,68,69]. Chemotherapy-induced cognitive impairment, commonly known as *chemobrain*, consists of damage in several cognitive domains, including impairment in working memory, attention, processing speed, concentration, and executive function [54,68]. Cognitive dysfunction is also related to cisplatin treatment, as it crosses the blood–brain barrier in low concentrations [52,70]. In the present study, repeated cisplatin treatment caused a decreased preference for the novel object, indicating impaired working memory and spatial recognition [54]. These results corroborate previous data showing that cisplatin induces cognitive impairment [52–54].

Pain and humour disorders, such as depression, may develop secondarily to each other or may coexist. In general, depression may cause increased pain perception by patients who may be more likely to develop chronic pain [71]. Cancer patients undergoing chemotherapy treatment present symptoms of depression and anxiety, in addition to neuropathic pain symptoms [72,73]. In our study, cisplatin caused neuropathic pain symptoms but not depressive- and anxiety-like behaviours since it altered neither the mice's immobility time in the forced swimming test nor thigmotaxis behaviour, unlike in other studies [74–76]. These discrepancies between the results may be due to the different administration schedules, doses of cisplatin, or differences between the animal strains tested [74–76]. Thus, it is important to better elucidate such conditions underlying chemotherapeutic treatment, as well as cognitive impairment and mood disorders, in experimental models, since they can influence or be influenced by chronic pain states [71,77].

The cisplatin dose used in this study promoted nociceptive responses without causing damage to the general health of the mice. On the other hand, higher doses of cisplatin result in weight loss accentuated after the second cisplatin administration [78]. Furthermore, cisplatin did not cause motor impairments, as evaluated by spontaneous and forced locomotor activity.

The pathological mechanisms underlying CIPN development have been widely debated [9,11,64,65]. Potential targets that might be involved in cisplatin-induced painful peripheral neuropathy pathophysiology are the kinin B_1 and B_2 receptors, which are involved in various painful conditions, including those induced by other chemotherapy drugs [27,31–33,39].

Kinins (bradykinin and kallidin), as well as their active metabolites (des-Arg^9-Bk and des-Arg^{10}-kallidin), are endogenous peptides that mediate inflammatory and painful processes via the kinin B_1 and B_2 receptors, respectively [79,80]. In the present study, pharmacological antagonism and gene silencing using antisense oligonucleotides for the kinin receptors attenuated cisplatin-induced mechanical allodynia. These findings indicate that cisplatin can promote the painful symptom characteristic of CIPN in male mice in a kinin B_1 and B_2 receptor-dependent manner. Since no study has shown discrepant kinin receptor effects on painful conditions in male and female experimental animals, we evaluated the antinociceptive effect of kinin B_1 and B_2 receptor antagonists only in male mice.

The systemic administration of peptide kinin B_1 and B_2 antagonists decreased mechanical allodynia in the therapeutic and preventive protocol. It is worth mentioning that nociceptive tests in the preventive protocol were carried out 24 h post administration of the antagonists, indicating a lasting effect of the peptide kinin B_1 and B_2 antagonists once efficacy was reached. In the therapeutic protocol, non-peptide kinin B_1 and B_2 receptor antagonists SSR240612 e FR173657 exerted a more prolonged antiallodynic effect than the peptide antagonists. Similarly, antinociceptive effects more prolonged from non-peptide antagonists than peptide antagonists were evidenced in a fibromyalgia model and paclitaxel-induced pain syndrome [23,27]. Notwithstanding the longer-lasting effect observed for non-peptide antagonists, the inhibition percentage of mechanical allodynia was similar to that caused by peptide antagonists. Therefore, their effects were not evaluated in the preventive protocol.

The ability of kinin antagonists to attenuate cisplatin-induced mechanical allodynia can be explained by the constitutive expression of kinin B_1 and B_2 receptors in structures important for nociceptive transmission, such as nociceptive neurons, the dorsal root ganglion, and spinal cord [25,26,28,81]. Still, immune cells, such as monocytes, neutrophils, and microglia, also express kinin receptors [80,82]. In this sense, microglia activation on the spinal cord was previously demonstrated in the cisplatin-induced peripheral neuropathy model [83].

Therefore, our results agree with previous studies that have linked kinin receptors to the pathogenesis of different acute and chronic pain models, highlighting the role of these receptors in pain hypersensitivity following mechanical stimulus [18,19,21–23,84]. In particular, kinin receptors also contribute to mechanical hypersensitivity induced by chemotherapeutic agents such as paclitaxel and vincristine [27,31,33].

To contribute to our hypothesis that kinin B_1 and B_2 receptors mediate cisplatin-induced painful symptoms, mice previously treated with cisplatin received sub-nociceptive doses of kinin B_1 and B_2 receptor agonists. Local exposure to agonists of kinin receptors (at doses that generally do not cause nociception) is associated with more prolonged and intensified nociceptive behaviours [18,23]. Kinin B_1 and B_2 receptor agonists—DABK and Bk, respectively—enhanced cisplatin-induced mechanical nociception. Similarly, chronic pain studies have reported hypersensitivity to sub-nociceptive doses of kinin B_1 and B_2 agonists [18,23]. The respective antagonist reduced this increased nociceptive response, providing additional evidence of the involvement of kinin B_1 and B_2 receptors in cisplatin-induced pain hypersensitivity.

The intrathecal administration of antisense oligonucleotides targeting kinin B_1 and B_2 receptors decreased cisplatin-induced mechanical allodynia. Our results are consistent with previous studies showing that genetic deletion of kinin receptors effectively reduces pain responses in different experimental models [18,85]. As mentioned before, in addition to their expression at the peripheral level, the kinin B_1 and B_2 receptors also are found or upregulated in the spinal cord, astrocytes, and microglia in the central nervous system, contributing to chronic pain states such as neuropathic pain [82,86,87]. This explains the ability of intrathecal antisense oligonucleotides targeting kinin B_1 and B_2 receptors to attenuate cisplatin-induced mechanical allodynia.

Although kinin receptor antagonists and antisense oligonucleotides reduced cisplatin-induced mechanical allodynia, in our study, they did not reduce cold hypersensitivity. These results are in agreement with a study by Gonçalves et al. (2021), which disregards the involvement of kinin receptors in cold hypersensitivity. Unlike our findings, kinin receptor antagonists attenuated the cold sensitivity in a spinal nerve ligation and fibromyalgia model [22,23]. However, considering that TRPA1 is a harmful cold sensor and that the activation of B_1 and B_2 receptors causes sensitization of TRP channels, including TRPA1 [25,39,88–92], kinin receptors may be indirectly involved in cold hypersensitivity. Therefore, it is essential to better elucidate the mechanisms of cold allodynia in the cisplatin-induced neuropathy model and define the role of kinin receptors in this condition.

In addition to neurotoxicity, cisplatin is also associated with nephrotoxic effects [6,8]. In this regard, cisplatin did not alter the urea and creatinine levels of animals in a previous study [93]. Interestingly, both kinin B_1 and B_2 receptors seem to be involved in cisplatin-induced nephrotoxicity once the deletion and blockage of kinin B_1 and B_2 receptors have been shown to protect against cisplatin-induced acute kidney injury [34,35]. Furthermore, Estrela et al. (2017) showed that the deletion and blockage of the kinin B_1 receptor prevented the downregulation of organic transporters in kidney cisplatin-induced toxicity, increasing the cisplatin efflux and consequently protecting against cisplatin nephrotoxicity [94]. Thus, using kinin receptor antagonists to relieve painful symptoms could also help to protect against cisplatin-induced renal toxicity. Kinin antagonists might also present additional beneficial effects, such as avoiding cancer cell proliferation since kinin antagonists alone or in association with chemotherapeutics, including cisplatin, inhibit the growth of ovarian and lung tumour cells [95–97]. In general, an ideal therapeutic strategy should act synergistically, aiding in antitumour action and protecting against neurotoxic and nephrotoxic effects. Thus, our study and previous studies support the potential of kinin antagonists in these conditions induced by cisplatin and a possible synergistic effect on antitumour activity.

Our findings show that the mechanisms mediated by kinin B_1 and B_2 receptors contribute to cisplatin-induced peripheral neuropathy symptoms, especially in mechanical nociception, indicating that kinin B_1 and B_2 receptors are potential pharmacological targets to relieve the pain symptoms associated with cisplatin. Furthermore, considering the safety and tolerability of the kinin B_2 receptor antagonist, Icatibant, which has already been approved for treatment of hereditary angioedema [98], our data suggest a possible clinical repositioning of Icatibant for patients with cancer undergoing chemotherapy with cisplatin. Therefore, regulating the activation of kinin B_1 and B_2 receptors is a promising alternative to avoid dose reduction or interruption of chemotherapy treatment, in addition to contributing to the treatment of painful symptoms of cancer survivors and re-establishing their quality of life.

Supplementary Materials: The following supporting information can be downloaded at: https://www.mdpi.com/article/10.3390/pharmaceutics15030852/s1, Table S1: Anxiety and depressive-like behaviours after cisplatin or vehicle injections. Table S2: Body weight and locomotor activity evaluations after cisplatin or vehicle injections. Table S3. Biochemical analysis after cisplatin or vehicle injections.

Author Contributions: All the authors contributed to this study. Study concept and design: G.B., I.B. and S.M.O. Acquisition of data: G.B. and M.F.P.F. Analysis and interpretation of data: G.B. and S.M.O. Drafting and revision the content of the manuscript: G.B., M.F.P.F., I.B. and S.M.O. Study supervision: S.M.O. All authors have read and agreed to the published version of the manuscript.

Funding: This study was financed in part by the Coordenação de Aperfeiçoamento de Pessoal de Nível Superior—Brasil (CAPES)—Finance Code 001; by the Fundação de Amparo à Pesquisa do Estado do Rio Grande do Sul-FAPERGS (Grant #21/2551-0001966-2) (Brazil); and by Conselho Nacional de Desenvolvimento Científico (CNPq). CAPES/PROEX (process #23038.002125/2021-

85; Grant: #0036/2021). Sara Marchesan Oliveira is the recipient of an award from CNPq (grant #304985/2020-1). Gabriela Becker, Maria Fernanda Pessano Fialho, and Indiara Brusco are recipients of a fellowship from CAPES/PROEX (processes #88887.568915/2020-00, #88882.182170/2018-01, and #88882.182148/2018-01, respectively).

Institutional Review Board Statement: The animal study protocol was approved by the Institutional Animal Care and Use Committee of the Federal University of Santa Maria (approval processes #7152261119/2020 and #6380261021/2022).

Informed Consent Statement: Not applicable.

Data Availability Statement: Not applicable.

Conflicts of Interest: The authors declare no conflict of interest.

References

1. Sung, H.; Ferlay, J.; Siegel, R.L.; Laversanne, M.; Soerjomataram, I.; Jemal, A.; Bray, F. Global Cancer Statistics 2020: GLOBOCAN Estimates of Incidence and Mortality Worldwide for 36 Cancers in 185 Countries. *CA Cancer J. Clin.* **2021**, *71*, 209–249. [CrossRef] [PubMed]
2. Kerns, S.L.; Fung, C.; Monahan, P.O.; Ardeshir-Rouhani-Fard, S.; Abu Zaid, M.I.; Williams, A.L.M.; Stump, T.E.; Sesso, H.D.; Feldman, D.R.; Hamilton, R.J.; et al. Cumulative Burden of Morbidity among Testicular Cancer Survivors after Standard Cisplatin-Based Chemotherapy: A Multi-Institutional Study. *J. Clin. Oncol.* **2018**, *36*, 1505–1512. [CrossRef] [PubMed]
3. Travis, L.B.; Fossa, S.D.; Sesso, H.D.; Frisina, R.D.; Herrmann, D.N.; Beard, C.J.; Feldman, D.R.; Pagliaro, L.C.; Miller, R.C.; Vaughn, D.J.; et al. Chemotherapy-Induced Peripheral Neurotoxicity and Ototoxicity: New Paradigms for Translational Genomics. *J. Natl. Cancer Inst.* **2014**, *106*, dju044. [CrossRef]
4. Miller, K.D.; Nogueira, L.; Devasia, T.; Mariotto, A.B.; Yabroff, K.R.; Jemal, A.; Kramer, J.; Siegel, R.L. Cancer Treatment and Survivorship Statistics, 2022. *CA Cancer J. Clin.* **2022**, *72*, 409–436. [CrossRef]
5. Colvin, L.A. Chemotherapy-Induced Peripheral Neuropathy: Where Are We Now? *Pain* **2019**, *160*, S1–S10. [CrossRef]
6. Starobova, H.; Vetter, I. Pathophysiology of Chemotherapy-Induced Peripheral Neuropathy. *Front. Mol. Neurosci.* **2017**, *10*, 174. [CrossRef]
7. Ibrahim, E.Y.; Ehrlich, B.E. Prevention of Chemotherapy-Induced Peripheral Neuropathy: A Review of Recent Findings. *Crit. Rev. Oncol. Hematol.* **2020**, *145*, 102831. [CrossRef] [PubMed]
8. Staff, N.P.; Grisold, A.; Grisold, W.; Windebank, A.J. Chemotherapy-Induced Peripheral Neuropathy: A Current Review. *Ann. Neurol.* **2017**, *81*, 772–781. [CrossRef]
9. Calls, A.; Carozzi, V.; Navarro, X.; Monza, L.; Bruna, J. Pathogenesis of Platinum-Induced Peripheral Neurotoxicity: Insights from Preclinical Studies. *Exp. Neurol.* **2020**, *325*, 113141. [CrossRef]
10. Seretny, M.; Currie, G.L.; Sena, E.S.; Ramnarine, S.; Grant, R.; Macleod, M.R.; Colvin, L.A.; Fallon, M. Incidence, Prevalence, and Predictors of Chemotherapy-Induced Peripheral Neuropathy: A Systematic Review and Meta-Analysis. *Pain* **2014**, *155*, 2461–2470. [CrossRef]
11. Staff, N.P.; Cavaletti, G.; Islam, B.; Lustberg, M.; Psimaras, D.; Tamburin, S. Platinum-Induced Peripheral Neurotoxicity: From Pathogenesis to Treatment. *J. Peripher. Nerv. Syst.* **2019**, *24*, S26–S39. [CrossRef] [PubMed]
12. Alberti, P. Platinum-Drugs Induced Peripheral Neurotoxicity: Clinical Course and Preclinical Evidence. *Expert Opin. Drug Metab. Toxicol.* **2019**, *15*, 487–497. [CrossRef] [PubMed]
13. Rathinam, R.; Ghosh, S.; Neumann, W.; Jamesdaniel, S. Cisplatin-Induced Apoptosis in Auditory, Renal, and Neuronal Cells Is Associated with Nitration and Downregulation of LMO4. *Cell Death Discov.* **2015**, *1*, 15052. [CrossRef]
14. Loprinzi, C.L.; Lacchetti, C.; Bleeker, J.; Cavaletti, G.; Chauhan, C.; Hertz, D.L.; Kelley, M.R.; Lavino, A.; Lustberg, M.B.; Paice, J.A.; et al. Prevention and Management of Chemotherapy-Induced Peripheral Neuropathy in Survivors of Adult Cancers: ASCO Guideline Update. *J. Clin. Oncol.* **2020**, *38*, 3325–3348. [CrossRef]
15. Smith, E.M.L.; Pang, H.; Cirrincione, C.; Fleishman, S.; Paskett, E.D.; Ahles, T.; Bressler, L.R.; Gilman, P.B.; Shapiro, C.L.; Chemotherapy-induced, W.; et al. Effect of Duloxetine on Pain, Function, and Quality of Life among Patients with Chemotherapy-Induced Painful Peripheral Neuropathy. *JAMA Psychiatry* **2013**, *309*, 1359–1367. [CrossRef]
16. Flatters, S.J.L.; Dougherty, P.M.; Colvin, L.A. Clinical and Preclinical Perspectives on Chemotherapy-Induced Peripheral Neuropathy (CIPN): A Narrative Review. *Br. J. Anaesth.* **2017**, *119*, 737–749. [CrossRef] [PubMed]
17. Ferreira, J.; Trichês, K.M.; Medeiros, R.; Cabrini, D.A.; Mori, M.A.S.; Pesquero, J.B.; Bader, M.; Calixto, J.B. The Role of Kinin B1 Receptors in the Nociception Produced by Peripheral Protein Kinase C Activation in Mice. *Neuropharmacology* **2008**, *54*, 597–604. [CrossRef]
18. Gonçalves, E.C.D.; Vieira, G.; Gonçalves, T.R.; Simões, R.R.; Brusco, I.; Oliveira, S.M.; Calixto, J.B.; Cola, M.; Santos, A.R.S.; Dutra, R.C. Bradykinin Receptors Play a Critical Role in the Chronic Post-Ischaemia Pain Model. *Cell. Mol. Neurobiol.* **2021**, *41*, 63–78. [CrossRef]

19. Quintão, N.L.M.; Rocha, L.W.; da Silva, G.F.; Paszcuk, A.F.; Manjavachi, M.N.; Bento, A.F.; da Silva, K.A.B.S.; Campos, M.M.; Calixto, J.B. The Kinin B_1 and B_2 Receptors and TNFR1/P55 Axis on Neuropathic Pain in the Mouse Brachial Plexus. *Inflammopharmacology* **2019**, *27*, 573–586. [CrossRef]
20. Quintão, N.L.M.; Passos, G.F.; Medeiros, R.; Paszcuk, A.F.; Motta, F.L.; Pesquero, J.B.; Campos, M.M.; Calixto, J.B. Neuropathic Pain-like Behavior after Brachial Plexus Avulsion in Mice: The Relevance of Kinin B_1 and B_2 Receptors. *J. Neurosci.* **2008**, *28*, 2856–2863. [CrossRef]
21. Silva, C.R.; Oliveira, S.M.; Hoffmeister, C.; Funck, V.; Guerra, G.P.; Trevisan, G.; Tonello, R.; Rossato, M.F.; Pesquero, J.B.; Bader, M.; et al. The Role of Kinin B1 Receptor and the Effect of Angiotensin I-Converting Enzyme Inhibition on Acute Gout Attacks in Rodents. *Ann. Rheum. Dis.* **2016**, *75*, 260–268. [CrossRef] [PubMed]
22. Werner, M.F.P.; Kassuya, C.A.L.; Ferreira, J.; Zampronio, A.R.; Calixto, J.B.; Rae, G.A. Peripheral Kinin B_1 and B_2 Receptor-Operated Mechanisms Are Implicated in Neuropathic Nociception Induced by Spinal Nerve Ligation in Rats. *Neuropharmacology* **2007**, *53*, 48–57. [CrossRef] [PubMed]
23. Brusco, I.; Benatti, A.; Regina, C.; Fischer, S.; Mattar, T.; Scussel, R.; Machado-de-ávila, R.A.; Ferreira, J.; Marchesan, S. Kinins and Their B 1 and B 2 Receptors Are Involved in Fibromyalgia-like Pain Symptoms in Mice. *Biochem. Pharmacol.* **2019**, *168*, 119–132. [CrossRef]
24. Ma, Q.P.; Heavens, R. Basal Expression of Bradykinin B1 Receptor in the Spinal Cord in Humans and Rats. *Neuroreport* **2001**, *12*, 2311–2314. [CrossRef] [PubMed]
25. Ma, Q.P. The Expression of Bradykinin B1 Receptors on Primary Sensory Neurones That Give Rise to Small Caliber Sciatic Nerve Fibres in Rats. *Neuroscience* **2001**, *107*, 665–673. [CrossRef] [PubMed]
26. Marceau, F.; Regoli, D. Bradykinin Receptor Ligands: Therapeutic Perspectives. *Nat. Rev. Drug Discov.* **2004**, *3*, 845–852. [CrossRef]
27. Brusco, I.; Silva, C.R.; Trevisan, G.; de Campos Velho Gewehr, C.; Rigo, F.K.; La Rocca Tamiozzo, L.; Rossato, M.F.; Tonello, R.; Dalmolin, G.D.; de Almeida Cabrini, D.; et al. Potentiation of Paclitaxel-Induced Pain Syndrome in Mice by Angiotensin I Converting Enzyme Inhibition and Involvement of Kinins. *Mol. Neurobiol.* **2017**, *54*, 7824–7837. [CrossRef]
28. Calixto, J.B.; Medeiros, R.; Fernandes, E.S.; Ferreira, J.; Cabrini, D.A.; Campos, M.M. Kinin B 1 Receptors: Key G-Protein-Coupled Receptors and Their Role in Inflammatory and Painful Processes. *Br. J. Pharmacol.* **2004**, *143*, 803–818. [CrossRef]
29. Ferreira, J.; Campos, M.M.; Araújo, R.; Bader, M.; Pesquero, J.B.; Calixto, J.B. The Use of Kinin B_1 and B_2 Receptor Knockout Mice and Selective Antagonists to Characterize the Nociceptive Responses Caused by Kinins at the Spinal Level. *Neuropharmacology* **2002**, *43*, 1188–1197. [CrossRef]
30. Quintão, N.L.M.; Santin, J.R.; Stoeberl, L.C.; Corrêa, T.P.; Melato, J.; Costa, R. Pharmacological Treatment of Chemotherapy-Induced Neuropathic Pain: PPARγ Agonists as a Promising Tool. *Front. Neurosci.* **2019**, *13*, 907. [CrossRef]
31. Bujalska, M.; Tatarkiewicz, J.; Gumułka, S.W. Effect of Bradykinin Receptor Antagonists on Vincristine- and Streptozotocin-Induced Hyperalgesia in a Rat Model of Chemotherapy-Induced and Diabetic Neuropathy. *Pharmacology* **2008**, *81*, 158–163. [CrossRef] [PubMed]
32. Bujalska, M.; Makulska-Nowak, H. Bradykinin Receptor Antagonists and Cyclooxygenase Inhibitors in Vincristine- and Streptozotocin-Induced Hyperalgesia. *Pharmacol. Rep.* **2009**, *61*, 631–640. [CrossRef]
33. Costa, R.; Motta, E.M.; Dutra, R.C.; Manjavachi, M.N.; Bento, A.F.; Malinsky, F.R.; Pesquero, J.B.; Calixto, J.B. Anti-nociceptive Effect of Kinin B_1 and B_2 Receptor Antagonists on Peripheral Neuropathy Induced by Paclitaxel in Mice. *Br. J. Pharmacol.* **2011**, *164*, 681–693. [CrossRef] [PubMed]
34. Estrela, G.R.; Wasinski, F.; Almeida, D.C.; Amano, M.T.; Castoldi, A.; Dias, C.C.; Malheiros, D.M.A.C.; Almeida, S.S.; Paredes-Gamero, E.J.; Pesquero, J.B.; et al. Kinin B1 Receptor Deficiency Attenuates Cisplatin-Induced Acute Kidney Injury by Modulating Immune Cell Migration. *J. Mol. Med.* **2014**, *92*, 399–409. [CrossRef] [PubMed]
35. Estrela, G.R.; Wasinski, F.; Bacurau, R.F.; Malheiros, D.M.A.C.; Câmara, N.O.S.; Araújo, R.C. Kinin B_2 Receptor Deletion and Blockage Ameliorates Cisplatin-Induced Acute Renal Injury. *Int. Immunopharmacol.* **2014**, *22*, 115–119. [CrossRef]
36. Brasil, M.; das, C.T. e I. Resolução Normativa n° 39, De 20 De Junho De 2018. *Diário Of. da União* **2018**, *120*, 7.
37. Zimmermann, M. Ethical Guidelines for Investigations of Experimental Pain in Conscious Animals. *Pain* **1983**, *16*, 109–110. [CrossRef]
38. McGrath, J.C.; Lilley, E. Implementing Guidelines on Reporting Research Using Animals (ARRIVE Etc.): New Requirements for Publication in BJP. *Br. J. Pharmacol.* **2015**, *172*, 3189–3193. [CrossRef]
39. Costa, R.; Bicca, M.A.; Manjavachi, M.N.; Segat, G.C.; Dias, F.C.; Fernandes, E.S.; Calixto, J.B. Kinin Receptors Sensitize TRPV4 Channel and Induce Mechanical Hyperalgesia: Relevance to Paclitaxel-Induced Peripheral Neuropathy in Mice. *Mol. Neurobiol.* **2018**, *55*, 2150–2161. [CrossRef]
40. Meotti, F.C.; Campos, R.; Da Silva, K.A.B.S.; Paszcuk, A.F.; Costa, R.; Calixto, J.B. Inflammatory Muscle Pain Is Dependent on the Activation of Kinin B_1 and B_2 Receptors and Intracellular Kinase Pathways. *Br. J. Pharmacol.* **2012**, *166*, 1127–1139. [CrossRef]
41. Park, H.J.; Stokes, J.A.; Corr, M.; Yaksh, T.L. Toll-like Receptor Signaling Regulates Cisplatin-Induced Mechanical Allodynia in Mice. *Cancer Chemother. Pharmacol.* **2014**, *73*, 25–34. [CrossRef] [PubMed]
42. Park, H.J.; Stokes, J.A.; Pirie, E.; Skahen, J.; Shtaerman, Y.; Yaksh, T.L. Persistent Hyperalgesia in the Cisplatin-Treated Mouse as Defined by Threshold Measures, the Conditioned Place Preference Paradigm, and Changes in Dorsal Root Ganglia Activated Transcription Factor 3: The Effects of Gabapentin, Ketorolac, and Etanercept. *Anesth. Analg.* **2013**, *116*, 224–231. [CrossRef]

43. John, T.; Lomeli, N.; Bota, D.A. Systemic Cisplatin Exposure during Infancy and Adolescence Causes Impaired Cognitive Function in Adulthood. *Behav. Brain Res.* **2017**, *319*, 200–206. [CrossRef]
44. Chaplan, S.R.; Bach, F.W.; Pogrel, J.W.; Chung, J.M.; Yaksh, T.L. Quantitative Assessment of Tactile Allodynia in the Rat Paw. *J. Neurosci. Methods* **1994**, *53*, 55–63. [CrossRef]
45. Oliveira, S.M.; Silva, C.R.; Ferreira, J. Critical Role of Protease-Activated Receptor 2 Activation by Mast Cell Tryptase in the Development of Postoperative Pain. *Anesthesiology* **2013**, *118*, 679–690. [CrossRef]
46. da Silva Brum, E.; Fialho, M.F.P.; Fischer, S.P.M.; Hartmann, D.D.; Gonçalves, D.F.; Scussel, R.; Machado-de-Ávila, R.A.; Dalla Corte, C.L.; Soares, F.A.A.; Oliveira, S.M. Relevance of Mitochondrial Dysfunction in the Reserpine-Induced Experimental Fibromyalgia Model. *Mol. Neurobiol.* **2020**, *57*, 4202–4217. [CrossRef] [PubMed]
47. Cobos, E.J.; Ghasemlou, N.; Araldi, D.; Segal, D.; Duong, K.; Woolf, C.J. Inflammation-Induced Decrease in Voluntary Wheel Running in Mice: A Non-Reflexive Test for Evaluating Inflammatory Pain and Analgesia. *Pain* **2012**, *153*, 876–884. [CrossRef]
48. Negus, S.S.; Neddenriep, B.; Altarifi, A.A.; Carroll, F.I.; Leitl, M.D.; Miller, L.L. Effects of Ketoprofen, Morphine, and Kappa Opioids On Pain- Related Depression of Nesting in Mice. *Pain* **2015**, *156*, 1153–1160. [CrossRef]
49. Hung, C.H.; Lee, C.H.; Tsai, M.H.; Chen, C.H.; Lin, H.F.; Hsu, C.Y.; Lai, C.L.; Chen, C.C. Activation of Acid-Sensing Ion Channel 3 by Lysophosphatidylcholine 16:0 Mediates Psychological Stress-Induced Fibromyalgia-like Pain. *Ann. Rheum. Dis.* **2020**, *79*, 1644–1656. [CrossRef]
50. Fischer, S.P.M.; Brusco, I.; Brum, E.S.; Fialho, M.F.P.; Camponogara, C.; Scussel, R.; Machado-de-Ávila, R.A.; Trevisan, G.; Oliveira, S.M. Involvement of TRPV1 and the Efficacy of α-Spinasterol on Experimental Fibromyalgia Symptoms in Mice. *Neurochem. Int.* **2020**, *134*, 104673. [CrossRef] [PubMed]
51. Yankelevitch-yahav, R.; Franko, M.; Huly, A.; Doron, R. The Forced Swim Test as a Model of Depressive-like Behavior. *J. Vis. Exp.* **2015**, *97*, e52587. [CrossRef]
52. Chiu, G.S.; Maj, M.A.; Rivzi, S.; Dantzer, R.; Vichaya, E.G.; Laumet, G.; Kavelaars, A.; Heijnen, C.J. Pifithrin-μ Prevents Cisplatin-Induced Chemobrain by Preserving Neuronal Mitochondrial Function. *Cancer Res.* **2017**, *3*, 742–752. [CrossRef]
53. Alexander, J.F.; Seua, A.V.; Arroyo, L.D.; Ray, P.R.; Wangzhou, A.; Heiβ-Lückemann, L.; Schedlowski, M.; Price, T.J.; Kavelaars, A.; Heijnen, C.J. Nasal Administration of Mitochondria Reverses Chemotherapy-Induced Cognitive Deficits. *Theranostics* **2021**, *11*, 3109–3130. [CrossRef]
54. Chiu, G.S.; Boukelmoune, N.; Chiang, A.C.A.; Peng, B.; Rao, V.; Kingsley, C.; Liu, H.L.; Kavelaars, A.; Kesler, S.R.; Heijnen, C.J. Nasal Administration of Mesenchymal Stem Cells Restores Cisplatin-Induced Cognitive Impairment and Brain Damage in Mice. *Oncotarget* **2018**, *9*, 35581–35597. [CrossRef]
55. Brum, S.; Moreira, R.; Regina, A.; Augusti, A.; Barbosa, F.; Linde, M.; Brandão, R.; Marchesan, S. Tabernaemontana Catharinensis Ethyl Acetate Fraction Presents Antinociceptive Activity without Causing Toxicological Effects in Mice. *J. Ethnopharmacol.* **2016**, *191*, 115–124. [CrossRef] [PubMed]
56. Zhang, M.; Du, W.; Acklin, S.; Jin, S.; Xia, F. SIRT2 Protects Peripheral Neurons from Cisplatin-Induced Injury by Enhancing Nucleotide Excision Repair. *J. Clin. Investig.* **2020**, *130*, 2953–2965. [CrossRef] [PubMed]
57. Cavaletti, G.; Marzorati, L.; Bogliun, G.; Colombo, N.; Marzola, M.; Pittelli, M.R.; Tredici, G. Cisplatin-lnduced Peripheral Neurotoxicity Is Dependent on Total-dose Intensity and Single-dose Intensity. *Cancer* **1992**, *69*, 203–207. [CrossRef] [PubMed]
58. Glendenning, J.L.; Barbachano, Y.; Norman, A.R.; Dearnaley, D.P.; Horwich, A.; Huddart, R.A. Long-Term Neurologic and Peripheral Vascular Toxicity after Chemotherapy Treatment of Testicular Cancer. *Cancer* **2010**, *116*, 2322–2331. [CrossRef] [PubMed]
59. Woller, S.A.; Corr, M.; Yaksh, T.L. Differences in Cisplatin-Induced Mechanical Allodynia in Male and Female Mice. *Eur. J. Pain* **2015**, *19*, 1476–1485. [CrossRef]
60. Khasabova, I.A.; Khasabov, S.G.; Olson, J.K.; Uhelski, M.L.; Kim, A.H.; Albino-Ramírez, A.M.; Wagner, C.L.; Seybold, V.S.; Simone, D.A. Pioglitazone, a PPARγ Agonist, Reduces Cisplatin-Evoked Neuropathic Pain by Protecting against Oxidative Stress. *Pain* **2019**, *160*, 688–701. [CrossRef]
61. Guindon, J.; Deng, L.; Fan, B.; Wager-miller, J.; Hohmann, A.G. Optimization of a Cisplatin Model of Chemotherapy-Induced Peripheral Neuropathy in Mice: Use of Vitamin C and Sodium Bicarbonate Pretreatments to Reduce Nephrotoxicity and Improve Animal Health Status. *Mol. Pain* **2014**, *10*, 1744-8069-10-56. [CrossRef] [PubMed]
62. Alotaibi, M.; Al-Aqil, F.; Alqahtani, F.; Alanazi, M.; Nadeem, A.; Ahmad, S.F.; Lapresa, R.; Alharbi, M.; Alshammari, A.; Alotaibi, M.; et al. Alleviation of Cisplatin-Induced Neuropathic Pain, Neuronal Apoptosis, and Systemic Inflammation in Mice by Rapamycin. *Front. Aging Neurosci.* **2022**, *14*, 891593. [CrossRef] [PubMed]
63. Singh, S.K.; Krukowski, K.; Laumet, G.O.; Weis, D.; Alexander, J.F.; Heijnen, C.J.; Kavelaars, A. CD8+ T Cell-Derived IL-13 Increases Macrophage IL-10 to Resolve Neuropathic Pain. *JCI Insight* **2022**, *7*, e154194. [CrossRef]
64. Boukelmoune, N.; Laumet, G.; Tang, Y.; Ma, J.; Mahant, I.; Singh, S.K.; Nijboer, C.; Benders, M.; Kavelaars, A.; Heijnen, C.J. Nasal Administration of Mesenchymal Stem Cells Reverses Chemotherapy-Induced Peripheral Neuropathy in Mice. *Brain Behav. Immun.* **2021**, *93*, 43–54. [CrossRef]
65. Laumet, G.; Edralin, J.D.; Dantzer, R.; Heijnen, C.J.; Kavelaars, A. Cisplatin Educates CD8+ T Cells to Prevent and Resolve Chemotherapy-Induced Peripheral Neuropathy in Mice. *Pain* **2019**, *160*, 1459–1468. [CrossRef]

66. González-Cano, R.; Montilla-García, Á.; Ruiz-Cantero, M.C.; Bravo-Caparrós, I.; Tejada, M.; Nieto, F.R.; Cobos, E.J. The Search for Translational Pain Outcomes to Refine Analgesic Development: Where Did We Come from and Where Are We Going? *Neurosci. Biobehav. Rev.* **2020**, *113*, 238–261. [CrossRef]
67. Griffiths, L.A.; Duggett, N.A.; Pitcher, A.L.; Flatters, S.J.L. Evoked and Ongoing Pain-Like Behaviours in a Rat Model of Paclitaxel-Induced Peripheral Neuropathy. *Pain Res. Manag.* **2018**, *2018*, 821763. [CrossRef]
68. Cauli, O. Oxidative Stress and Cognitive Alterations Induced by Cancer Chemotherapy Drugs: A Scoping Review. *Antioxidants* **2021**, *10*, 1116. [CrossRef]
69. Stouten-Kemperman, M.M.; de Ruiter, M.B.; Caan, M.W.A.; Boogerd, W.; Kerst, M.J.; Reneman, L.; Schagen, S.B. Lower Cognitive Performance and White Matter Changes in Testicular Cancer Survivors 10 Years after Chemotherapy. *Hum. Brain Mapp.* **2015**, *36*, 4638–4647. [CrossRef] [PubMed]
70. Fumagalli, G.; Monza, L.; Cavaletti, G.; Rigolio, R.; Meregalli, C. Neuroinflammatory Process Involved in Different Preclinical Models of Chemotherapy-Induced Peripheral Neuropathy. *Front. Immunol.* **2021**, *11*, 626687. [CrossRef]
71. Surah, A.; Baranidharan, G.; Morley, S. Chronic Pain and Depression. *Contin. Educ. Anaesth. Crit. Care Pain* **2014**, *14*, 85–89. [CrossRef]
72. Linden, W.; Vodermaier, A.; MacKenzie, R.; Greig, D. Anxiety and Depression after Cancer Diagnosis: Prevalence Rates by Cancer Type, Gender, and Age. *J. Affect. Disord.* **2012**, *141*, 343–351. [CrossRef] [PubMed]
73. Naser, A.Y.; Hameed, A.N.; Mustafa, N.; Alwafi, H.; Dahmash, E.Z.; Alyami, H.S.; Khalil, H. Depression and Anxiety in Patients with Cancer: A Cross-Sectional Study. *Front. Psychol.* **2021**, *12*, 585534. [CrossRef] [PubMed]
74. Mu, L.; Wang, J.; Cao, B.; Jelfs, B.; Chan, R.H.M.; Xu, X.; Hasan, M.; Zhang, X.; Li, Y. Impairment of Cognitive Function by Chemotherapy: Association with the Disruption of Phase-Locking and Synchronization in Anterior Cingulate Cortex. *Mol. Brain* **2015**, *8*, 32. [CrossRef]
75. Abdelkader, N.F.; Saad, M.A.; Abdelsalam, R.M. Neuroprotective Effect of Nebivolol against Cisplatin-Associated Depressive-like Behavior in Rats. *J. Neurochem.* **2017**, *141*, 449–460. [CrossRef]
76. Saadati, H.; Noroozzadeh, S.; Esmaeili, H.; Amirshahrokhi, K.; Shadman, J.; Niapour, A. The Neuroprotective Effect of Mesna on Cisplatin-Induced Neurotoxicity: Behavioral, Electrophysiological, and Molecular Studies. *Neurotox. Res.* **2021**, *39*, 826–840. [CrossRef]
77. da Silva, M.D.; Guginski, G.; Sato, K.L.; Sanada, L.S.; Sluka, K.A.; Santos, A.R.S. Persistent Pain Induces Mood Problems and Memory Loss by the Involvement of Cytokines, Growth Factors, and Supraspinal Glial Cells. *Brain Behav. Immun. Health* **2020**, *7*, 100118. [CrossRef]
78. Calls, A.; Torres-Espin, A.; Navarro, X.; Yuste, V.J.; Udina, E.; Bruna, J. Cisplatin-Induced Peripheral Neuropathy Is Associated with Neuronal Senescence-like Response. *Neuro. Oncol.* **2021**, *23*, 88–99. [CrossRef]
79. Moreau, M.E.; Garbacki, N.; Molinaro, G.; Brown, N.J.; Marceau, F.; Adam, A. The Kallikrein-Kinin System: Current and Future Pharmacological Targets. *J. Pharmacol. Sci.* **2005**, *99*, 6–38. [CrossRef]
80. Dutra, R.C. Kinin Receptors: Key Regulators of Autoimmunity. *Autoimmun. Rev.* **2017**, *16*, 192–207. [CrossRef]
81. Couture, R.; Harrisson, M.; Vianna, R.M.; Cloutier, F. Kinin Receptors in Pain and Inflammation. *Eur. J. Pharmacol.* **2001**, *429*, 161–176. [CrossRef]
82. Noda, M.; Kariura, Y.; Amano, T.; Manago, Y.; Nishikawa, K.; Aoki, S.; Wada, K. Kinin Receptors in Cultured Rat Microglia. *Neurochem. Int.* **2004**, *45*, 437–442. [CrossRef]
83. Hu, L.Y.; Zhou, Y.; Cui, W.Q.; Hu, X.M.; Du, L.X.; Mi, W.L.; Chu, Y.X.; Wu, G.C.; Wang, Y.Q.; Mao-Ying, Q.L. Triggering Receptor Expressed on Myeloid Cells 2 (TREM2) Dependent Microglial Activation Promotes Cisplatin-Induced Peripheral Neuropathy in Mice. *Brain. Behav. Immun.* **2018**, *68*, 132–145. [CrossRef]
84. Brusco, I.; Justino, A.B.; Silva, C.R.; Scussel, R.; Machado-de-Ávila, R.A.; Oliveira, S.M. Inhibitors of Angiotensin I Converting Enzyme Potentiate Fibromyalgia-like Pain Symptoms via Kinin Receptors in Mice. *Eur. J. Pharmacol.* **2021**, *895*, 173870. [CrossRef]
85. Rashid, H.; Inoue, M.; Matsumoto, M.; Ueda, H. Switching of Bradykinin-Mediated Nociception Following Partial Sciatic Nerve Injury in Mice. 2004, 308, 1158–1164. *J. Pharmacol. Exp. Ther.* **2004**, *308*, 1158–1164. [CrossRef] [PubMed]
86. Cernit, V.; Sénécal, J.; Othman, R.; Couture, R. Reciprocal Regulatory Interaction between TRPV1 and Kinin B1 Receptor in a Rat Neuropathic Pain Model. *Int. J. Mol. Sci.* **2020**, *21*, 821. [CrossRef] [PubMed]
87. Talbot, S.; Chahmi, E.; Dias, J.P.; Couture, R. Key Role for Spinal Dorsal Horn Microglial Kinin B1 receptor in Early Diabetic Pain Neuropathy. *J. Neuroinflammation* **2010**, *7*, 36. [CrossRef]
88. Story, G.M.; Peier, A.M.; Reeve, A.J.; Eid, S.R.; Mosbacher, J.; Hricik, T.R.; Earley, T.J.; Hergarden, A.C.; Andersson, D.A.; Hwang, S.W.; et al. ANKTM1, a TRP-like Channel Expressed in Nociceptive Neurons, Is Activated by Cold Temperatures. *Cell* **2003**, *112*, 819–829. [CrossRef] [PubMed]
89. Jordt, S.E.; Bautista, D.M.; Chuang, H.H.; McKemy, D.D.; Zygmunt, P.M.; Högestätt, E.D.; Meng, I.D.; Julius, D. Mustard Oils and Cannabinoids Excite Sensory Nerve Fibres through the TRP Channel ANKTM1. *Nature* **2004**, *427*, 260–265. [CrossRef]
90. Bandell, M.; Story, G.M.; Hwang, S.W.; Viswanath, V.; Eid, S.R.; Petrus, M.J.; Earley, T.J.; Patapoutian, A. Noxious Cold Ion Channel TRPA1 Is Activated by Pungent Compounds and Bradykinin. *Neuron* **2004**, *41*, 849–857. [CrossRef]
91. Ferreira, J.; Da Silva, G.L.; Calixto, J.B. Contribution of Vanilloid Receptors to the Overt Nociception Induced by B 2 Kinin Receptor Activation in Mice. *Br. J. Pharmacol.* **2004**, *141*, 787–794. [CrossRef] [PubMed]

92. Bautista, D.M.; Jordt, S.E.; Nikai, T.; Tsuruda, P.R.; Read, A.J.; Poblete, J.; Yamoah, E.N.; Basbaum, A.I.; Julius, D. TRPA1 Mediates the Inflammatory Actions of Environmental Irritants and Proalgesic Agents. *Cell* **2006**, *124*, 1269–1282. [CrossRef]
93. Ta, L.E.; Low, P.A.; Windebank, A.J. Mice with Cisplatin and Oxaliplatin-Induced Painful Neuropathy Develop Distinct Early Responses to Thermal Stimuli. *Mol. Pain* **2009**, *5*, 1744-8069-5-9. [CrossRef]
94. Estrela, G.R.; Wasinski, F.; Felizardo, R.J.F.; Souza, L.L.; Câmara, N.O.S.; Bader, M.; Araujo, R.C. MATE-1 Modulation by Kinin B1 Receptor Enhances Cisplatin Efflux from Renal Cells. *Mol. Cell. Biochem.* **2017**, *428*, 101–108. [CrossRef]
95. Chan, D.C.; Gera, L.; Stewart, J.M.; Helfrich, B.; Zhao, T.L.; Feng, W.Y.; Chan, K.K.; Covey, J.M.; Bunn, P.A. Bradykinin Antagonist Dimer, CU201, Inhibits the Growth of Human Lung Cancer Cell Lines in Vitro and in Vivo and Produces Synergistic Growth Inhibition in Combination with Other Antitumor Agents. *Clin. Cancer Res.* **2002**, *8*, 1280–1287. [PubMed]
96. da Costa, P.L.N.; Sirois, P.; Tannock, I.F.; Chammas, R. The Role of Kinin Receptors in Cancer and Therapeutic Opportunities. *Cancer Lett.* **2014**, *345*, 27–38. [CrossRef]
97. Jutras, S.; Bachvarova, M.; Keita, M.; Bascands, J.L.; Mes-Masson, A.M.; Stewart, J.M.; Bachvarov, D. Strong Cytotoxic Effect of the Bradykinin Antagonist BKM-570 in Ovarian Cancer Cells—Analysis of the Molecular Mechanisms of Its Antiproliferative Action. *FEBS J.* **2010**, *277*, 5146–5160. [CrossRef] [PubMed]
98. Farkas, H.; Kőhalmi, K.V. Icatibant for the Treatment of Hereditary Angioedema with C1-Inhibitor Deficiency in Adolescents and in Children Aged over 2 Years. *Expert Rev. Clin. Immunol.* **2018**, *14*, 447–460. [CrossRef]

Disclaimer/Publisher's Note: The statements, opinions and data contained in all publications are solely those of the individual author(s) and contributor(s) and not of MDPI and/or the editor(s). MDPI and/or the editor(s) disclaim responsibility for any injury to people or property resulting from any ideas, methods, instructions or products referred to in the content.

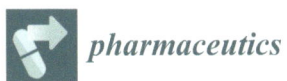

Article

Clinical and Electrophysiological Changes in Pediatric Spinal Muscular Atrophy after 2 Years of Nusinersen Treatment

Mihaela Axente [1,2], Andrada Mirea [2,3,*], Corina Sporea [2,3,*], Liliana Pădure [2,3], Cristina Manuela Drăgoi [4], Alina Crenguța Nicolae [4] and Daniela Adriana Ion [5]

1. Faculty of Medicine, University of Medicine and Pharmacy "Carol Davila", 37 Dionisie Lupu Street, 020021 Bucharest, Romania
2. National University Center for Children Neurorehabilitation "Dr. Nicolae Robanescu", 44 Dumitru Minca Street, 041408 Bucharest, Romania
3. Faculty of Midwifery and Nursing, University of Medicine and Pharmacy "Carol Davila", 37 Dionisie Lupu Street, 020021 Bucharest, Romania
4. Department of Biochemistry, Faculty of Pharmacy, "Carol Davila" University of Medicine and Pharmacy, 020956 Bucharest, Romania
5. Department of Pathophysiology, National Institute for Infectious Diseases Prof. Dr. Matei Balș, Carol Davila University of Medicine and Pharmacy, 1 Calistrat Grozovici Street, 021105 Bucharest, Romania
* Correspondence: andrada.mirea@gmail.com (A.M.); corina.sporea@gmail.com (C.S.)

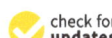

Citation: Axente, M.; Mirea, A.; Sporea, C.; Pădure, L.; Drăgoi, C.M.; Nicolae, A.C.; Ion, D.A. Clinical and Electrophysiological Changes in Pediatric Spinal Muscular Atrophy after 2 Years of Nusinersen Treatment. *Pharmaceutics* 2022, 14, 2074. https://doi.org/10.3390/pharmaceutics14102074

Academic Editor: Pedro Dorado

Received: 24 August 2022
Accepted: 27 September 2022
Published: 29 September 2022

Publisher's Note: MDPI stays neutral with regard to jurisdictional claims in published maps and institutional affiliations.

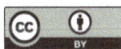

Copyright: © 2022 by the authors. Licensee MDPI, Basel, Switzerland. This article is an open access article distributed under the terms and conditions of the Creative Commons Attribution (CC BY) license (https://creativecommons.org/licenses/by/4.0/).

Abstract: In the new therapeutic era, disease-modifying treatment (nusinersen) has changed the natural evolution of spinal muscular atrophy (SMA), creating new phenotypes. The main purpose of the retrospective observational study was to explore changes in clinical evolution and electrophysiological data after 2 years of nusinersen treatment. We assessed distal compound motor action potential (CMAP) on the ulnar nerve and motor abilities in 34 SMA patients, aged between 1 and 16 years old, under nusinersen treatment, using specific motor scales for types 1, 2 and 3. The evaluations were performed at treatment initiation and 26 months later. There were registered increased values for CMAP amplitudes after 2 years of nusinersen, significantly correlated with motor function evolution in SMA type 1 patients ($p < 0.005$, $r = 0.667$). In total, 45% of non-sitters became sitters and 25% of sitters became walkers. For SMA types 1 and 2, the age at the treatment initialization is highly significant ($p < 0.0001$) and correlated with treatment yield. A strong negative correlation ($r = -0.633$) was observed for SMA type 1 and a very strong negative correlation ($r = -0.813$) for SMA type 2. In treated SMA cases, the distal amplitude of the CMAP and motor functional scales are important prognostic factors, and early diagnosis and treatment are essential for a better outcome.

Keywords: spinal muscular atrophy; compound motor action potential; the children's hospital of Philadelphia infant test of neuromuscular disorders; hammersmith functional motor scale expanded

1. Introduction

Spinal muscular atrophy (SMA) is a degenerative neuromuscular genetic disorder with autosomal recessive transmission characterized by progressive loss of spinal and brainstem motor neurons with severe hypotonia, muscle weakness, atrophy, swallowing, and respiratory dysfunction [1,2].

Weakness is predominantly in the girdles and truncal, with greater involvement of the lower limbs and areflexia on examination. Bulbar and respiratory muscle weakness can occur in infantile type 1, particularly in more severe cases. Facial and ocular muscles are generally spared [3].

About 95% of the cases result from decreased amounts of survival motor neuron (SMN) protein due to deletions or mutations in the SMN1 gene, on chromosome 5q.

Most cases of SMA (95%) are caused by the biallelic homozygous deletion mutation in the SMN1 gene at 5q [4], with subsequently decreased amounts of survival motor neuron (SMN) protein. There are rare situations with compound heterozygous variants or punctiform mutations. The allelic SMN2 gene, also present on chromosome 5, contributes to a small extent to the production of SMN protein and thus to the phenotypic aspect of the disease [5]. The SMN2 gene differs from the SMN1 gene by only five nucleotides. The substitution cytosine-thymine in the sixth position of exon 7 disturbs splicing, resulting in exon 7 exclusion and a rapid degradation of SMN2 protein. The SMN2 gene produces up to 10% of full-length SMN protein due to normal splicing. The number of copies of the SMN2 gene varies from zero to eight, correlating directly with the amount of functional SMN protein and predicting disease severity.

Antisense oligonucleotides therapy of SMA is directed towards increasing the inclusion of exon 7 in the mRNA of the SMN2 gene to increase functional SMN protein [6].

SMA includes a wide range of phenotypes that are classified into clinical groups based on onset and maximum motor function achieved (untreated patients): very weak infants unable to sit unsupported (type 1) [7]; non-ambulant patients able to sit independently, and even walk with support (type 2); ambulant patients, with normal neurological development during early childhood, but with progressive loss of muscle strength (type 3) [8]. Approximately 95% of SMA type 1 patients have two SMN2 gene copies; 80% of SMA type 2 patients have three copies and 97% of type 3 patients have three to four copies. Recent recommendations [6] subdivided the functional classification from the original consensus statement document into three groups: non-sitters, sitters, and walkers.

1.1. Electrophysiology

CMAP represents motor fiber action potential summation in a motor area. It is obtained by the supramaximal stimulation of a peripheral motor nerve [9]. It is easy to obtain but a non-specific parameter, which does not provide enough information about chronic reinnervation mechanisms. CMAP amplitude decrease is observed in most of the symptomatic patients, as SMA is a degenerative peripheral motoneuron disease. Nevertheless, due to compensatory changes (collateral reinnervation), CMAP amplitude can be maintained. With the development of innovative therapies, in clinical trials, CMAP was introduced as a monitoring parameter and prognostic factor of the patients' evolution [10]. A sharp decrease in it was also noticed with the installation of motor regression, especially in the first form of SMA [11].

1.2. Treatment

The development of nusinersen, a synthetic, stabilized antisense oligonucleotide (ASO) that targets the splicing of SMN2 and increases the formation of a more stable protein product, has transformed the fatal type of SMA (type 1) into a stable condition. The first approved SMN2 pre-mRNA targeted therapy consisted of modified ASO, which was designed to bind to the intronic splice silencer site located in intron 7 of SMN-2 pre-messenger RNA, promoting exon 7 inclusion at the SMN2 messenger RNA level [12–15]. Earlier treatment leads to better outcomes, and initiation before symptom onset is associated with nearly normal early motor development in some infants [16].

In Romania, the first nusinersen administration was in October 2018 in the National University Center for Children Neurorehabilitation "Dr. Nicolae Robanescu". This procedure followed all the legal regulations for the patients' safety [17].

Table 1 shows the functional scales used based on the patient's age, SMA type, and neurological condition. Examinations using scales should be carried out by physiotherapists or physicians, employing tests based on the standard neurological examination [18].

The primary study objective was to examine the relationship between clinical evolution and electrophysiological data in SMA patients after two years of nusinersen treatment, investigating the distal ulnar CMAP amplitude and assessing CHOP/HFMSE/6MWT score at nusinersen initiation (T0) and every 4 months up to 26 months later (T26). Our working hypothesis was that there are statistically relevant correlations between clinical and electrophysiological data after 2 years of nusinersen in our cohort of SMA patients.

Table 1. Recommended functional scales according to patient's functional status.

Patient's Functional Status	Recommended Functional Scales
Non-sitter	CHOP INTEND
Sitter	HFMSE
Walker	6 MWT, HFMSE

1.3. Ethical Approval

The study was conducted according to the guidelines of the Declaration of Helsinki and approved by the Ethics Committee of National University Center for Children Neurorehabilitation "Dr. Nicolae Robanescu" No. 7465/01.10.2018. Data were collected during periodic evaluations, in accordance with our drug administration protocols, and all patients' parents signed informed consents.

2. Materials and Methods

We assessed motor abilities in 34 SMA patients diagnosed with types 1, 2, and 3, aged between 1 and 16 years old. 33 patients had biallelic deletion of SMN1 and 1 compound heterozygous, with 2 or 3 SMN2 copies, under nusinersen treatment. The assessments were performed at treatment initiation (T0) and every 4 months up to 26 months (T26). Assessments were performed at nusinersen administration time (Injection 1–Injection 10) using The Children's Hospital of Philadelphia Infant Test of Neuromuscular Disorders (CHOP INTEND) for type 1 and Hammersmith Functional Motor Scale Expanded (HFMSE) for SMA types 2 and 3. Simultaneously, the distal CMAP on the ulnar nerve was recorded. The study was carried out between October 2018 and October 2021.

Patients with genetic confirmation of SMA, pediatric age (0–18 years old) and 2 or more copies of SMN2 were included in the study.

Patients who were currently receiving another medication (risdiplam or onasemnogene abeparvovec-xioi) or who were agitated or uncooperative were excluded.

CMAP was recorded in the distal ulnar nerve, by supramaximal stimulation. Electrophysiological examinations were conducted using a 6-channel EMG Keypoint. No sedation was administered. According to good standing practice [19], a pleasant atmosphere was created to ensure the child's and the family's relaxation to facilitate the best possible approach. The recorded distal skin temperature was between 36.5 and 37 degrees in all children. We used surface pediatric electrodes placed on the hypothenar eminence. The electrical stimulation was performed distally (wrist) on the ulnar nerve, using progressive intensities ranged between 10 and 90 mA to obtain maximal amplitude. The CMAP was feasible and reproductible (electrical stimulation was repeated 3 times).

CHOP INTEND was developed to assess the motor abilities of patients with SMA type 1 before the age of six months who never achieve independent sitting [20–23]. Each of the 16 items on this scale is graded on a scale from 0 (no response) to 4, with 0 being the lowest grade and 4 being the highest (complete response). The total number of possible points ranges from 0 to 64.

HFMSE allows for the assessment of high-functioning SMA type 2 and includes 20 items from the Hammersmith Functional Motor Scale (a tool for evaluation of motor function in pediatric patients with SMA type 2, not designed for ambulatory patients), and 13 items from Gross Motor Function Measure. HFMSE can distinguish between ambulatory SMA type 3 patients and allows for the inclusion of a broader range of intermediate and mild SMA patients [23–27]. The score ranges between 0 and 66.

A 6 min walk test (6 MWT) [28] is a submaximal exercise test used to assess aerobic capacity and endurance. The distance covered over 6 min is used as the outcome by which to compare changes in performance capacity.

The percentage yields for CHOP/HFMSE scores' evolution were calculated based on SMA type. The percent yield is calculated by multiplying the actual yield (the actual improvement in motor development after 26 months of nusinersen treatment) by the theoretical yield (the maximum possible value of motor development).

Simultaneously, we tracked the evolution of CMAP under treatment at the same time intervals, 26 months.

The statistical data processing was performed using the Statistical Package for the Social Sciences IBM SPSS Statistics 24 and Excel 2021 software. The data processing for the analysis of the potential correlations between the collected data followed-up on two statistical indicators: statistical significance (p) and Pearson correlation coefficient (r) [29,30]. The Pearson correlation coefficient is a measure of linear correlation between two sets of data. It returns a value between -1 and 1, where 1 indicates a strong positive relationship, 0 indicates no relationship at all, and -1 indicates a strong negative relationship. The r value indicates a moderate correlation if $0.40 < r < 0.70$, a strong correlation if $0.70 < r < 0.90$ and a very strong one if $r > 0.90$.

3. Results

At the start of treatment (T0), the SMA type I group consisted of 11 non-sitter patients. After 10 administrations of nusinersen (T26), 45.45% became sitters (Table 2), with their CMAP amplitude increasing from 0.53 ± 0.23 to 1.85 ± 1.05. The other 54.55% patients who remained non-sitters showed an increase in CMAP from 0.26 ± 0.23 to 1.19 ± 0.66.

Table 2. Clinical data before and after 26 months of nusinersen in SMA type 1, 2, and 3.

Variables	Non-Sitters		Sitters		Walkers	
Time	T0	T26	T0	T26	T0	T26
Age at treatment initiation (months)	2–76		13–196		30–185	
SMA subtype						
- SMA 1	11 (100%)	6 (54.55%)		5 (45.45%)		
- SMA 2			16 (100%)	12 (75%)		4 (25%)
- SMA 3			4 (57.14%)	4 (57.14%)	3 (42.8%)	3 (42.8%)
SMN2 copies						
- 2 copies	11 (100%)			3 (18.75%)		2 (28.57%)
- 3 copies				13 (81.25%)		5 (71.43%)

At T0, the type II SMA group consisted of 16 sitters. At T26, 25% of the patients became walkers (Table 2), with their CMAP amplitude increasing from 2.73 ± 2.08 to 3.65 ± 1.55. The other 75% of patients who remained sitters showed an increase in CMAP from 0.99 ± 0.91 to 1.73 ± 1.18.

The SMA type III group consisted of four sitters and three walkers, both at T0 and T26 (Table 2). The CMAP of the sitters increased from 1.25 ± 0.55 to 2.05 ± 0.66, while the CMAP of the walkers increased from 2.73 ± 2.38 to 3.66 ± 2.85.

Figure 1 presents the motor and electrophysiological changes in the first 26 months after starting nusinersen treatment for each patient with SMA types 1, 2 and 3.

There is a significant increase in CHOP, consistent with CMAP in 5 patients for SMA type 1. In SMA type 2 patients, HFMSE is generally stationary, with only two of them having significant variations in CMAP (above the group average). In SMA type 3 patients, CMAP/HFMSE show a stationary trend between T0 and T26.

Motor function evolution after 26 months of nusinersen treatment is shown in Figure 2.

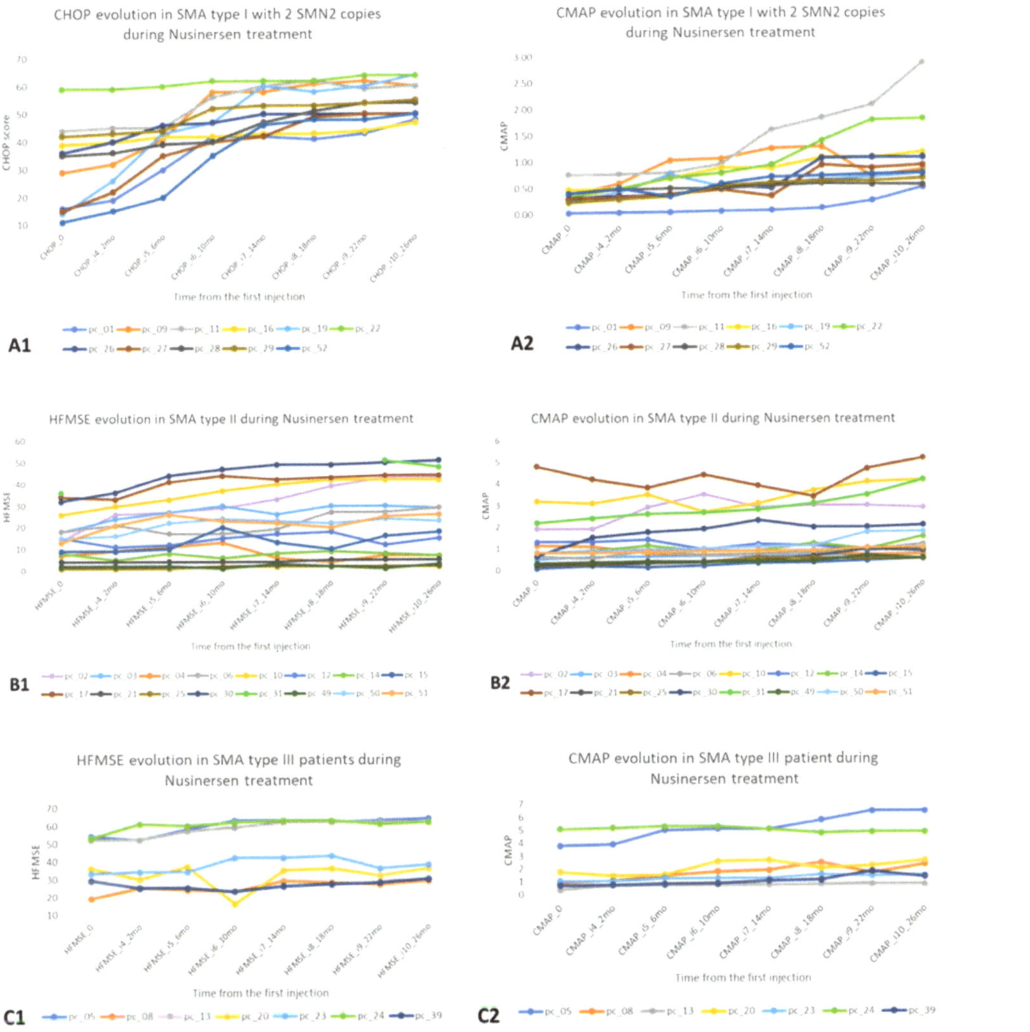

Figure 1. Motor and electrophysiological evolution in the first 26 months after starting nusinersen treatment for patients with SMA types 1, 2 and 3. (**A1**)—CHOP evolution in SMA type 1 with 2 copies of SMN; (**A2**)—CMAP evolution in SMA type 1 with 2 copies of SMN; (**B1**)—HFMSE evolution in SMA type 2; (**B2**)—CMAP evolution in SMA type 2; (**C1**)—HFMSE evolution in SMA type 3; (**C2**)—CMAP evolution in SMA type 3.

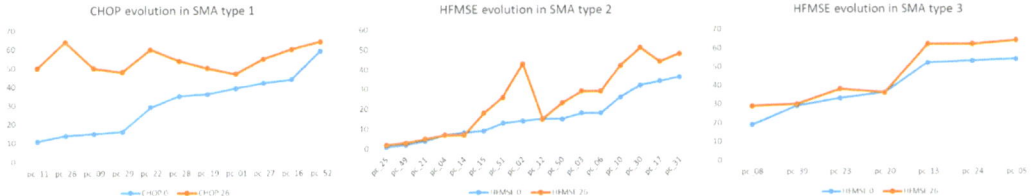

Figure 2. CHOP and HFMSE evolution at T0 and T26 for each type of SMA.

In SMA type 1, we observed CHOP increase between T0 and T26. In SMA type 2, there were two patients with a better outcome than the others who had differences between T0 and T26, and whose evaluations slightly increased. In SMA type 3, no regression was registered, but very close values were obtained in both evaluations, with a single patient having the same HFMSE score at T0/T26.

Electrophysiological changes in ulnar nerve conduction at T0 and T26 are illustrated in Figure 3.

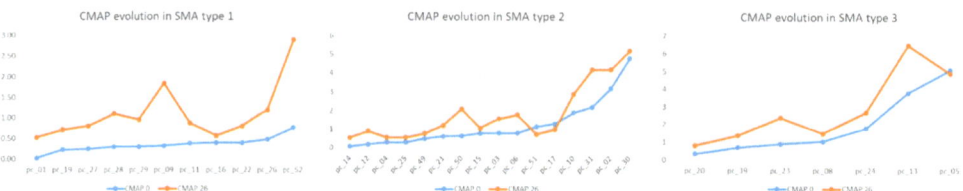

Figure 3. CMAP evolution at T26 for each type of SMA.

The most significant increase in distal CMAP amplitude was recorded in SMA type 1 patients, statistically correlated with scores on CHOP scales ($p < 0.001$).

Most of the SMA type 2 patients started treatment long after symptom onset (13–96 months) and presented stationary CMAP amplitude and HFMSE scores.

The majority (four out of seven patients) of SMA type 3 patients were non-ambulant at T0. They started treatment several years after losing gait, remaining non-ambulant at T26.

Low values of CMAP amplitude at the distal ulnar nerve were observed. CMAP amplitude is shown to be significantly ($p < 0.005$) strongly correlated ($r = 0.667$) with motor function evolution only in SMA type 1. For SMA types 2 and 3 there are no significant statistical correlations.

4. Discussion

According to the obtained results, there is a correlation between the increase in the score on the functional scales and an increase in CMAP in patients with SMA type 1 who have passed into a higher motor stage; this is correlated with the early start of treatment (shortly after the onset of motor regression).

Patients who were diagnosed a few months after the loss of motor acquisitions regained them in the first months after starting treatment. Additionally, the children with borderline shapes passed in superior form, with some acquiring the sitting position and others assisted/independent walking. The favorable evolution depends on a complex of factors—some proven (compliance with standards of care—physical therapy [31], respiratory nursing [32], early treatment of secondary scoliosis [33,34]), others still under research—such as genetic factors (number of SMN2 copies or other yet undiscovered aspects) and biochemical factors (level of cerebrospinal fluid neurofilaments).

Patients who had a higher amplitude of CMAP (number of motoneurons/axons) at the beginning of treatment had a better clinical evolution, thus demonstrating that CMAP is a marker of the degenerative process.

We had a particular case, a compound heterozygous case, aged 9 years, who started treatment with nusinersen at the age of 7. In particular, there was a discrepancy between motor level (ambulatory) and extremely low level (<1 mV) of CMAP amplitude at the level of the ulnar nerve, which increased slightly during 2 years of treatment. Further research is needed on biomarkers (genetic, biochemical) to investigate particular clinical and electrophysiological responses in each case.

A relevant correlation was found between the number of SMN2 copies and the disease phenotype, with patients with fewer SMN2 copies having a more modest clinical evolution and an extremely low CMAP.

Nusinersen treatment has changed the paradigm of this disease evolution; early forms with neonatal onset or in the first months of life, with severe bulbar dysfunction, are no longer fatal, and in late forms have significantly improved motor performance and quality of life. We found a clinically significant improvement in patients who started treatment as soon as possible [35] at the time of the first signs of the disease (motor regression), both in the early and late forms.

5. Conclusions

After 2 years of nusinersen treatment, children with SMA types 1, 2 and 3 had a favorable clinical evolution, as shown by the scores on the motor scales. Clinical data were correlated with electrophysiological data, with statistical significance in SMA type 1. However, it is important to follow up CMAP as an electrophysiological marker to capture motor regression [36], but also as a prognostic factor.

Author Contributions: Conceptualization, M.A., A.M. and C.S.; methodology, M.A., A.M. and C.S.; software, A.M. and C.S.; validation, M.A., A.M. and C.S.; formal analysis, M.A., A.M. and C.S.; investigation, M.A. and A.M.; resources, M.A., A.M., C.S., L.P., C.M.D. and A.C.N.; data curation, M.A., A.M. and C.S.; writing—original draft preparation, M.A., A.M., C.S., C.M.D. and A.C.N.; writing—review and editing, M.A., A.M., C.S., L.P., C.M.D., A.C.N. and D.A.I.; visualization, M.A., A.M., C.S., L.P., C.M.D., A.C.N. and D.A.I.; supervision, M.A., A.M. and C.S.; project administration, M.A. All authors have read and agreed to the published version of the manuscript.

Funding: This research received no external funding.

Institutional Review Board Statement: The study was conducted in accordance with the Declaration of Helsinki, and approved by the Ethics Committee of National University Center for Children Neurorehabilitation "Dr. Nicolae Robanescu" (protocol code 7465, date of approval 1 October 2018).

Informed Consent Statement: Informed consent was obtained from all subjects' parents, involved in the study.

Data Availability Statement: The data presented in this study are available on request from the corresponding author.

Acknowledgments: We are grateful to all our colleagues (physical therapists, occupational therapists, nurses) for their support in drafting this lecture.

Conflicts of Interest: The authors declare no conflict of interest.

References

1. Kariyawasam, D.S.T.; D'silva, A.; Lin, C.; Ryan, M.M.; Farrar, M.A. Biomarkers and the development of a personalized medicine approach in spinal muscular atrophy. *Front. Neurol.* **2019**, *10*, 1–12. [CrossRef] [PubMed]
2. Yonekawa, T.; Komaki, H.; Saito, Y.; Sugai, K.; Sasaki, M. Peripheral nerve abnormalities in pediatric patients with spinal muscular atrophy. *Brain Dev.* **2013**, *35*, 165–171. [CrossRef] [PubMed]
3. Keinath, M.C.; Prior, D.E.; Prior, T.W. Spinal Muscular Atrophy: Mutations, Testing, and Clinical Relevance. *Appl. Clin. Genet.* **2021**, *14*, 11. [CrossRef] [PubMed]
4. Lefebvre, S.; Bürglen, L.; Reboullet, S.; Clermont, O.; Burlet, P.; Viollet, L.; Benichou, B.; Cruaud, C.; Millasseau, P.; Zeviani, M.; et al. Identification and characterization of a spinal muscular atrophy-determining gene. *Cell* **1995**, *80*, 155–165. [CrossRef]
5. Farrar, M.A.; Kiernan, M.C. The Genetics of Spinal Muscular Atrophy: Progress and Challenges. *Neurotherapeutics* **2015**, *12*, 290–302. [CrossRef]
6. Sansone, V.A.; Walter, M.C.; Attarian, S.; Delstanche, S.; Mercuri, E.; Lochmüller, H.; Neuwirth, C.; Vazquez-Costa, J.F.; Kleinschnitz, C.; Hagenacker, T. Measuring Outcomes in Adults with Spinal Muscular Atrophy–Challenges and Future Directions–Meeting Report. *J. Neuromuscul. Dis.* **2020**, *7*, 523–534. [CrossRef]
7. Al-Zaidy, S.A.; Mendell, J.R. From Clinical Trials to Clinical Practice: Practical Considerations for Gene Replacement Therapy in SMA Type 1. *Pediatr. Neurol.* **2019**, *100*, 3–11. [CrossRef]
8. Chabanon, A.; Seferian, A.M.; Daron, A.; Péréon, Y.; Cances, C.; Vuillerot, C.; De Waele, L.; Cuisset, J.-M.; Laugel, V.; Schara, U. Prospective and longitudinal natural history study of patients with type 2 and 3 spinal muscular atrophy: Baseline data NatHis-SMA study. *PLoS ONE* **2018**, *13*, e0201004. [CrossRef] [PubMed]

9. Lewelt, A.; Krosschell, K.J.; Scott, C.; Sakonju, A.; Kissel, J.T.; Crawford, T.O.; Acsadi, G.; D'Anjou, G.; Elsheikh, B.; Reyna, S.P.; et al. Compound muscle action potential and motor function in children with spinal muscular atrophy. *Muscle Nerve* **2010**, *42*, 703–708. [CrossRef]
10. A Study of Multiple Doses of Nusinersen (ISIS 396443) Delivered to Infants with Genetically Diagnosed and Presymptomatic Spinal Muscular Atrophy (NURTURE). Available online: https://clinicaltrials.gov/ct2/show/NCT02386553 (accessed on 15 May 2021).
11. Arnold, W.D.; Simard, L.R.; Rutkove, S.B.; Kolb, S.J. Development and testing of biomarkers in spinal muscular atrophy. In *Spinal Muscular Atrophy*; Elsevier: Amsterdam, The Netherlands, 2017; pp. 383–397.
12. European Medicines Agency. Annex 1. Summary of Product Characteristics. Available online: https://www.ema.europa.eu/en/documents/product-information/spinraza-epar-product-information_en.pdf (accessed on 17 May 2021).
13. American Society of Health-System Pharmacists. Spinraza (nusinersen) Approved. Available online: https://www.ahfsdruginformation.com/spinraza-nusinersen-approved/ (accessed on 17 May 2021).
14. European Medicines Agency. EU/3/12/976: Orphan Designation for the Treatment of 5q Spinal Muscular Atrophy. Available online: https://www.ema.europa.eu/en/medicines/human/orphan-designations/eu312976 (accessed on 17 May 2021).
15. Hua, Y.; Sahashi, K.; Hung, G.; Rigo, F.; Passini, M.A.; Bennett, C.F.; Krainer, A.R. Antisense correction of SMN2 splicing in the CNS rescues necrosis in a type III SMA mouse model. *Genes Dev.* **2010**, *24*, 1634–1644. [CrossRef]
16. Fay, A.J. Neuromuscular Diseases of the Newborn. *Semin. Pediatr. Neurol.* **2019**, *32*, 100771. [CrossRef]
17. Bîrsanu, S.; Banu, O.; Nanu, C. Assessing legal responsibility in romanian pharmaceutical practice. *Farmacia* **2022**, *70*, 557–564. [CrossRef]
18. Pierzchlewicz, K.; Kępa, I.; Podogrodzki, J.; Kotulska, K. Spinal muscular atrophy: The use of functional motor scales in the era of disease-modifying treatment. *Child Neurol. Open* **2021**, *8*, 2329048X211008725. [CrossRef]
19. Pitt, M.C. Nerve conduction studies and needle EMG in very small children. *Eur. J. Paediatr. Neurol.* **2012**, *16*, 285–291. [CrossRef]
20. Glanzman, A.M.; Mazzone, E.; Main, M.; Pelliccioni, M.; Wood, J.; Swoboda, K.J.; Scott, C.; Pane, M.; Messina, S.; Bertini, E. The Children's Hospital of Philadelphia infant test of neuromuscular disorders (CHOP INTEND): Test development and reliability. *Neuromuscul. Disord.* **2010**, *20*, 155–161. [CrossRef] [PubMed]
21. Kichula, E.; Duong, T.; Glanzman, A.; Pasternak, A.; Darras, B.; Finkel, R.; De Vivo, D.; Zolkipli-Cunningham, Z.; Day, J. *Children's Hospital of Philadelphia Infant Test of Neuromuscular Disorders (CHOP INTEND) Feasibility for Individuals with Severe Spinal Muscular Atrophy II (S46. 004)*; AAN Enterprises: Apex, NC, USA, 2018.
22. CHOP INTEND (Children's Hospital of Philadelphia Infant Test of Neuromuscular Disorders). Available online: https://smauk.org.uk/files/files/Research/CHOPINTEND.pdf (accessed on 29 May 2021).
23. Physical Assessments for Individuals with Spinal Muscular Atrophy (SMA). Biogen. Together in SMA. Available online: https://www.togetherinsma.com/en_us/home/introduction-to-sma/physical-assessment.html?tabKey=tab21 (accessed on 25 June 2021).
24. O'Hagen, J.M.; Glanzman, A.M.; McDermott, M.P.; Ryan, P.A.; Flickinger, J.; Quigley, J.; Riley, S.; Sanborn, E.; Irvine, C.; Martens, W.B. An expanded version of the Hammersmith Functional Motor Scale for SMA II and III patients. *Neuromuscul. Disord.* **2007**, *17*, 693–697. [CrossRef]
25. Glanzman, A.M.; O'Hagen, J.M.; McDermott, M.P.; Martens, W.B.; Flickinger, J.; Riley, S.; Quigley, J.; Montes, J.; Dunaway, S.; Deng, L. Validation of the Expanded Hammersmith Functional Motor Scale in spinal muscular atrophy type II and III. *J. Child Neurol.* **2011**, *26*, 1499–1507. [CrossRef] [PubMed]
26. HFMSE—Hammersmith Functional Motor Scale—Expanded. Spinal Muscular Atrophy UK. Available online: https://smauk.org.uk/files/files/Research/HFMSEscale.pdf (accessed on 29 May 2021).
27. Hammersmith Functional Motor Scale Expanded for SMA (HFMSE). Available online: http://columbiasma.org/docs/HFMSE_2019_Manual.pdf (accessed on 29 May 2021).
28. Six Minute Walk Test. Available online: https://www.physio-pedia.com/Six_Minute_Walk_Test_/_6_Minute_Walk_Test (accessed on 29 May 2021).
29. Williams, F.; Monge, P. *Reasoning with Statistics: How to Read Quantitative Research*, 5th ed.; Harcourt College Publishers: Orlando, FL, USA, 2001; ISBN 978-0155068155.
30. Pearson's Correlation Coefficient. Available online: https://www.statisticssolutions.com/free-resources/directory-of-statistical-analyses/pearsons-correlation-coefficient/ (accessed on 17 June 2021).
31. Mirea, A.; Leanca, M.C.; Onose, G.; Sporea, C.; Padure, L.; Shelby, E.-S.; Dima, V.; Daia, C. Physical Therapy and Nusinersen Impact on Spinal Muscular Atrophy Rehabilitative Outcome. *FBL* **2022**, *27*, 179. [CrossRef]
32. Fauroux, B.; Griffon, L.; Amaddeo, A.; Stremler, N.; Mazenq, J.; Khirani, S.; Baravalle-Einaudi, M. Respiratory management of children with spinal muscular atrophy (SMA). *Arch. Pédiatrie* **2020**, *27*, 7S29–7S34. [CrossRef]
33. Farber, H.J.; Phillips, W.A.; Kocab, K.L.; Hanson, D.S.; Heydemann, J.A.; Dahl, B.T.; Spoede, E.T.; Jefferson, L.S. Impact of scoliosis surgery on pulmonary function in patients with muscular dystrophies and spinal muscular atrophy. *Pediatr. Pulmonol.* **2020**, *55*, 1037–1042. [CrossRef]
34. Swarup, I.; MacAlpine, E.M.; Mayer, O.H.; Lark, R.K.; Smith, J.T.; Vitale, M.G.; Flynn, J.M.; Anari, J.B.; Cahill, P.J. Impact of growth friendly interventions on spine and pulmonary outcomes of patients with spinal muscular atrophy. *Eur. Spine J.* **2021**, *30*, 768–774. [CrossRef] [PubMed]

35. Mirea, A.; Shelby, E.-S.; Axente, M.; Badina, M.; Padure, L.; Leanca, M.; Dima, V.; Sporea, C. Combination Therapy with Nusinersen and Onasemnogene Abeparvovec-xioi in Spinal Muscular Atrophy Type I. *J. Clin. Med.* **2021**, *10*, 5540. [CrossRef] [PubMed]
36. Weng, W.-C.; Hsu, Y.-K.; Chang, F.-M.; Lin, C.-Y.; Hwu, W.-L.; Lee, W.-T.; Lee, N.-C.; Chien, Y.-H. CMAP changes upon symptom onset and during treatment in spinal muscular atrophy patients: Lessons learned from newborn screening. *Genet. Med.* **2021**, *23*, 415–420. [CrossRef] [PubMed]

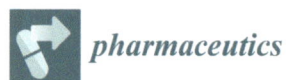 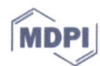

Review

Applications of Exosomes in Diagnosing Muscle Invasive Bladder Cancer

Jillian Marie Walker [1], Padraic O'Malley [2] and Mei He [1,*]

1 Department of Pharmaceutics, College of Pharmacy, University of Florida, Gainesville, FL 32611, USA
2 Department of Urology, College of Medicine, University of Florida, Gainesville, FL 32611, USA
* Correspondence: mhe@cop.ufl.edu

Abstract: Muscle Invasive Bladder Cancer (MIBC) is a subset of bladder cancer with a significant risk for metastases and death. It accounts for nearly 25% of bladder cancer diagnoses. A diagnostic work-up for MIBC is inclusive of urologic evaluation, radiographic imaging with a CT scan, urinalysis, and cystoscopy. These evaluations, especially cystoscopy, are invasive and carry the risk of secondary health concerns. Non-invasive diagnostics such as urine cytology are an attractive alternative currently being investigated to mitigate the requirement for cystoscopy. A pitfall in urine cytology is the lack of available options with high reliability, specificity, and sensitivity to malignant bladder cells. Exosomes are a novel biomarker source which could resolve some of the concerns with urine cytology, due to the high specificity as the surrogates of tumor cells. This review serves to define muscle invasive bladder cancer, current urine cytology methods, the role of exosomes in MIBC, and exosomes application as a diagnostic tool in MIBC. Urinary exosomes as the specific populations of extracellular vesicles could provide additional biomarkers with specificity and sensitivity to bladder malignancies, which are a consistent source of cellular information to direct clinicians for developing treatment strategies. Given its strong presence and differentiation ability between normal and cancerous cells, exosome-based urine cytology is highly promising in providing a perspective of a patient's bladder cancer.

Keywords: muscle invasive bladder cancer; exosomes; biomarkers; bladder cancer screening; bladder cancer diagnosis

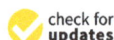

Citation: Walker, J.M.; O'Malley, P.; He, M. Applications of Exosomes in Diagnosing Muscle Invasive Bladder Cancer. *Pharmaceutics* 2022, 14, 2027. https://doi.org/10.3390/pharmaceutics14102027

Academic Editors: Cristina Manuela Drăgoi, Alina Crenguța Nicolae and Ion-Bogdan Dumitrescu

Received: 22 August 2022
Accepted: 20 September 2022
Published: 23 September 2022

Publisher's Note: MDPI stays neutral with regard to jurisdictional claims in published maps and institutional affiliations.

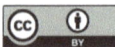

Copyright: © 2022 by the authors. Licensee MDPI, Basel, Switzerland. This article is an open access article distributed under the terms and conditions of the Creative Commons Attribution (CC BY) license (https://creativecommons.org/licenses/by/4.0/).

1. Introduction

The bladder is part of the urinary system, located in the pelvic cavity, and serves as a short-term reservoir for urine [1–3]. The bladder is comprised of four layers as depicted in Figure 1. The innermost layer is the transitional epithelium [4]. This tissue type is important in bladder structure due to flexible stretching ability. Transitional epithelium's high elasticity allows for substantial surface area to store urine. The next layer out is the lamina propria which serves to reinforce the inner lining and is made of elastic connective tissue. The third layer of the bladder is the smooth muscle layer also known as the detrusor muscle, which is three layers thick and contracts to evacuate urine. The fourth outermost layer of the bladder is the serosal layer, which serves as a barrier to decrease friction between the bladder and surrounding organs.

Bladder cancer manifests as two broad classifications, non-muscle invasive bladder cancer (NMIBC) and muscle invasive bladder cancer (MIBC). The pathophysiology of bladder cancer is described as a dual pathway and can be best defined by the presence of papillary and nonpapillary lesions [3,4]. NMIBC accounts for 75% of all bladder cancer cases, it does not extend beyond the first layer of the bladder [5]. Papillary lesions typically indicate non-muscle invasive bladder cancer (NMIBC), which accounts for most bladder cancer diagnose. NMIBC is characterized by chromosome nine deletion, which holds the CDKN2A gene that codes for tumor suppressor proteins [6]. Additionally, mutations arise on fibroblast growth factor receptor 3 (FGFR3), PI3K, and telomerase reverse transcriptase (TERT) [7–10]. Muscle invasive bladder cancer is the second route of the dual pathway as illustrated in Figure 1. It is defined by tumor infiltration beyond the epithelial layers of the bladder and into the detrusor muscle. MIBC also has a deletion of chromosome 9 and mutations in FGFR3, PI3K, TERT [11–13]. Additionally, retinoblastoma protein 1 (Rb1) and p53 are mutated and/or deleted [14–18]. In MIBC, Rb1 is truncated which promotes tumorigenesis. There is also an ~50% increase in p53 mutations in muscle invasive bladder cancer which leads to impaired DNA repair capabilities and loss of function in p53 associated tumor suppressor genes [17]. MIBC accounts for 25% of all bladder cancers and, depending on the aggravating factors, has a five-year survival of 70% [19]. The dual pathway of this malignancy contributes to the intricacies in presentation, diagnosis, and treatment.

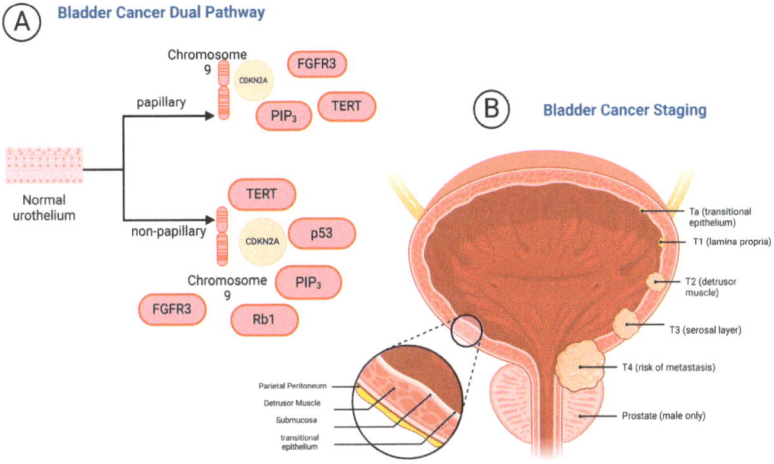

Figure 1. (**A**) The bladder cancer dual pathway involves the presence of papillary or non-papillary lesions. papillary lesions harbor mutations in FGFR3, TERT, PIP3, and deletion of CDKN2A on Chromosome 9. Papillary lesions typically present as NMIBC. Non-papillary lesions include mutation of TERT, PIP3, FGFR3, p53, Rb1, and deletion of CDKN2A on chromosome 9. Non-papillary lesions typically describe MIBC. (**B**) The bladder consists of four layers: the epithelium, submucosa, detrusor muscle, and parietal peritoneum. Staging for bladder cancer is depicted in this figure. Tumors are classified based on the TNM grading system where T describes the primary tumor in terms of its size and tissue penetration. N characterizes the involvement, or lack thereof, lymph nodes. M describes the presence of absence of metastasis. MIBC is characterized by being T2 and can present with or without nodal or metastatic involvement.

In 2022, there will be approximately 81,000 new cases of bladder cancer in America [19]. Of those cases, 25% will be MIBC. Muscle invasive bladder cancer is more predominant in men than women with a median age at diagnosis of 73. It is also twice as common in White men than Black or Latino men. Modifiable risk factors for muscle invasive bladder cancer include environmental exposures to aromatic amines, cigarette smoke, and chronic bladder infections. Non-modifiable risk factors for muscle invasive bladder cancer include a family history of bladder cancer and being diagnosed with Lynch syndrome [20].

MIBC often presents with a myriad of symptoms such as hematuria, dysuria, and general constitutional symptoms. These symptoms may be transient, and it should be noted that it can be observed in other non-malignant urogenital disease states. Due to the ambiguity of bladder cancer presentative symptoms, delayed diagnosis is often among patients. The later a patient is diagnosed, the higher the risk for initial diagnosis with MIBC.

Patients presenting with concerning symptoms will undergo a comprehensive clinical work-up. A work-up may include a urologic evaluation, radiographic imaging with a CT scan, urinalysis, and cystoscopy. Of the available diagnostic methods, cystoscopy is currently the standard for bladder cancer diagnosis [21–23]. Once a diagnosis is confirmed, bladder cancer will be staged using the TNM staging system. Bladder cancer is considered MIBC once it is determined a T2 lesion is present. A T2 lesion or higher indicates the invasion of the cancer into the muscular layer of the bladder. The associated risk for metastasis is higher with muscle invasive bladder cancer and metastatic sites can be local or distant. Local metastatic sites include adipose tissue, lymph nodes, and the peritoneum. Distant sites include the patient's bones, liver, and lungs [24]. The gold standard of care treatment for muscle invasive bladder cancer is cisplatin-based neoadjuvant chemotherapy with radical cystectomy.

2. Biomarkers in Bladder Cancer Diagnosis

Liquid biopsy is popular in cancer diagnostics because samples are collected with less invasive means than solid tissue biopsy. Liquid biopsy can be employed for diagnostics, prognosis, and theragnostic [22,23,25–27]. There are several types of samples which can be used for biopsy, including blood, urine, and cerebrospinal fluid (CSF) [21,28]. Biomarkers are biological molecules found within a given biopsy specimen used to detect and monitor illnesses and/or conditions. Popular biomarkers of interest in cancer include circulating free DNA (cfDNA), circulating tumor cells (CTAs), circulating proteins and cytokines, circulating extracellular vesicles and exosomes, and T-cells [29,30]. The generation and unique clinical utility of exosomes are the focus of this review. Of the types of liquid biopsy, urine samples are optimal for application in bladder cancer, because urine is stored in the bladder and has the most direct source connecting with bladder cancerous cells [31,32]. There are several urinary biomarker tests approved by the FDA which will be discussed in this review. However, none of them can achieve all the qualities required for a clinically useful urinary biomarker test for bladder cancer diagnosis. An ideal urinary biomarker test needs to incorporate several components including specificity, sensitivity, cost-effectiveness, and ease of interpretation [26,27,33]. The low false-positive rate and low risk of false negatives and undiagnosed disease progression are essential. The cost-effectiveness is critical for both health systems to employ on a large scale and for patients to pay for.

3. Exosomes in Muscle Invasive Bladder Cancer

3.1. Exosomes Defined

Exosomes are a subgroup of extracellular vesicles (EVs) in size range < 200nm, and derived from the membranes of multivesicular bodies [34,35]. They are released from several cell types, including diseased, malignant, and normal cells. Across the cell types, exosomes communicate and influence physiology at local and distant sites within the body. Exosomes are enriched with CD63, and can be found in blood, breast milk, urine, serum, saliva, mesenchymal, tumor, and dendritic cell samples [36–39]. They can also cross several internal barriers such as the blood-brain-barrier, the retinal barrier, stromal barrier, placental barrier, and cerebral spinal fluid barrier [40–43]. Exosomes are heterogenous by their surface molecules and cargos such as proteins, lipids, mRNA, miRNA, lncRNA, and DNA [44]. mRNA is implicated in tumor progression and metastasis through the abnormal upregulation of anion transport, cell growth factors, and the MAPK cascade [45]. Exosome miRNAs have roles in regulation of gene expression and tumor microenvironment in both healthy and malignant cells [46]. lncRNA contributes to the growth and survival of tumors [47]. Exosome DNA may protect tumor cells from regulatory inflammation processes, in turn supporting tumor survival [48]. Exosome biogenesis is largely supported by the endosomal sorting complex required for transport (ESCRT) and micro-vesicular bodies (MVB) [49–51]. Prior to exosome release, they are loaded with cargos which may consist of miRNA, proteins, and/or lipids. Once loaded with cargo, further release is regulated via synergistic ESCRT dependent and independent pathways [52]. They are selectively up-taken into cells via endocytosis, receptor–ligand interaction, or cellular membrane fusion [52]. Within the scope of cancer, exosomes are implicated in cancer development and survival [53–56].

Exosomes have a prominent role in cellular communication, which may lead to the promotion of malignancies as tumors release exosomes carrying pro-tumor genetic information. These pro-tumor exosomes mediated actions are illustrated in Figure 2. Through autocrine interaction, exosomes can change the direction of exosome releasing cells leading to tumor promotion [53,55,57–59]. Via paracrine interactions, exosomes can modulate intracellular interaction and the microenvironment of the cells. Angiogenesis is promoted by exosomes, especially in hypoxic conditions [60–62], which leads to downstream signaling cascades that can promote malignancies [62]. Cancer promoting histological changes are also influenced by exosomes. They are thought to be highly involved in the epithelial to mesenchymal transition (EMT) malignant lesions undergo as cancer develops [63]. Lastly, exosomes are impactful in angiogenesis to grow and maintain tumor survival. Cells under stress or in hypoxic conditions often release more exosomes [64,65]. Cancerous cells are under stress and experience hypoxic conditions, in turn, an increased release of exosome and signaling is observed [66,67]. Exosomes also contribute to pre-metastatic environments and metastasis. In pre-metastatic environments, exosomes are released from tumors and sent to distant sites to condition the environment into a suitable tumor micro-environment [68–70].

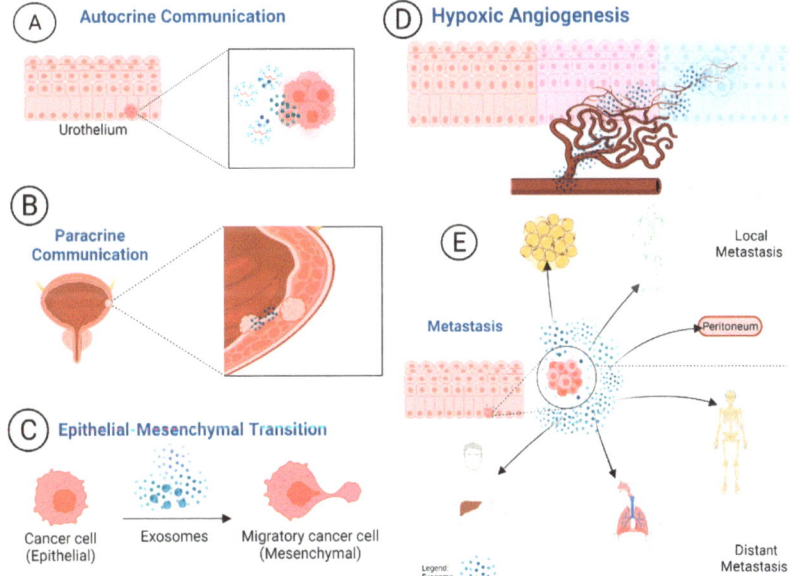

Figure 2. Exosomes are involved in cancer cell development, proliferation, and survival. (**A**) Through autocrine communication, exosomes communicate to the cells they are released from to promote a suitable microenvironment for tumors and contribute to the activation of pro-tumor mutations within their host cell. (**B**) Paracrine communication allows exosomes to communicate to nearby cells. They can modify the signaling pathways leading to changes in gene expression of surrounding cells. (**C**) Exosome's role in the epithelial to mesenchymal transition (EMT). (**D**) In hypoxic conditions exosomes can promote the growth of new blood vessels, often called angiogenesis. Through this process, nutrients can be sent to malformed cells to support their growth and proliferation into cancer cells. (**E**) Through exosome regulation of cellular communication, changing the histology of the tissue could

create a more suitable tumor microenvironment. This process supports more malignant forms of cancer. The cellular communication of exosomes to distant sites allows them to prepare distant organs for later infiltration of tum or cells.

3.2. Exosomes Involvement in MIBC Progression

The role of exosomes in MIBC progression is not fully understood in current literature. It has been suggested that high quantity of exosomes from MIBC may attribute from the pro-cancer actions such as increased tumor growth, invasion, and angiogenesis [71–73]. Starting with proliferation, tumor-derived extracellular vesicles (TEVs) and exosomes alter the operations of tumor suppressor genes to create a protumor microenvironment [74]. The accompanying hypoxia often found in tumor microenvironments further supports the actions of TEVs [75–78]. A key role of exosomes in high grade tumors and eventual MIBC is promoting metastasis. Exosomes support metastasis by carrying, transferring oncogenic cargoes, and hindering tumor suppressor exosomes [75]. Examples of such activity are evident in bladder cancer exosomes activating the ERK1/2 MAP kinase signaling pathway to promote malignancy of low tumor grade bladder cancer cells [79]. As bladder cancer metastasis continues, the tumor has a higher chance of developing into MIBC. A cornerstone characteristic of muscle invasive bladder cancer is the epithelial to mesenchymal transition (EMT). EMT describes the process of epithelial, urothelial cells in the case of bladder cancer, transforming into mesenchymal tissue (Figure 2C). Mesenchymal tissue can support carcinogenesis which contributes to larger, faster-growing tumors. The clinical significance of the processes from EMT is the development into higher grade aggressive tumors as MIBC. Due to the fast-growing nature of bladder cancer tumors, especially with upregulated pro-tumor EVs and exosomes, MIBC could lead to a complicated clinical picture.

Exosomes are highly implicated in the development and progression of muscle invasive bladder cancer [75,76]. Several in vitro studies have described the presence of carcinogenic activity being mediated by exosomes. In vitro exosomes demonstrate cellular communication between cancerous bladder cells and histologically diverse tissue, supporting the proposal of exosome mediated metastasis [80,81]. Carcinogenic exosomes had an increase in unfolded endoplasmic reticulum proteins, which leads to the oxidative stress response mechanism within cells when they are proliferating quickly [82]. This oxidative stress phenomenon was observed in mice models utilizing bladder cancer cells [83,84]. Demonstrated using muscle invasive bladder cancer cells, the presence of EMT underscores the impact exosomes have in the setting of MIBC [84]. It was observed that exosomes induce and promote the upregulation of mesenchymal markers in urothelial cells [73,85]. Lastly, exosomes have been documented as upregulating Bcl2 and Cyclin D which promote tumorigenesis [84]. These findings support the role of exosomes in cancer as well as the specific contributions in muscle invasive bladder cancer [82,85,86]. Additionally, to the above findings, there are several exosome biomarkers implicated in bladder cancer tumorigenesis [85,87–89]. These urine-based markers are characterized in Table 1. Exosomes established role in muscle invasive bladder cancer and documented urine biomarkers yield opportunity for an exosome-based urine biomarker test for MIBC diagnosis.

3.3. Exosome Biomarkers for Muscle Invasive Bladder Cancer Diagnosis

Urinary exosome biomarkers are not currently used as diagnostic tools for MIBC detection. However, exosomes would make an excellent source for biomarkers for several reasons. Exosomes participate in cell-to-cell communication and stimulation of immune responses [90,91]. They can receive feedback and respond to their cellular environment. This quality can be manipulated to identify biomarkers to detect tumors. Additionally, exosomes are reported to be released in a larger quantity in malignant cells than healthy cells [92,93]. So, exosome biomarkers used in a biomarker test would reveal clear results segregating healthy from diseased areas of the bladder. Table 1 lists the biomarkers that are present in urinary exosomes and are implicated in the promotion of bladder cancer. It should be noted that several of these biomarkers are found in other tumor types and therefore not unique to bladder cancer, such as EDIL-3 found also in sarcomas exosomes modulating angiogenesis [94]. The main modes of action for these biomarkers include an increase in tumor cell migration, proliferation of tumor cells, angiogenesis, decreased apoptosis of cancer cells, and pro-tumor microenvironment support. Although this table list is not an exhaustive list of all the discovered biomarkers, it is inclusive of well described urinary exosomes derived biomarkers. Current research suggests there are many more urinary exosome biomarkers to be discovered.

Table 1. Identified Urinary Biomarkers for Bladder Cancer.

Urinary Biomarkers	EV Source	Mechanism of Action	Effect	Reference
CD36	Urine protein	Increases fatty acid uptake	Increase migration, proliferation, and angiogenesis	[84,95,96]
CD73	Urine protein	Regulates cellular signaling	Increase migration, proliferation, and angiogenesis	[84,95,96]
CD44	Urine protein	Docks proteases on cell membrane	Increase migration, proliferation, and angiogenesis	[84,95,96]
CD9	Urine protein	Exosome mediation of metastasis in conjunction with NUGC-3 and OCUM-12	Promotion of tumor invasion and metastasis	[96,97]
TSG101	Urine protein	regulates ubiquitin-mediated protein degradation, cellular transcription, cell proliferation, and division.	Promotes an increase in downstream cellular stress	[98]
EDIL-3	Urine protein gene	Promotes angiogenesis and metastasis in malignant environments	Enhances the aggressiveness and growth of the tumor/s	[76]
Alpha 1-antitrypsin	Urine protein	Immunity regulation	Decrease apoptosis	[99]
MUC1	Urine protein gene	Promotes histological morphologies and metastasis through several routes of cellular communication	Cancer progression and metastasis	[100]
MUC4	Urine protein gene	Enhances the EMT process and influences immunomodulation	Promotes aggressive metastatic cancers	[101]
MAGE-B4	Urine protein	Increase tumorigenesis and proliferation	Increase ubiquiation and degradation of p53	[89,95]
miR-21	Urine miRNA	Decrease AKT and MAPK pathways	Increase invasion	[77,84,95]
GALNT1	Urine RNAs, lncRNAs	Mediates O-linked glycosylation of sonic hedgehog to promote its activation	Maintains bladder cancer stem cells and bladder tumorigenesis	[95,102–104]
UCA1	Urine RNAs, lncRNAs	Regulates CREB	Increase proliferation	[95,102–104]
MALAT-1	Urine RNAs, lncRNAs	Antagonize miR-125b	Decrease apoptosis	[95,102–104]
UCA 201	Urine RNAs, lncRNAs	Increase the expression levels of ZEB1 and ZEB2 decrease the expression of hsa-miR-145 and the downstream actin-binding protein FSCN1	Increase migration and invasion	[95,102–104]

4. FDA Approved Urine-Biomarker Tests for Bladder Cancer

In addition to the standard of care in bladder cancer for diagnosis as cystoscopy, there are several urine based methods for bladder cancer diagnosis, including florescence cystoscopy, urine cytology, urine-based marker detection, and urinary tract imaging as the well-recognized methods to support cystoscopy findings [105]. Urine-based markers are comprised of proteins emitted from tumors, DNA, RNA, exosomes, or other cellular components. They are of particular interest because the collection is inexpensive and non-invasive in terms of developing detection methods with good sensitivity even in low-grade tumors. Currently, six FDA approved urine biomarker tests for bladder cancer have been depicted and summarized in Table 2.

The NMP22BC test kit is a protein-based immunoassay test for bladder cancer diagnosis which utilizes the biomarker nuclear matrix protein 22 (NMP-22). NMP-22 is a cellular protein, which after bladder cell apoptosis, is increased in its release into the urine. Its median sensitivity is ~61% and its specificity is 71% [106]. The NMP-22 BladderChek has an advantage over the NMP22 test because it can be rapidly completed in 30 min. NMP-22 BladderChek is approximately 55.7% specific and approximately 85.7% sensitive at the 95% confidence interval. Both the NMP-22 BladderChek and NMP22BC test kit are affected by tumor grade, staging and concurrent genitourinary pathologies.

The BTA TRAK and BTA stat are quantitative and qualitative tests, respectively. BTA stat is an adjunctive rapid immunochromatographic assay to cystoscopy. It utilizes monoclonal antibodies to identify complement-factor H-related protein, associated with bladder cancer, to identify malignancy. The BTA stat sensitivity is 67% and the specificity is 70% [107], and both values are influenced by the presence of other urinary conditions because it can confound the results of the test. BTA TRAK is not as widely used as its stat counterpart, which may be due to its high false-positive and negative rate. BTA Trak's median sensitivity is ~75.5% and its median specificity is 53.5%.

ImmunoCyt/uCyt+ is used as an adjunctive test to cystoscopy for monitoring recurrent bladder cancer. It is an immunocytochemical test that utilizes three fluorescent antibodies. The corresponding antigens include two mucins associated with bladder cancer and one carcinoembryonic antigen which are only found in exfoliated cancerous bladder cancer cells. Their sensitivity and specificity are both 78% [96].

Lastly, UroVysion utilizes fluorescence in situ hybridization (FISH) to detect bladder cancer. It has a clinical sensitivity of 75% and specificity of 93% [108]. It should be noted that this assay has a profound anticipatory effect due to its sensitivity. Thus, it is imperative that positive test using this method are closely monitored. There are several options available for cytological bladder cancer detection. However, as described with each available test, further improvement regarding sensitivity and specificity of the measurements is needed. Table 2 listed the six FDA approved urinary biomarker tests for bladder cancer. None of these tests are used alone for bladder cancer diagnosis due to their low sensitivity and specificity. The ideal urinary biomarker tests for bladder cancer would need to have high specificity, high sensitivity, being cost-effective, and easy to replicate.

Table 2. FDA Approved Urine Biomarker Tests for Bladder Cancer.

Test	Type of Test	Biomarker Tested	Sensitivity	Specificity	Reference
NMP22 BC test kit	Sandwich ELISA	NMP22	61%	71%	[106]
NMP22 Bladder Check	Sandwich ELISA	NMP22	55.7%	85.7%	[106,109]
BTA TRAK	ELISA	Complement factor H-related protein	75.5%	53.5%	[106]
BTA stat	Sandwich ELISA	Complement factor H-related protein	67%	70%	[106,110]
ImmunoCyt/uCyt	Immunofluorescent cytology	Monoclonal antibodies	78%	78%	[106,111,112]
UroVysion	FISH	DNA of malignant urothelial cells	75%	93%	[106,113–115]

5. Muscle Invasive Bladder Cancer Diagnostic Tests in Clinical Trials

Presently, only two exosome-based biomarker diagnosis for muscle invasive bladder cancer clinical trials currently being conducted as summarized in Table 3. However, a few more clinical trials are investigating other circulating biomarkers including cell free DNAs in muscle invasive bladder cancer. An American multi-facility observational cohort study called Clinical Performance Evaluation of the C2i-Test, MIBC patients are submitting blood samples for detection of molecular residual disease via ctDNA analysis [116]. The measured primary outcome is predicting three-year recurrence free survival post definitive treatment. The AURORAX-0093A: Glycosaminoglycan Profiling for Prognostication of Muscle-invasive Bladder Cancer—a Pilot Study (AUR93A) is an observational cohort study based in Italy and Sweden, which is utilizing glycosaminoglycan profiling scores to determine the prognosis of MIBC. The primary outcome is the proportion of patients who have complete response at the first post-radical cystectomy visit. The Samsung Medical Center in Seoul, Republic of Korea is conducting an observational cohort study called Clinical Utility of VI-RADS in Diagnosis of MIBC, which is studying the application of Vesical Imaging Report and Data System (VI-RADS) in Diagnosis of Muscle Invasive Bladder Cancer. The primary endpoint is measuring the accuracy of the VI-RADS scoring system in MIBC diagnosis [117]. Currently, there are 92 in total as the pioneer clinical trials utilizing exosomes for diagnosing cancers mainly including lung cancer, breast cancer, pancreatic cancer, prostate cancer, and colorectal cancer. The absence of clinical trials involving exosomes in MIBC diagnosis indicates the need for more research in this area.

Table 3. Clinical Trials Utilizing Extracellular Vesicles and Exosomes as Biomarkers for Bladder Cancer Diagnosis. Information is from searching via clinicaltrials.gov.

ClinicalTrials.Gov Identifier	Trial Status	Cancer Type	Primary Endpoint
NCT04155359	Recruiting	Bladder Cancer	The test measures up to 280 sncRNA present in urine exosomes and produces a dichotomized assessment of "−1" (no cancer) and "+1" (cancer) based on the expression profiles of the exosomal sncRNAs
NCT05270174	Not yet recruiting	Preoperative Diagnosis of Lymphatic Metastasis in Patients with Bladder Cancer	Explore Whether lncRNA-ElNAT1 in Urine Exosomes Can be Used as a New Target for Preoperative Diagnosis of Lymph Node Metastasis

6. Discussion

The bladder is a urinary reservoir consisting of four distinct layers: (1) the transitional epithelium; (2) lamina propria; (3) detrusor muscle; (4) and serosal layer. Bladder cancer can develop into non-muscle invasive bladder cancer or muscle invasive bladder cancer. These tumor growth patterns are best described in the dual development pathway of bladder cancer. Papillary lesions have mutations and cellular disorders, however, there is no infiltration to the bladder tissue beyond epithelium. Non-papillary lesions have further disorder due to deletion of p53 and Rb1. These lesions extend to the detrusor muscle and are considered a higher risk version of bladder cancer. Bladder cancer is highly prevalent in the United States and 25% of all bladder cancer cases will be muscle invasive bladder cancer. This cancer mainly affects elderly white men. Modifiable risk factors for developing ladder cancer include environmental exposures to aromatic amines, cigarette smoke, and chronic bladder infections. To diagnose bladder cancer, patients will undergo a work-up inclusive of a urologic evaluation, radiographic imaging with a CT scan, urinalysis, and cystoscopy. Many efforts have been made to replace this procedure with a less invasive method of diagnosis, such as urine biomarker tests. However, due to the low sensitivity and specificity of currently available tests, urinary biomarkers have not been able to replace cystoscopy in bladder cancer diagnosis. Urinary exosomes are the promising alternative. Exosomes are a key biological player in the development of MIBC and implicate several pro-tumor actions such as tumor proliferation, metastasis, and survival. Exosome's largest role in muscle invasive bladder cancer is the epithelial to mesenchymal transition, which has been observed that exosomes induce and promote the upregulation of mesenchymal markers in urothelial cells [118]. This transition leads to a strong pro-tumor microenvironment within the layers of the bladder. EMT supported tumor growth, which can lead to more invasive bladder cancer such as muscle invasive bladder cancer. Identifying exosome biomarkers strongly associated with the EMT process, which will progress the strategies employed to diagnose invasive bladder cancers early and save patients' lives.

EVs and Exosomes are a promising source of biomarkers for muscle invasive bladder cancer. However, they are not without flaws. Exosomes have pitfalls in their isolation and purification methods. The Minimal information for studies of extracellular vesicles 2018 ([119,120]) describes several isolation and purification techniques [121]. The consensus is ultracentrifugation and ultrafiltration may have the largest amount of yield, however, it will co-isolate other membrane particles and protein aggregate. As described by Doyle and Wang, these two methods have a high risk of destroying exosomes in the process of isolation and purification leading to low yield amounts of pure exosomes [91]. From a clinical standpoint, it is imperative that standards be established for exosome biomarker characteristics to accommodate for the variety of patient populations [122] and to accommodate for the natural heterogeneity of patient populations. Therefore, the isolation and purification methods for extracting exosomes from various clinical fluids are critical. The EVs and exosomes isolation techniques have been intensively developed in the past decade. Vast amount of review papers regarding EV isolation techniques have been reported [123–136]. The well-documented methods for isolating exosomes from biological samples include, but not limited to, differential ultracentrifugation, size-exclusion chromatography and immunoaffinity capture [137]. The MISEV describes the application of the exosomes as the deciding factor in the type of separation to use [121]. The downstream characterization of EV and exosome quality and biomarker expression is also challenging. The well accepted nanoparticle tracking analysis suffers from largely scattered variations [138]. In the case of clinical research and for application in biomarker identification, collecting the purest EV population is imperative. It is recommended to employ ultracentrifugation in conjunction with ultrafiltration as a conventional approach, due to their wide accessibility and cost-effectiveness compared to other isolation methods. However, ultracentrifugation has a low recovery rate of 2–25%. Note that recovery and purity of exosomes are dependent on the density, size, quantity, and molecular relevance of the sample [91]. Ultrafiltration is subject to EV destruction due to the shear force of membrane filtration. Currently, affinity purification such as immunomagnetic beads and affinity column are getting more recognition in terms of homogeneous population and purity relevant to interests [139]. Due to variance in EV isolation and variable return of results from widely accepted methods, it is important that highly specific and sensitive isolation techniques are developed in the future for improving diagnostic outcomes.

The tests currently approved by the Food and Drug Administration (FDA) for bladder cancer diagnosis do not unlock the power of exosomes. Given the vast array of exosome biomarkers identified in the development and survival of bladder cancer, the huge needs of exosome biomarker diagnostic test are presented. For developing exosome based diagnostic test, the well-established exosome isolation and characterization are critical and need to be standardized. Some pioneer research work has been reported recently to overcome the isolation challenge and ensure the exosome purity and specificity [84,96,139]. However, clinical translation is still lacking. More efforts on clinical translation will be needed in the future research.

Author Contributions: Conceptualization, J.M.W., P.O. and M.H.; writing—original draft preparation, J.M.W.; writing—review and editing, P.O. and M.H. All authors have read and agreed to the published version of the manuscript.

Funding: This research is supported by UFHCC Cancer Center GU pilot grant and NIH NIGMS 1R35GM133794.

Institutional Review Board Statement: Not applicable.

Informed Consent Statement: Not applicable.

Data Availability Statement: Not applicable.

Conflicts of Interest: The authors declare no conflict of interest.

References

1. Matuszczak, M.; Kiljańczyk, A.; Salagierski, M. A Liquid Biopsy in Bladder Cancer—The Current Landscape in Urinary Biomarkers. *Int. J. Mol. Sci.* **2022**, *23*, 8597. [CrossRef]
2. Lokeshwar, S.D.; Lopez, M.; Sarcan, S.; Aguilar, K.; Morera, D.S.; Shaheen, D.M.; Lokeshwar, B.L.; Lokeshwar, V.B. Molecular Oncology of Bladder Cancer from Inception to Modern Perspective. *Cancers* **2022**, *14*, 2578. [CrossRef]
3. Lonati, C.; Simeone, C.; Suardi, N.; Briganti, A.; Montorsi, F.; Moschini, M. Micropapillary bladder cancer: An evolving biology. *Curr. Opin. Urol.* **2022**, *32*, 504–510. [CrossRef]
4. Šoipi, S.; Vučić, M.; Spajić, B.; Krušlin, B.; Tomić, M.; Ulamec, M. Review of the Bladder Cancer Molecular Classification Proposed: A New Era—New Taxonomy. *Acta Clin. Croat.* **2021**, *60*, 519–523. [CrossRef] [PubMed]
5. Czerniak, B.; Dinney, C.; McConkey, D. Origins of Bladder Cancer. *Annu. Rev. Pathol. Mech. Dis.* **2016**, *11*, 149–174. [CrossRef]
6. Sangster, A.G.; Gooding, R.J.; Garven, A.; Ghaedi, H.; Berman, D.M.; Davey, S.K. Mutually exclusive mutation profiles define functionally related genes in muscle invasive bladder cancer. *PLoS ONE* **2022**, *17*, e0259992. [CrossRef]
7. Zuiverloon, T.C.; Tjin, S.S.; Busstra, M.; Bangma, C.H.; Boevé, E.R.; Zwarthoff, E.C. Optimization of Nonmuscle Invasive Bladder Cancer Recurrence Detection Using a Urine Based FGFR3 Mutation Assay. *J. Urol.* **2011**, *186*, 707–712. [CrossRef]
8. Zuiverloon, T.C.; van der Aa, M.N.; van der Kwast, T.H.; Steyerberg, E.W.; Lingsma, H.F.; Bangma, C.H.; Zwarthoff, E.C. *Fibroblast Growth Factor Receptor 3* Mutation Analysis on Voided Urine for Surveillance of Patients with Low-Grade Non-Muscle–Invasive Bladder Cancer. *Clin. Cancer Res.* **2010**, *16*, 3011–3018. [CrossRef]
9. Wu, H.; Zhang, Z.-Y.; Zhang, Z.; Xiao, X.-Y.; Gao, S.-L.; Lu, C.; Zuo, L.; Zhang, L.-F. Prediction of bladder cancer outcome by identifying and validating a mutation-derived genomic instability-associated long noncoding RNA (lncRNA) signature. *Bioengineered* **2021**, *12*, 1725–1738. [CrossRef]
10. van Rhijn, B.W.; van der Kwast, T.H.; Liu, L.; Fleshner, N.E.; Bostrom, P.J.; Vis, A.N.; Alkhateeb, S.S.; Bangma, C.H.; Jewett, M.A.; Zwarthoff, E.C.; et al. The FGFR3 mutation is related to favorable pT1 bladder cancer. *J Urol.* **2012**, *187*, 310–314. [CrossRef]
11. Hurst, C.D.; Platt, F.M.; Knowles, M.A. Comprehensive Mutation Analysis of the TERT Promoter in Bladder Cancer and Detection of Mutations in Voided Urine. *Eur. Urol.* **2014**, *65*, 367–369. [CrossRef] [PubMed]
12. Cheng, L.; Zhang, S.; Wang, M.; Lopez-Beltran, A. Biological and clinical perspectives of TERT promoter mutation detection on bladder cancer diagnosis and management. *Hum. Pathol.* **2022**. [CrossRef] [PubMed]
13. Ahmad, F.; Mahal, V.; Verma, G.; Bhatia, S.; Das, B.R. Molecular investigation ofFGFR3gene mutation and its correlation with clinicopathological findings in Indian bladder cancer patients. *Cancer Rep.* **2018**, *1*, e1130. [CrossRef]
14. Ding, Q.; Zhang, Y.; Sun, X. The study of p53 gene mutation in human bladder cancer. *Chin. J. Surg. J* **1995**, *33*, 684–686. [PubMed]
15. Jahnson, S.; Söderkvist, P.; Aljabery, F.; Olsson, H. Telomerase reverse transcriptase mutation and the p53 pathway in T1 urinary bladder cancer. *Br. J. Urol.* **2021**, *129*, 601–609. [CrossRef]
16. Liu, Y.; Kwiatkowski, D.J. Combined CDKN1A/TP53 Mutation in Bladder Cancer Is a Therapeutic Target. *Mol. Cancer Ther.* **2015**, *14*, 174–182. [CrossRef] [PubMed]
17. Payton, S. Bladder cancer: Mutation found in >70% of tumours. *Nat. Rev. Urol.* **2013**, *10*, 616. [PubMed]
18. Noel, N.; Couteau, J.; Maillet, G.; Gobet, F.; D'Aloisio, F.; Minier, C.; Pfister, C. TP53 and FGFR3 Gene Mutation Assessment in Urine: Pilot Study for Bladder Cancer Diagnosis. *Anticancer Res.* **2015**, *35*, 4915–4921.
19. Witjes, J.A. Follow-up in non-muscle invasive bladder cancer: Facts and future. *World J. Urol.* **2021**, *39*, 4047–4053. [CrossRef]
20. Guillaume, L.; Guy, L. Epidemiology of and risk factors for bladder cancer and for urothelial tumors. *Rev. Prat.* **2014**, *64*, 1372–1374.
21. Hu, X.; Li, G.; Wu, S. Advances in Diagnosis and Therapy for Bladder Cancer. *Cancers* **2022**, *14*, 3181. [CrossRef]
22. Ahmadi, H.; Duddalwar, V.; Daneshmand, S. Diagnosis and Staging of Bladder Cancer. *Hematol. Clin. N. Am.* **2021**, *35*, 531–541. [CrossRef] [PubMed]
23. DeGeorge, K.C.; Holt, H.R.; Hodges, S.C. Bladder Cancer: Diagnosis and Treatment. *Am. Fam. Physician* **2017**, *96*, 507–514. [PubMed]
24. Sun, M.; Trinh, Q.-D. Diagnosis and Staging of Bladder Cancer. *Hematol. Clin. N. Am.* **2015**, *29*, 205–218. [CrossRef]
25. Lodewijk, I.; Dueñas, M.; Rubio, C.; Munera-Maravilla, E.; Segovia, C.; Bernardini, A.; Teijeira, A.; Paramio, J.M.; Suárez-Cabrera, C. Liquid Biopsy Biomarkers in Bladder Cancer: A Current Need for Patient Diagnosis and Monitoring. *Int. J. Mol. Sci.* **2018**, *19*, 2514. [CrossRef]
26. Chan, K.M.; Gleadle, J.; Li, J.; Vasilev, K.; MacGregor, M. Shedding Light on Bladder Cancer Diagnosis in Urine. *Diagnostics* **2020**, *10*, 383. [CrossRef]
27. Ferro, M.; La Civita, E.; Liotti, A.; Cennamo, M.; Tortora, F.; Buonerba, C.; Crocetto, F.; Lucarelli, G.; Busetto, G.; Del Giudice, F.; et al. Liquid Biopsy Biomarkers in Urine: A Route towards Molecular Diagnosis and Personalized Medicine of Bladder Cancer. *J. Pers. Med.* **2021**, *11*, 237. [CrossRef]
28. Jeong, S.-H.; Ku, J.H. Urinary Markers for Bladder Cancer Diagnosis and Monitoring. *Front. Cell Dev. Biol.* **2022**, *10*, 892067. [CrossRef]
29. Jaiswal, P.K.; Goel, A.; Mittal, R.D. Survivin: A molecular biomarker in cancer. *Indian J. Med. Res.* **2015**, *141*, 389–397. [CrossRef]
30. Sawyers, C.L. The cancer biomarker problem. *Nat.* **2008**, *452*, 548–552. [CrossRef]
31. Piao, X.-M.; Cha, E.-J.; Yun, S.J.; Kim, W.-J. Role of Exosomal miRNA in Bladder Cancer: A Promising Liquid Biopsy Biomarker. *Int. J. Mol. Sci.* **2021**, *22*, 1713. [CrossRef]

32. Ku, J.H.; Godoy, G.; Amiel, G.E.; Lerner, S.P. Urine survivin as a diagnostic biomarker for bladder cancer: A systematic review. *Br. J. Urol.* **2012**, *110*, 630–636. [CrossRef] [PubMed]
33. Mowatt, G.; Zhu, S.; Kilonzo, M.; Boachie, C.; Fraser, C.; Griffiths, T.R.L.; N'Dow, J.; Nabi, G.; Cook, J.; Vale, L. Systematic review of the clinical effectiveness and cost-effectiveness of photodynamic diagnosis and urine biomarkers (FISH, ImmunoCyt, NMP22) and cytology for the detection and follow-up of bladder cancer. *Health Technol. Assess.* **2010**, *14*, 1–331. [CrossRef] [PubMed]
34. Bebelman, M.P.; Smit, M.J.; Pegtel, D.M.; Baglio, S.R. Biogenesis and function of extracellular vesicles in cancer. *Pharmacol. Ther.* **2018**, *188*, 1–11. [CrossRef] [PubMed]
35. Dreyer, F.; Baur, A. Biogenesis and Functions of Exosomes and Extracellular Vesicles. *Methods Mol. Biol.* **2016**, *1448*, 201–216. [CrossRef] [PubMed]
36. Li, Y.; Meng, L.; Li, B.; Li, Y.; Shen, T.; Zhao, B. The Exosome Journey: From Biogenesis to Regulation and Function in Cancers. *J. Oncol.* **2022**, *2022*, 9356807. [CrossRef]
37. Hariharan, H.; Kesavan, Y.; Raja, N.S. Impact of native and external factors on exosome release: Understanding reactive exosome secretion and its biogenesis. *Mol. Biol. Rep.* **2021**, *48*, 7559–7573. [CrossRef]
38. Gurung, S.; Perocheau, D.; Touramanidou, L.; Baruteau, J. The exosome journey: From biogenesis to uptake and intracellular signalling. *Cell Commun. Signal.* **2021**, *19*, 47. [CrossRef]
39. Hessvik, N.P.; Llorente, A. Current knowledge on exosome biogenesis and release. *Cell. Mol. Life Sci.* **2018**, *75*, 193–208. [CrossRef]
40. Das, C.K.; Jena, B.C.; Banerjee, I.; Das, S.; Parekh, A.; Bhutia, S.K.; Mandal, M. Exosome as a Novel Shuttle for Delivery of Therapeutics across Biological Barriers. *Mol. Pharm.* **2018**, *16*, 24–40. [CrossRef]
41. Elliott, R.; He, M. Unlocking the Power of Exosomes for Crossing Biological Barriers in Drug Delivery. *Pharmaceutics* **2021**, *13*, 122. [CrossRef]
42. Ramos-Zaldívar, H.M.; Polakovicova, I.; Salas-Huenuleo, E.; Corvalán, A.H.; Kogan, M.J.; Yefi, C.P.; Andia, M.E. Extracellular vesicles through the blood–brain barrier: A review. *Fluids Barriers CNS* **2022**, *19*, 60. [CrossRef] [PubMed]
43. Krämer-Albers, E.-M. Extracellular Vesicles at CNS barriers: Mode of action. *Curr. Opin. Neurobiol.* **2022**, *75*, 102569. [CrossRef]
44. Zeng, Y.; Qiu, Y.; Jiang, W.; Shen, J.; Yao, X.; He, X.; Li, L.; Fu, B.; Liu, X. Biological Features of Extracellular Vesicles and Challenges. *Front. Cell Dev. Biol.* **2022**, *10*, 816698. [CrossRef]
45. Schulz-Siegmund, M.; Aigner, A. Nucleic acid delivery with extracellular vesicles. *Adv. Drug Deliv. Rev.* **2021**, *173*, 89–111. [CrossRef]
46. Vu, L.T.; Gong, J.; Pham, T.T.; Kim, Y.; Le, M.T.N. microRNA exchange via extracellular vesicles in cancer. *Cell Prolif.* **2020**, *53*, e12877. [CrossRef] [PubMed]
47. Abramowicz, A.; Story, M.D. The Long and Short of It: The Emerging Roles of Non-Coding RNA in Small Extracellular Vesicles. *Cancers* **2020**, *12*, 1445. [CrossRef]
48. Veziroglu, E.M.; Mias, G.I. Characterizing Extracellular Vesicles and Their Diverse RNA Contents. *Front. Genet.* **2020**, *11*, 700. [CrossRef] [PubMed]
49. Groot, M.; Lee, H. Sorting Mechanisms for MicroRNAs into Extracellular Vesicles and Their Associated Diseases. *Cells* **2020**, *9*, 1044. [CrossRef]
50. Ageta, H.; Tsuchida, K. Post-translational modification and protein sorting to small extracellular vesicles including exosomes by ubiquitin and UBLs. *Experientia* **2019**, *76*, 4829–4848. [CrossRef]
51. Anand, S.; Samuel, M.; Kumar, S.; Mathivanan, S. Ticket to a bubble ride: Cargo sorting into exosomes and extracellular vesicles. *Biochim. Biophys. Acta Proteins Proteom.* **2019**, *1867*, 140203. [CrossRef] [PubMed]
52. Zhang, L.; Yu, D. Exosomes in cancer development, metastasis, and immunity. *Biochim Biophys Acta Rev. Cancer.* **2019**, *1871*, 455–468. [CrossRef] [PubMed]
53. Takahashi, R.-U.; Prieto-Vila, M.; Hironaka, A.; Ochiya, T. The role of extracellular vesicle microRNAs in cancer biology. *Clin. Chem. Lab. Med. CCLM* **2017**, *55*, 648–656. [CrossRef] [PubMed]
54. Willms, E.; Cabañas, C.; Mäger, I.; Wood, M.J.A.; Vader, P. Extracellular Vesicle Heterogeneity: Subpopulations, Isolation Techniques, and Diverse Functions in Cancer Progression. *Front. Immunol.* **2018**, *9*, 738. [CrossRef]
55. Fujita, Y.; Yoshioka, Y.; Ochiya, T. Extracellular vesicle transfer of cancer pathogenic components. *Cancer Sci.* **2016**, *107*, 385–390. [CrossRef]
56. Yamamoto, T.; Yamamoto, Y.; Ochiya, T. Extracellular vesicle-mediated immunoregulation in cancer. *Int. J. Hematol.* **2022**, 1–7. [CrossRef]
57. Li, Z.; Zhu, X.; Huang, S. Extracellular vesicle long non-coding RNAs and circular RNAs: Biology, functions and applications in cancer. *Cancer Lett.* **2020**, *489*, 111–120. [CrossRef]
58. Bebelman, M.P.; Janssen, E.; Pegtel, D.M.; Crudden, C. The forces driving cancer extracellular vesicle secretion. *Neoplasia* **2020**, *23*, 149–157. [CrossRef]
59. Carles-Fontana, R.; Heaton, N.; Palma, E.; Khorsandi, S.E. Extracellular Vesicle-Mediated Mitochondrial Reprogramming in Cancer. *Cancers* **2022**, *14*, 1865. [CrossRef]
60. Gai, C.; Carpanetto, A.; Deregibus, M.C.; Camussi, G. Extracellular vesicle-mediated modulation of angiogenesis. *Histol. Histopathol.* **2016**, *31*, 379–391. [CrossRef]
61. Ko, S.Y.; Naora, H. Extracellular Vesicle Membrane-Associated Proteins: Emerging Roles in Tumor Angiogenesis and Anti-Angiogenesis Therapy Resistance. *Int. J. Mol. Sci.* **2020**, *21*, 5418. [CrossRef]

62. Zhang, S.; Yang, J.; Shen, L. Extracellular vesicle-mediated regulation of tumor angiogenesis- implications for anti-angiogenesis therapy. *J. Cell Mol. Med.* **2021**, *25*, 2776–2785. [CrossRef] [PubMed]
63. Mukherjee, S.; Pillai, P.P. Current insights on extracellular vesicle-mediated glioblastoma progression: Implications in drug resistance and epithelial-mesenchymal transition. *Biochim. Biophys. Acta BBA-Gen. Subj.* **2022**, *1866*, 130065. [CrossRef]
64. Eitan, E.; Suire, C.; Zhang, S.; Mattson, M.P. Impact of lysosome status on extracellular vesicle content and release. *Ageing Res. Rev.* **2016**, *32*, 65–74. [CrossRef] [PubMed]
65. Hao, Y.; Song, H.; Zhou, Z.; Chen, X.; Li, H.; Zhang, Y.; Wang, J.; Ren, X.; Wang, X. Promotion or inhibition of extracellular vesicle release: Emerging therapeutic opportunities. *J. Control. Release* **2021**, *340*, 136–148. [CrossRef]
66. Xi, L.; Peng, M.; Liu, S.; Liu, Y.; Wan, X.; Hou, Y.; Qin, Y.; Yang, L.; Chen, S.; Zeng, H.; et al. Hypoxia-stimulated ATM activation regulates autophagy-associated exosome release from cancer-associated fibroblasts to promote cancer cell invasion. *J. Extracell. Vesicles* **2021**, *10*, e12146. [CrossRef]
67. Moloudizargari, M.; Asghari, M.H.; Abdollahi, M. Modifying exosome release in cancer therapy: How can it help? *Pharmacol. Res.* **2018**, *134*, 246–256. [CrossRef]
68. Parayath, N.N.; Padmakumar, S.; Amiji, M.M. Extracellular vesicle-mediated nucleic acid transfer and reprogramming in the tumor microenvironment. *Cancer Lett.* **2020**, *482*, 33–43. [CrossRef]
69. Brena, D.; Huang, M.-B.; Bond, V. Extracellular vesicle-mediated transport: Reprogramming a tumor microenvironment conducive with breast cancer progression and metastasis. *Transl. Oncol.* **2021**, *15*, 101286. [CrossRef]
70. Li, Y.; Zhao, W.; Wang, Y.; Wang, H.; Liu, S. Extracellular vesicle-mediated crosstalk between pancreatic cancer and stromal cells in the tumor microenvironment. *J. Nanobiotechnol.* **2022**, *20*, 208. [CrossRef]
71. Geng, H.; Zhou, Q.; Guo, W.; Lu, L.; Bi, L.; Wang, Y.; Min, J.; Yu, D.; Liang, Z. Exosomes in bladder cancer: Novel biomarkers and targets. *J. Zhejiang Univ. Sci. B* **2021**, *22*, 341–347. [CrossRef] [PubMed]
72. Hiltbrunner, S.; Mints, M.; Eldh, M.; Rosenblatt, R.; Holmström, B.; Alamdari, F.; Johansson, M.; Veerman, R.E.; Winqvist, O.; Sherif, A.; et al. Urinary Exosomes from Bladder Cancer Patients Show a Residual Cancer Phenotype despite Complete Pathological Downstaging. *Sci. Rep.* **2020**, *10*, 5960. [CrossRef] [PubMed]
73. Liu, Y.-R.; Ortiz-Bonilla, C.J.; Lee, Y.-F. Extracellular Vesicles in Bladder Cancer: Biomarkers and Beyond. *Int. J. Mol. Sci.* **2018**, *19*, 2822. [CrossRef]
74. Santos, N.L.; Bustos, S.O.; Bhatt, D.; Chammas, R.; Andrade, L.N.D.S. Tumor-Derived Extracellular Vesicles: Modulation of Cellular Functional Dynamics in Tumor Microenvironment and Its Clinical Implications. *Front. Cell Dev. Biol.* **2021**, *9*, 737449. [CrossRef] [PubMed]
75. Silvers, C.R.; Liu, Y.-R.; Wu, C.-H.; Miyamoto, H.; Messing, E.M.; Lee, Y.-F. Identification of extracellular vesicle-borne periostin as a feature of muscle-invasive bladder cancer. *Oncotarget* **2016**, *7*, 23335–23345. [CrossRef] [PubMed]
76. Silvers, C.R.; Miyamoto, H.; Messing, E.M.; Netto, G.J.; Lee, Y.-F. Characterization of urinary extracellular vesicle proteins in muscle-invasive bladder cancer. *Oncotarget* **2017**, *8*, 91199–91208. [CrossRef] [PubMed]
77. Baumgart, S.; Meschkat, P.; Edelmann, P.; Heinzelmann, J.; Pryalukhin, A.; Bohle, R.; Heinzelbecker, J.; Stöckle, M.; Junker, K. MicroRNAs in tumor samples and urinary extracellular vesicles as a putative diagnostic tool for muscle-invasive bladder cancer. *J. Cancer Res. Clin. Oncol.* **2019**, *145*, 2725–2736. [CrossRef]
78. Silvers, C.R.; Messing, E.M.; Miyamoto, H.; Lee, Y.-F. Tenascin-C expression in the lymph node pre-metastatic niche in muscle-invasive bladder cancer. *Br. J. Cancer* **2021**, *125*, 1399–1407. [CrossRef]
79. Yu, E.Y.-W.; Zhang, H.; Fu, Y.; Chen, Y.-T.; Tang, Q.-Y.; Liu, Y.-X.; Zhang, Y.-X.; Wang, S.-Z.; Wesselius, A.; Li, W.-C.; et al. Integrative Multi-Omics Analysis for the Determination of Non-Muscle Invasive vs. Muscle Invasive Bladder Cancer: A Pilot Study. *Curr. Oncol.* **2022**, *29*, 5442–5456. [CrossRef]
80. Tong, Y.; Liu, X.; Xia, D.; Peng, E.; Yang, X.; Liu, H.; Ye, T.; Wang, X.; He, Y.; Xu, H.; et al. Biological Roles and Clinical Significance of Exosome-Derived Noncoding RNAs in Bladder Cancer. *Front. Oncol.* **2021**, *11*, 704703. [CrossRef]
81. Xue, M.; Chen, W.; Li, X. Extracellular vesicle-transferred long noncoding RNAs in bladder cancer. *Clin. Chim. Acta* **2021**, *516*, 34–45. [CrossRef] [PubMed]
82. Andreu, Z.; Oshiro, R.O.; Redruello, A.; López-Martín, S.; Gutiérrez-Vázquez, C.; Morato, E.; Marina, A.I.; Gómez, C.O.; Yáñez-Mó, M. Extracellular vesicles as a source for non-invasive biomarkers in bladder cancer progression. *Eur. J. Pharm. Sci.* **2017**, *98*, 70–79. [CrossRef] [PubMed]
83. Urabe, F.; Kimura, T.; Ito, K.; Yamamoto, Y.; Tsuzuki, S.; Miki, J.; Ochiya, T.; Egawa, S. Urinary extracellular vesicles: A rising star in bladder cancer management. *Transl. Androl. Urol.* **2021**, *10*, 1878–1889. [CrossRef] [PubMed]
84. Georgantzoglou, N.; Pergaris, A.; Masaoutis, C.; Theocharis, S. Extracellular Vesicles as Biomarkers Carriers in Bladder Cancer: Diagnosis, Surveillance, and Treatment. *Int. J. Mol. Sci.* **2021**, *22*, 2744. [CrossRef]
85. Wu, C.-H.; Silvers, C.R.; Messing, E.M.; Lee, Y.-F. Bladder cancer extracellular vesicles drive tumorigenesis by inducing the unfolded protein response in endoplasmic reticulum of nonmalignant cells. *J. Biol. Chem.* **2019**, *294*, 3207–3218. [CrossRef]
86. Xu, Y.; Zhang, P.; Tan, Y.; Jia, Z.; Chen, G.; Niu, Y.; Xiao, J.; Sun, S.; Zhang, X. A potential panel of five mRNAs in urinary extracellular vesicles for the detection of bladder cancer. *Transl. Androl. Urol.* **2021**, *10*, 809–820. [CrossRef]
87. Xiang, Y.; Lv, D.; Song, T.; Niu, C.; Wang, Y. Tumor suppressive role of microRNA-139-5p in bone marrow mesenchymal stem cells-derived extracellular vesicles in bladder cancer through regulation of the KIF3A/p21 axis. *Cell Death Dis.* **2022**, *13*, 599. [CrossRef]

88. Igami, K.; Uchiumi, T.; Shiota, M.; Ueda, S.; Tsukahara, S.; Akimoto, M.; Eto, M.; Kang, D. Extracellular vesicles expressing CEACAM proteins in the urine of bladder cancer patients. *Cancer Sci.* **2022**, *113*, 3120–3133. [CrossRef]
89. Tomiyama, E.; Matsuzaki, K.; Fujita, K.; Shiromizu, T.; Narumi, R.; Jingushi, K.; Koh, Y.; Matsushita, M.; Nakano, K.; Hayashi, Y.; et al. Proteomic analysis of urinary and tissue-exudative extracellular vesicles to discover novel bladder cancer biomarkers. *Cancer Sci.* **2021**, *112*, 2033–2045. [CrossRef]
90. Di Bella, M.A. Overview and Update on Extracellular Vesicles: Considerations on Exosomes and Their Application in Modern Medicine. *Biology* **2022**, *11*, 804. [CrossRef]
91. Doyle, L.; Wang, M. Overview of Extracellular Vesicles, Their Origin, Composition, Purpose, and Methods for Exosome Isolation and Analysis. *Cells* **2019**, *8*, 727. [CrossRef]
92. Bin Zha, Q.; Yao, Y.F.; Ren, Z.J.; Li, X.J.; Tang, J.H. Extracellular vesicles: An overview of biogenesis, function, and role in breast cancer. *Tumor Biol.* **2017**, *39*, 1010428317691182. [CrossRef]
93. Shang, M.; Ji, J.S.; Song, C.; Gao, B.J.; Jin, J.G.; Kuo, W.P.; Kang, H. Extracellular Vesicles: A Brief Overview and Its Role in Precision Medicine. *Methods Mol. Biol.* **2017**, *1660*, 1–14. [PubMed]
94. Palinski, W.; Monti, M.; Camerlingo, R.; Iacobucci, I.; Bocella, S.; Pinto, F.; Iannuzzi, C.; Mansueto, G.; Pignatiello, S.; Fazioli, F.; et al. Lysosome purinergic receptor P2X4 regulates neoangiogenesis induced by microvesicles from sarcoma patients. *Cell Death Dis.* **2021**, *12*, 797. [CrossRef]
95. De Oliveira, M.C.; Caires, H.R.; Oliveira, M.J.; Fraga, A.; Vasconcelos, M.H.; Ribeiro, R. Urinary Biomarkers in Bladder Cancer: Where Do We Stand and Potential Role of Extracellular Vesicles. *Cancers* **2020**, *12*, 1400. [CrossRef]
96. Oeyen, E.; Hoekx, L.; De Wachter, S.; Baldewijns, M.; Ameye, F.; Mertens, I. Bladder Cancer Diagnosis and Follow-Up: The Current Status and Possible Role of Extracellular Vesicles. *Int. J. Mol. Sci.* **2019**, *20*, 821. [CrossRef]
97. Ruan, S.; Greenberg, Z.; Pan, X.; Zhuang, P.; Erwin, N.; He, M. Extracellular Vesicles as an Advanced Delivery Biomaterial for Precision Cancer Immunotherapy. *Adv. Health Mater.* **2022**, *11*, e2100650. [CrossRef]
98. Ferraiuolo, R.-M.; Manthey, K.C.; Stanton, M.J.; Triplett, A.A.; Wagner, K.-U. The Multifaceted Roles of the Tumor Susceptibility Gene 101 (TSG101) in Normal Development and Disease. *Cancers* **2020**, *12*, 450. [CrossRef]
99. Yazarlou, F.; Mowla, S.J.; Oskooei, V.K.; Motevaseli, E.; Tooli, L.F.; Afsharpad, M.; Nekoohesh, L.; Sanikhani, N.S.; Ghafouri-Fard, S.; Modarressi, M.H. Urine exosome gene expression of cancer-testis antigens for prediction of bladder carcinoma. *Cancer Manag. Res.* **2018**, *10*, 5373–5381. [CrossRef]
100. Jeppesen, D.K.; Nawrocki, A.; Jensen, S.G.; Thorsen, K.; Whitehead, B.; Howard, K.A.; Dyrskjøt, L.; Ørntoft, T.F.; Larsen, M.R.; Ostenfeld, M.S. Quantitative proteomics of fractionated membrane and lumen exosome proteins from isogenic metastatic and nonmetastatic bladder cancer cells reveal differential expression of EMT factors. *Proteomics* **2014**, *14*, 699–712. [CrossRef]
101. Gao, X.P.; Dong, J.J.; Xie, Y.; Guan, X. Integrative Analysis of MUC4 to Prognosis and Immune Infiltration in Pan-Cancer: Friend or Foe? *Front. Cell Dev. Biol.* **2021**, *9*, 695544. [CrossRef] [PubMed]
102. Liu, Q. The emerging roles of exosomal long non-coding RNAs in bladder cancer. *J. Cell. Mol. Med.* **2022**, *26*, 966–976. [CrossRef] [PubMed]
103. Su, Q.; Wu, H.; Zhang, Z.; Lu, C.; Zhang, L.; Zuo, L. Exosome-Derived Long Non-Coding RNAs as Non-Invasive Biomarkers of Bladder Cancer. *Front. Oncol.* **2021**, *11*, 719863. [CrossRef]
104. Abbastabar, M.; Sarfi, M.; Golestani, A.; Karimi, A.; Pourmand, G.; Khalili, E. Tumor-derived urinary exosomal long non-coding RNAs as diagnostic biomarkers for bladder cancer. *Excli J.* **2020**, *19*, 301–310. [CrossRef] [PubMed]
105. Oktem, G.C.; Kocaaslan, R.; Karadag, M.A.; Bagcioglu, M.; Demir, A.; Cecen, K.; Unluer, E. The role of transcavitary ultrasonography in diagnosis and staging of nonmuscle-invasive bladder cancer: A prospective non-randomized clinical study. *Springerplus* **2014**, *3*, 519. [CrossRef] [PubMed]
106. Zuiverloon, T.C.M.; De Jong, F.C.; Theodorescu, D. Clinical Decision Making in Surveillance of Non-Muscle-Invasive Bladder Cancer: The Evolving Roles of Urinary Cytology and Molecular Markers. *Oncology* **2017**, *31*, 855–862. [PubMed]
107. D'Andrea, D.; Soria, F.; Zehetmayer, S.; Gust, K.M.; Korn, S.; Witjes, J.A.; Shariat, S.F. Diagnostic accuracy, clinical utility and influence on decision-making of a methylation urine biomarker test in the surveillance of non-muscle-invasive bladder cancer. *Br. J. Urol.* **2019**, *123*, 959–967. [CrossRef] [PubMed]
108. Powles, T.; Bellmunt, J.; Comperat, E.; De Santis, M.; Huddart, R.; Loriot, Y.; Necchi, A.; Valderrama, B.; Ravaud, A.; Shariat, S.; et al. Bladder cancer: ESMO Clinical Practice Guideline for diagnosis, treatment and follow-up. *Ann. Oncol.* **2021**, *33*, 244–258. [CrossRef]
109. Wang, Z.; Que, H.; Suo, C.; Han, Z.; Tao, J.; Huang, Z.; Ju, X.; Tan, R.; Gu, M. Evaluation of the NMP22 BladderChek test for detecting bladder cancer: A systematic review and meta-analysis. *Oncotarget* **2017**, *8*, 100648–100656. [CrossRef]
110. Guo, A.; Wang, X.; Shi, J.; Sun, C.; Wan, Z. Bladder tumour antigen (BTA stat) test compared to the urine cytology in the diagnosis of bladder cancer: A meta-analysis. *Can. Urol. Assoc. J.* **2014**, *8*, 347–352. [CrossRef]
111. Comploj, E.; Mian, C.; Ambrosini-Spaltro, A.; Dechet, C.; Palermo, S.; Trenti, E.; Lodde, M.; Horninger, W.; Pycha, A. uCyt+/ImmunoCyt and cytology in the detection of urothelial carcinoma: An update on 7422 analyses. *Cancer Cytopathol.* **2013**, *121*, 392–397. [CrossRef] [PubMed]
112. He, H.; Han, C.; Hao, L.; Zang, G. ImmunoCyt test compared to cytology in the diagnosis of bladder cancer: A meta-analysis. *Oncol. Lett.* **2016**, *12*, 83–88. [CrossRef] [PubMed]

113. Ainthachot, S.; Sa-Ngiamwibool, P.; Thanee, M.; Watcharadetwittaya, S.; Chamgramol, Y.; Pairojkul, C.; Deenonpoe, R. Chromosomal aberrations, visualized using UroVysion® fluorescence in-situ hybridization assay, can predict poor prognosis in formalin-fixed paraffin-embedded tissues of cholangiocarcinoma patients. *Hum. Pathol.* **2022**, *126*, 31–44. [CrossRef] [PubMed]
114. Mettman, D.; Saeed, A.; Shold, J.; Laury, R.; Ly, A.; Khan, I.; Golem, S.; Olyaee, M.; O'Neil, M. Refined pancreatobiliary UroVysion criteria and an approach for further optimization. *Cancer Med.* **2021**, *10*, 5725–5738. [CrossRef]
115. Hu, Z.; Ke, C.; Liu, Z.; Zeng, X.; Li, S.; Xu, H.; Yang, C. Evaluation of UroVysion for Urachal Carcinoma Detection. *Front. Med.* **2020**, *7*, 437. [CrossRef]
116. Weinstock, C.; Agrawal, S.; Chang, E. Optimizing Clinical Trial Design for Patients with Non–muscle-invasive Bladder Cancer. *Eur. Urol.* **2022**, *82*, 47–48. [CrossRef]
117. El-Karamany, T.M.; Al-Adl, A.M.; Hosny, M.M.; Eldeep, H.A.; El-Hamshary, S.A. Clinical utility of vesical imaging-reporting and data system (VI-RADS) in non−muscle invasive bladder cancer (NMIBC) patients candidate for en-bloc transurethral resection: A prospective study. *Urol. Oncol. Semin. Orig. Investig.* **2022**. [CrossRef]
118. Huang, C.-S.; Ho, J.-Y.; Chiang, J.-H.; Yu, C.-P.; Yu, D.-S. Exosome-Derived LINC00960 and LINC02470 Promote the Epithelial-Mesenchymal Transition and Aggressiveness of Bladder Cancer Cells. *Cells* **2020**, *9*, 1419. [CrossRef]
119. Longjohn, M.N.; Christian, S.L. Characterizing Extracellular Vesicles Using Nanoparticle-Tracking Analysis. *Methods Mol. Biol.* **2022**, *2508*, 353–373. [CrossRef]
120. Vestad, B.; Llorente, A.; Neurauter, A.; Phuyal, S.; Kierulf, B.; Kierulf, P.; Skotland, T.; Sandvig, K.; Haug, K.B.F.; Øvstebø, R. Size and concentration analyses of extracellular vesicles by nanoparticle tracking analysis: A variation study. *J. Extracell. Vesicles* **2017**, *6*, 1344087. [CrossRef]
121. Théry, C.; Witwer, K.W.; Aikawa, E.; Alcaraz, M.J.; Anderson, J.D.; Andriantsitohaina, R.; Antoniou, A.; Arab, T.; Archer, F.; Atkin-Smith, G.K.; et al. Minimal information for studies of extracellular vesicles 2018 (MISEV2018): A position statement of the International Society for Extracellular Vesicles and update of the MISEV2014 guidelines. *J. Extracell. Vesicles* **2018**, *7*, 1535750. [CrossRef] [PubMed]
122. Thietart, S.; Rautou, P.E. Extracellular vesicles as biomarkers in liver diseases: A clinician's point of view. *J. Hepatol.* **2020**, *73*, 1507–1525. [CrossRef] [PubMed]
123. Liu, W.-Z.; Ma, Z.-J.; Kang, X.-W. Current status and outlook of advances in exosome isolation. *Anal. Bioanal. Chem.* **2022**, *414*, 7123–7141. [CrossRef] [PubMed]
124. Liga, A.; Vliegenthart, A.D.B.; Oosthuyzen, W.; Dear, J.W.; Kersaudy-Kerhoas, M. Exosome isolation: A microfluidic road-map. *Lab a Chip* **2015**, *15*, 2388–2394. [CrossRef]
125. Hou, R.; Li, Y.; Sui, Z.; Yuan, H.; Yang, K.; Liang, Z.; Zhang, L.; Zhang, Y. Advances in exosome isolation methods and their applications in proteomic analysis of biological samples. *Anal. Bioanal. Chem.* **2019**, *411*, 5351–5361. [CrossRef] [PubMed]
126. Ludwig, N.; Whiteside, T.L.; Reichert, T.E. Challenges in Exosome Isolation and Analysis in Health and Disease. *Int. J. Mol. Sci.* **2019**, *20*, 4684. [CrossRef]
127. Boriachek, K.; Islam, M.N.; Möller, A.; Salomon, C.; Nguyen, N.-T.; Hossain, M.S.A.; Yamauchi, Y.; Shiddiky, M.J.A. Biological Functions and Current Advances in Isolation and Detection Strategies for Exosome Nanovesicles. *Small* **2018**, *14*, 1702153. [CrossRef]
128. Zhang, Y.; Bi, J.; Huang, J.; Tang, Y.; Du, S.; Li, P. Exosome: A Review of Its Classification, Isolation Techniques, Storage, Diagnostic and Targeted Therapy Applications. *Int. J. Nanomed.* **2020**, *15*, 6917–6934. [CrossRef]
129. Li, P.; Kaslan, M.; Lee, S.H.; Yao, J.; Gao, Z. Progress in Exosome Isolation Techniques. *Theranostics* **2017**, *7*, 789–804. [CrossRef]
130. Yang, D.; Zhang, W.; Zhang, H.; Zhang, F.; Chen, L.; Ma, L.; Larcher, L.M.; Chen, S.; Liu, N.; Zhao, Q.; et al. Progress, opportunity, and perspective on exosome isolation—Efforts for efficient exosome-based theranostics. *Theranostics* **2020**, *10*, 3684–3707. [CrossRef]
131. Xu, K.; Jin, Y.; Li, Y.; Huang, Y.; Zhao, R. Recent Progress of Exosome Isolation and Peptide Recognition-Guided Strategies for Exosome Research. *Front. Chem.* **2022**, *10*, 844124. [CrossRef] [PubMed]
132. Martins, T.S.; Vaz, M.; Henriques, A.G. A review on comparative studies addressing exosome isolation methods from body fluids. *Anal. Bioanal. Chem.* **2022**, 1–25. [CrossRef] [PubMed]
133. Chen, J.; Li, P.; Zhang, T.; Xu, Z.; Huang, X.; Wang, R.; Du, L. Review on Strategies and Technologies for Exosome Isolation and Purification. *Front. Bioeng. Biotechnol.* **2022**, *9*, 811971. [CrossRef] [PubMed]
134. Singh, K.; Nalabotala, R.; Koo, K.M.; Bose, S.; Nayak, R.; Shiddiky, M.J.A. Separation of distinct exosome subpopulations: Isolation and characterization approaches and their associated challenges. *Analyst* **2021**, *146*, 3731–3749. [CrossRef] [PubMed]
135. Sharma, S.; Salomon, C. Techniques Associated with Exosome Isolation for Biomarker Development: Liquid Biopsies for Ovarian Cancer Detection. *Methods Mol. Biol.* **2019**, *2055*, 181–199. [CrossRef]
136. Shirejini, S.Z.; Inci, F. The Yin and Yang of exosome isolation methods: Conventional practice, microfluidics, and commercial kits. *Biotechnol. Adv.* **2021**, *54*, 107814. [CrossRef]
137. Sidhom, K.; Obi, P.O.; Saleem, A. A Review of Exosomal Isolation Methods: Is Size Exclusion Chromatography the Best Option? *Int. J. Mol. Sci.* **2020**, *21*, 6466. [CrossRef]

138. Witwer, K.W.; Soekmadji, C.; Hill, A.F.; Wauben, M.H.; Buzas, E.I.; Di Vizio, D.; Falcon-Perez, J.M.; Gardiner, C.; Hochberg, F.; Kurochkin, I.V.; et al. Updating the MISEV minimal requirements for extracellular vesicle studies: Building bridges to reproducibility. *J. Extracell Vesicles.* **2017**, *6*, 1396823. [CrossRef]
139. He, N.; Thippabhotla, S.; Zhong, C.; Greenberg, Z.; Xu, L.; Pessetto, Z.; Godwin, A.K.; Zeng, Y.; He, M. Nano pom-poms prepared exosomes enable highly specific cancer biomarker detection. *Commun. Biol.* **2022**, *5*, 660. [CrossRef]

MDPI AG
Grosspeteranlage 5
4052 Basel
Switzerland
Tel.: +41 61 683 77 34

Pharmaceutics Editorial Office
E-mail: pharmaceutics@mdpi.com
www.mdpi.com/journal/pharmaceutics

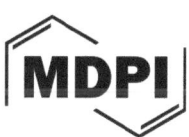

Disclaimer/Publisher's Note: The statements, opinions and data contained in all publications are solely those of the individual author(s) and contributor(s) and not of MDPI and/or the editor(s). MDPI and/or the editor(s) disclaim responsibility for any injury to people or property resulting from any ideas, methods, instructions or products referred to in the content.